WRITTEN IN THE FLESH: A HISTORY OF DESIRE

Written in the Flesh is a history of sexual desire – a provocative chronicle of the changing nature of what people yearn to do sexually.

The desire for sexual pleasure and total body sex – that is, the expansion of sexuality from a limited focus on the face and genitals to include the entire body – is certainly not a new phenomenon: the ancient Greeks, Romans, and Chinese, among others, were quite familiar with an eroticism that went beyond the strictly heterosexual and procreational. In the long centuries of Christian Europe, when the miserable conditions of life and religious repression conspired to minimize the expression of sexual longing, desire was driven underground. Yet in the late nineteenth century, increasing privacy, prosperity, and good health again permitted the underlying biological urge for total body sex to express itself, and encouraged a shift of erotic pleasure toward new and unexplored body zones: the mouth, nipples, anus, and further.

This new work by renowned medical historian Edward Shorter demonstrates that desire is hard-wired into the brain, expressing itself in remarkably similar ways in men and women, adolescent and adult, and in gays, lesbians, and straights alike. Drawing from a wide array of sources, including memoirs, novels, collections of letters, diaries, and indeed a large pornographic corpus, Shorter explores the widening of Western society's sexual repertoire.

Written in the Flesh is a history of what people like to do in bed and how that has changed. The change is relentless: human sexuality continually seeks new means of liberation in its expression of pleasure.

EDWARD SHORTER holds the Jason A. Hannah Chair in the History of Medicine at the University of Toronto.

Written in the Flesh

A History of Desire

EDWARD SHORTER

UNIVERSITY OF TORONTO PRESS
Toronto Buffalo London

© Edward L. Shorter 2005
University of Toronto Press
Toronto Buffalo London
Printed in Canada

Reprinted in paperback 2006

ISBN 0-8020-3843-3 (cloth)
ISBN 0-8020-9452-X (paper)

Printed on acid-free paper

Library and Archives Canada Cataloguing in Publication

Shorter, Edward
Written in the flesh : a history of desire / Edward Shorter.

Includes bibliographical references and index.
ISBN 0-8020-3843-3 (bound). – ISBN 0-8020-9452-X (pbk.)

1. Sex – Western countries – History.   2. Desire – History.
3. Sensuality – History.   I. Title.

HQ21.S482 2005   306.7′09   C2005-900164-X

Every effort has been made to obtain permission to reproduce the
illustrations in this book. Any omissions brought to our attention
will be rectified in future printings of this book.

University of Toronto Press acknowledges the financial assistance
to its publishing program of the Canada Council for the Arts and
the Ontario Arts Council.

University of Toronto Press acknowledges the financial support for
its publishing activities of the Government of Canada through the
Book Publishing Industry Development Program (BPIDP).

For my dearest Anne Marie

Contents

Illustrations follow pages 86 and 166

Acknowledgments

I must thank my secretary, Andrea Clark, for the many services and courtesies that have eased the writing of this book. Susan Bélanger, my long-time research assistant, has once again been indispensable, in her tidy, thoughtful, and industrious manner. The Interlibrary Loan service of the University of Toronto, whose staff toil anonymously, has been a great help. And I have particularly to thank Meg Masters for some timely editorial help. My dear friend and agent, Beverly Slopen, found, in the University of Toronto Press, a perfect publisher – and Len Husband and Margaret Allen, my editors there, have been a pleasure to work with. Frederick Crews, who read an earlier version and reread a later one for the Press, offered some very reflective comments and has emerged more as a debating partner than an impersonal critic. As the book germinated, one faithful hound that lay at the side of my word processor, the golden shepherd Becky, has now passed on, and as I labour now, it is the Chesapeake Bay retriever Bruna who lies panting in her place.

Edward Shorter
Toronto
September 2004

WRITTEN IN THE FLESH: A HISTORY OF DESIRE

CHAPTER ONE

Introduction

This book is a history not of sex but of sexual desire. A history of sex would include what was thought about it, media attitudes, and its role in marriage and the family. These are all worthy subjects, but none of them is in this book. It is a history of desire, of longing, of what people yearn to do in their heart of hearts. This is the first book of this nature ever written. Yes, it is audacious to take on the whole ball of wax, desire from the ancients to the present. But it is only in the long perspective that we see how completely unlike past times our own patterns of sexual desire are.

From the ancients to the present the world of desire has changed. Not necessarily in the sense of 'progress,' for what one thinks of these changes is an intensely personal matter. But, for better or worse, it has changed. Centuries down the road, the descendants of people who lived in pain and sorrow now relish the sexual force that lies inherent in their bodies. There is a powerful story here, but it's important to separate eternal themes in the history of desire from the narrative arc, so that we do not attribute novelty where there is none, or slide over epochal transformations in the view that there is nothing new under the sun.

What Drives What?

This book argues that sexual behaviour and sensual pleasure are the product of biologically driven desire rather than of fashion or social conditioning. It is in capital letters nature not nurture that drives desire. Just as our bodies tell us what we might like to eat, or when we should go to sleep, they lay down for us our pattern of lust: whether gay or straight, whether total body sex or the missionary position, it is biology, decked out to be sure in the tastes of the era but nonetheless brain driven, that impels us forward. This point of view has only recently started to command attention. In gay studies it is now almost universally assumed that sexual orientation is inborn. In the study of drugs that increase sexual potency, such as apomorphine ('Uprima' of Takeda Abbott Pharmaceuticals),[1] it is clear that the drug acts directly on some kind of desire centre in the brain. One can train rats to administer repeatedly to themselves small electrical doses that excite the brain. So there clearly is some kind of biological, brain-based component in desire that presumably is part of the basic wiring of our nervous systems. And if that is the case, why has it not always been historically visible, in the way that it is manifestly visible in social behaviour today? That is the main question of the book, and it gives the story a central narrative that emerges with overpowering clarity: the history of desire is the history of the almost biological liberation of the brain to free up the mind in the direction of total body sex.

By 'total body sex' one understands the body as a whole as an instrument or a receptacle of desire, not just the face and genitals. Total body sex implicates all of the orifices, the long muscles of the arms and legs, the vee-ness of the torso. It means that the entire body is capable of giving and receiving pleasure, and this is the goalpost towards which desire is racing today.

Desire is a brain-driven longing for sensuality, one that ultimately prevails over all previous social limitations, pushing us ever more relentlessly towards the maximization of the positive sensations that come from the external nerve endings on our bodies. The history of desire is the history of the brain's efforts to drive the mind to create a world in which the peripheral receptors from head to foot send back pleasurable sensations to the brain. The tongue, the nose, the skin, the genitals – all have sensory receptors. Responding to these peripheral receptors, the brain becomes the engine of hedonism, maximizing the inbound pleasurable sensations that reach it and minimizing the nocive. This is the essence of desire.

The story breaks into three parts, with a preface. The preface is the free-and-easy sexuality of classical antiquity, not unlike our own. In part one, night falls over Christian Europe. Then an initial breakout from these long weary centuries occurs around the turn of the twentieth century, as people begin an early exploration of the sexual possibilities of the entire body, strictly taboo before. In part three, after the 1960s a vast acceleration of experimenting with sexual zones and sexual styles occurs, leading in the direction of total body sex.

So the tale is a straightforward one, but its implications are significant. Desire is what the conservative philosophers of yore feared: that the drive for pleasure may indeed be in charge of the human condition. And today it's clear that biological rules govern human behaviour much more tightly than anyone had feared, or hoped. Yet society today ardently aspires to these results rather than hating and fearing them. Our liberal hedonic rules – for better or worse – valorize the physical pleasures without quite coming to grips with the price that must be paid as eroticized couples withdraw from community life in order to pursue private pleasures.

Some of this will be bad news for those who prefer society to retain its moral base in religion. But asserting that the brain is in charge and that pleasure seeking is the result of a constant neural drive rather than the oscillations of fashion also goes against the conventional wisdom about the history of pleasure. Until recently, historians have tended to see the history of sexuality as a pendular movement, going from liberal to conservative and back across the ages. Indeed, those who believe sexuality is socially constructed avoid the term 'desire' altogether as smacking of 'innate drives.' In those circles, the correct term is 'pleasure,' meaning that society determines what you like. This strikes the present author as unlikely. Instead, this book argues something quite different. First, that people in past times experienced a much narrower range of desire than we do. This in itself is unsurprising: they were poorer.

Further, this book suggests that people once placed sexual desire much farther down the list of priorities than we do. This requires more demonstration. The sceptic asks, 'Haven't we always had more or less the same attitudes to sensuality? Haven't we always desired the same things in such a basic human experience?'

No, we haven't. The reason that the desire for physically sensuous experiences comes to the surface so dramatically at the end of the nineteenth century is that the external limits on desire's range and depth are removed. A sensualization takes place of sexuality because private life becomes less mean, more anonymous, and less subject to the scolding of the village elders.

Let's be clear about how this works. The physical brain is the substrate of the mind. Our genes wire the brain in a certain way. The underlying neural circuits of desire themselves probably do not change. Indeed, much of this desire of the brain – hard-wired via genetics – is likely a historical constant. To understand change in history, we must understand how external limitations on this drive are abolished. The history of human sensuality may therefore be understood as the steady removal in the external world of those circumstances that limit the brain's desire for pleasure.

The implication for our own time is this: once the external constraints come off the brain's ability to drive the mind, the search for pleasure is unopposed. After 1900, the drive towards sensuality becomes unilinear, continuous, and irreversible. After the 1960s – as the last vestiges of the former constraints fall away – the drive for pleasure accelerates sharply, producing in this twenty-first century a world of hedonism that has dramatically changed the social landscape.

To be sure, what people actually experience is always a mixture of biology and social conditioning: desire surges from the body, the mind interprets what society will accept and what not, and the rest of the signals are edited out by culture. In this book we see the interplay of biology and society, for example, in the rise of the homosexual 'queen' or the post-1960s isolation from the community that permits cocooning. Yet it is not true, as so many social constructionists maintain, that we recognize our desires only when society tells us what they are; it is not true that a homosexual subculture – just to continue with that example – is made possible by the sex doctors at the end of the nineteenth century. Homosexual subcultures go far back in history.

Or look at the elderly. In the past, it was society that told the elderly the pleasures of the flesh were no longer appropriate for them. In 1759 Lady Mary Wortley Montagu, then seventy years old and living in self-imposed exile in Italy, sighed to a friend, 'The Alps were once mole-hills in my sight when they interposed between me and the slightest inclination; now age begins to freeze.' Once, everything had seemed possible to her; now 'a stove in winter, a garden in summer bounds all our desires.'[2] Today, by contrast, our culture stipulates that the experience of old age may be a time of sexual fulfilment. It is the culture, not the brain, that has changed.

Thus much of the story is an intertwining of body and culture, yet with an emphasis on the physicality of desire rather than the moulding of it. Any student of hedonics will be impressed by the phenomenon: we don't choose desire; desire chooses us. We have relatively little rational control over the pleasures we seek out. Instead, we are driven to them. Anyone who recalls the recurring nature of his or her first masturbatory fantasies realizes the truth of this. It is the deeper neural circuits of desire that push us towards the pleasures we select. Rationality plays little role in what we fantasize about in the bathtub, regard on the street, or undertake in bed.

So, how do we choose pleasure? The brain decides. Then

culture tweaks at the mind. What else influences the mind beyond culture? There is the idiosyncrasy of one's personal development. We all have special private experiences of pleasure that others do not share, rules we elaborate ourselves for figuring out what feels good. For the eighteenth-century romantic writer Jean-Jacques Rousseau, merely kissing the hand of his longed-for Mme d'Houdetot offered the most exquisite satisfaction. He would ease up to it after long preliminaries. 'Those of you who read this will probably laugh about my sex life,' he later wrote; 'But dear readers, please don't deceive yourselves. I probably had more pleasure in my love life, ending with this hand kissing, than you will ever have in yours, which begin at that point.'[3] It was doubtless Rousseau's own distinctive personal development, rather than the surrounding culture, that made hand kissing seem to him the summit of erotic experience. Yet Rousseau dwelt in an emotionally very conservative world, in which he stood out like a sore thumb (giving all his children to a foundling hospital, for example). A less driven man would have been ground into obeisance by the culture of provincial Switzerland and small-town France.

With all this talk about culture, the reader may well ask, Where is the non-Western part of the story? Did desire among the Chinese or the Peruvians not evolve differently? Today, every group may not have achieved the hedonic heights of Western culture, or even aspire to do so. Many Islamic readers will smile at these lines. A cursory knowledge of the Latino or the Vietnamese worlds will demonstrate much relinquishing of pleasure for community values. Many religious fundamentalists will find the narrative related in this book a horrifying one; and where – one might ask – lies the world of pleasure for the AIDS victim or the battered woman?

Two points in response. First, non-Western cultures are absent in this book simply because the present author does not know enough about them. Europe and the Anglo-Saxon world come to the fore because that is the world he is familiar with. This is not a universal history of desire; it's very much a

Western history. Yet that piece of the human experience is worth knowing. Second, the book dwells on the sexually more innovative segments of our own culture rather than the religious conservatives because it is the sexual innovators who seem to be the wave of the future. The following pages capture the central tendency, and sooner or later most other groups will get there too. Even though other parts of the world are absent from this book, a massive convergence in sexual styles, as in so much else, is currently in progress. Dispatches from Japan, for example, confirm this on an almost daily basis. We are, in other words, not portraying a representative cross-section of the world as it is today, or was five hundred years ago, but average lives as they were yesterday and may be tomorrow.

Who Says So?

That men and women are desire driven has, of course, always been known. It was the fourth-century BC Greek philosopher Epicurus who articulated the 'pleasure principle,' declaring to one correspondent, 'We call pleasure the beginning and end of the blessed life.' And in Epicurus's 'calculus of desires,' sex – though not as necessary as warmth – was natural indeed.[4] On a December night in 1662 Samuel Pepys, an administrator in the English Navy Office, crept away from a sociable dinner to see a ribald play and possibly to meet women as well: 'I ought not to do [this] without my wife,' he confided to his diary. 'But Lord, to consider how my natural desire is to pleasure ...' Pepys thanked God for the will power to remain on the straight and narrow (one of the few times in his life that he actually did so).[5]

Yet we are talking about something more than the age-old conflict between the temptation of the flesh and the redemption of the spirit. Rather, people have always realized that the body's desires themselves are the force that drives events forward, whatever the pious wishes of the spirit may dictate. And this awareness of body-centredness goes back, again, to the ancient Greeks. Plato in his *Symposium* celebrated the sexual origin of social relations. He allows Diotima to say that Eros propels the desire for physical beauty, for 'the beauty of one body is akin to the beauty of another.' Ultimately, the psyche arises from this love of physical beauty.'[6] For the ancients, there was no doubt that sexual desire led to praise of beauty, which in turn led to everything else.

During the Middle Ages, the urgings of the body were seen as evidence of sin. But as later generations of writers reflected about the mind and what drives it forward, they returned to the dark secrets of physicality that the ancients had once explored. The English philosopher John Locke drifted near this dangerous water in his *Essay Concerning Human Understanding* (1690), claiming that 'the mind very often sets itself on work in search of some hidden idea ...' Where are these ideas hidden? 'Sometimes they start up in our minds of their own accord, and offer themselves to the understanding, and very often are roused and tumbled out of their dark cells into open daylight, by turbulent and tempestuous passion.'[7] What dark cells could he have possibly meant save the desires of the brain itself? Locke thought that the passions unlocked deeper desires, which would rush from below to flagellate the mind.

Several decades later, Lady Mary Wortley Montagu, contemplating, as we have seen, an old age that would confine her to her 'boat and easy chair,' told her friends that she believed her choices to be in the hands of some inexorable biological destiny. 'I am much inclined to think we are no more free agents than the queen of clubs when she victoriously takes prisoner the knave of hearts ...' We are as incapable of escaping our destiny 'as a card that sticks to a glove when the gamester is determined to throw it on the table.'[8] She had an intuitive sense of the brain urging on the mind, but in this case it was the aging brain forcing the mind to limit activity and seek out the fireside. What Lady Mary viscerally perceived, English philosopher Jeremy Bentham elevated to the status of a philosophical law in 1789 in his

Introduction to the Principles of Morals and Legislation: 'Nature has placed mankind under the governance of two sovereign masters, pain and pleasure. It is for them alone to point out what we ought to do, as well as to determine what we shall do.'[9]

Thus the notion that events are brain or body driven rather than the outcome of logical choice or socially dictated has been with us across the years. As Lord Byron drifted through northern Italy towards his final appointment in Greece, he wrote early in 1822, apparently discouraged about his years spent in the pursuit of pleasure, 'Man is born *passionate* of body – but with an innate though secret tendency to the love of Good in his Main-spring of Mind. – But God help us all! – It is at present a sad jar of atoms.'[10] Hence, free will and choice were nothing amid this jar of atoms.

After the late nineteenth century, when the surrounding world truly does start to become more hedonistic, observations about the brain-driven nature of passion fairly rush forth. D.H. Lawrence, in a postscript that he wrote in 1928 to his novel *Lady Chatterley's Lover*, fulminated against the 'puritan hush! hush! which produces the sexual moron.' But Lawrence was equally uneasy about 'the modern young jazzy and high-brow person who ... just "does as she likes."' He snubbed young women for not experiencing the profound emotions that he himself felt. Yet of interest is where Lawrence believed these emotions to originate: 'The body feels real hunger, real thirst ... real passion, real hate, real grief. All the emotions belong to the body, and are only recognised by the mind.'[11]

Meanwhile across London, Virginia Woolf was as far removed from Lawrence in terms of social class and attitude as it was possible to get. Yet in 1930, she too rejected the conceit that desire concerned mainly the mind, refusing to accept 'that the body is a sheet of plain glass through which the soul looks straight and clear.' Indeed, she said, 'The very opposite is true. All day, all night the body intervenes; blunts or sharpens, colours or discolours ... The creature within can only gaze through the pane – smudged or rosy.' She spoke of 'Those great wars which the body wages with the mind a slave to it, in the solitude of the bedrooms against the assault of fever or the outcome of melancholia ... Of all this daily drama of the body there is no record.' The Bloomsbury crowd were not known for being creatures of the flesh. Yet here their most brilliant member articulated what had become commonly accepted by the twentieth century: that the body encroached heavily upon the autonomy of the mind.[12]

Recognition of human motivation as somehow body driven runs throughout modern letters. There is a long tradition of intuiting the existence of physical sensuality as something separate from the mind, without agonizing about whether it is culturally determined.

It was the Freudian psychoanalysts who started to codify this background intuition into a formal doctrine: the notion of 'polymorphous perversity.' The child's entire body virtually tingles with sexuality, they thought, and thus is 'polymorphously perverse,' in the moral judgment of the day. In 1905, Freud attributed this pan-sexuality to early seduction experiences: 'It is instructive that under the influence of seduction the child can become polymorphously perverse, and can be led to every conceivable sexual deviation.' He thought these perverse impulses were later reactivated in adult life in the form of the kinds of behaviour that prostitutes indulge in. (Freud may have had anal intercourse in mind, without mentioning it.)[13] In 1906 he generalized these views, assuming polymorphous perversity to be present in all children, who then repress in adult life this latent capacity to enjoy pleasure all over the body. 'The child's constitutional predisposition in the area of sexuality is far more variegated than previously assumed; it might be called "polymorphously perverse." From this predisposition, as a result of the repression of certain components, so-called normal sexual behaviour emerges [in adults].'[14]

Freud had initially tiptoed rather nervously about such themes as oral and anal sex. Yet there later emerged among psychoanalytic writers an enthusiasm about sex of all kinds except the homosexual version. The American Freudian Norman O. Brown conceived the polymorphous perversity of early infancy as a kind of undifferentiated sexuality in which all body parts and all sexual practices were equally erotic.[15]

Support from the big guns of psychoanalysis reinforced popular belief that sexual ambitions were motivated by dark underlying forces over which the rational being had little control (except that the analysts saw the dark forces as situated in the unconscious mind rather than in the substance of the brain itself). Salvador Dali believed his own sex life to be the very incarnation of the principle of polymorphous perversity. Writing in 1942 of his childhood he said, 'I was to become the prototype *par excellence* of the phenomenally retarded "polymorphous perverse," having kept almost intact all the reminiscences of the nursling's erogenous paradise: I clutched at pleasure with boundless, selfish eagerness ...'[16] With psychoanalysis, therefore, the notion that we are driven relentlessly towards pleasure by subrational forces acquired wide currency.

The point is that over the centuries in Western society there has been a powerful endorsement of the view that sensual tastes and sexual desires rush directly from deeper sources in the body, rather than being generated by fashion and custom. It is a view that some have always articulated – however much to the dissatisfaction of the church. And it received a compelling affirmation in the twentieth century from the doctrine of psychoanalysis, though the analysts saw the process as psychogenic rather than neurogenic: arising from the mind rather than from the brain.

More recently, opinion in the neurosciences has also swung behind this neurogenic version of the experience of sensuality. For many years, elite opinion had maintained otherwise: that the mind was free to choose good or evil, as the teaching of the church insisted; or that human affairs were capable of the guidance of sweet reason, as liberal political opinion believed in the eighteenth-century Enlightenment and after.

Yet science has stressed for many years the importance of heredity in the forming of the human personality and desire. 'In humanity, it is heredity that determines the disposition of all emotions,' stated French psychiatrist Prosper Lucas in 1847.[17] This kind of genetic thinking became the basis for some hugely inadvised social policies (such as the sterilization of those with mental retardation). After the 1940s it went out of style, then began to return with studies of personality traits and psychiatric illnesses in twins. Since the 1960s it has become apparent that a good deal of human character does have a major genetic component. Hereditary factors are now thought to account for 30 to 60 per cent of the variance in personality traits; as well, half or more of the major psychiatric illnesses seem to involve a family genetic history.[18] Under these circumstances, it would be naive to claim that something as basic to the human constitution as desire does not have a brain-driven basis: sensuality is no more under the control of culture and of free will than any other aspect of our emotional metabolism.

Since the Second World War, the neurosciences have succeeded in identifying pleasure centres in the brain and in linking them to other brain pathways. In 1954, James Olds and Peter Milner of McGill University first began research in the neurophysiology of desire. They found that when certain areas of the rat brain were attached to electrodes, rats would stimulate those areas ceaselessly to derive gratification. (The rats avoided the stimulation of pain-producing areas; still other areas were neutral and produced no hedonic response.)[19] Four years later, in 1958, Olds showed that such brain centres as the hypothalamus responded to psychopharmaceuticals, and thus that desire had a chemistry of its own.[20]

By the beginning of the twenty-first century, research on the brain and pleasure had acquired a leading edge. According to physical anthropologist Helen Fisher at Rutgers University, mating and reproduction seem to be broken down into three separate brain centres: (1) the sex drive itself, associated with the sex hormones – the estrogens and androgens;

(2) the attraction system, which determines specific partner choice, associated with the catecholamines (dopamine, noradrenalin); (3) the attachment system (for nest-building), connected with the neuropeptide hormones vasopressin and oxytocin.[21] This book is mainly about desire and its objects, thus the sex drive and the attraction system, but the point is that these very human urgings have solid neurophysiological underpinnings. The concept of 'brain driven' is not a metaphor.

As psychologist Jaak Panksepp at Bowling Green State University comments ironically, 'It was a remarkable feat of nature to weave powerful sexual feelings and desires in the fabric of the brain, without also revealing the reproductive purposes of those feelings to the eager participants.'[22] That's right. The participants want mainly to have fun. Yet how about homosexuality, consensual sadomasochism, and fetishism? Why not deep neural circuits for these kinds of desire? Nobody knows yet.

Thus the argument of this book, while incapable of definitive proof, can at least be made plausible. There are reasonable grounds to think that the brain might drive the mind forward towards pleasure, (a) because people have always intuitively believed this, and (b) because recent research in the neurosciences gives cause to think that it might be so. The present work adds (c): that, historically, people in Western society have evidenced a relentless and irreversible effort to gratify sexual desires once traditional society's hindrances to gratification were removed.

These perspectives help us weigh in just measure the long tradition that believes mind is independent of brain and body. Harvard philosopher William James spoke in 1902 for those generations of observers who find it unacceptable to contemplate the mind's indenture to the brain. James sneered at the 'medical materialism' of the day that assumed that 'the dependence of mental states upon bodily conditions must be thoroughgoing and complete.' 'So of all our raptures and our drynesses,' he jibed, 'our longings and pantings, our questions and beliefs. They are equally organically founded.' Of course, he believed the opposite. In James's view, there must be higher truths and beliefs independent of body states. 'Otherwise none of our thoughts and feelings ... could retain any value as revelations of the truth, for every one of them without exception flows from the state of its possessor's body at the time.'[23]

Had James lived in our own time he doubtless would have opposed current genetic and biological approaches just as he thundered against the medical materialism of his day. Yet since James's era we have had evidence that turns us in revulsion from the free-will argument. Are we free to choose good over evil? The events of the recently past twentieth century – perhaps the most discouraging century in human history from some points of view – have certainly shown us that pious, God-fearing people can do wrong, as the Germans demonstrated in the Holocaust. We know now that supposedly intelligent and enlightened voters are capable of hideous political choices and that the confidence shown by the liberals of the nineteenth century in human reason was dreadfully misplaced.

May we, through an act of will, rise above desire and choose morally for ourselves and our society? The message of this book is that it's a lot harder than liberal political philosophers once believed. Oscar Wilde agreed. In Wilde's novel *The Picture of Dorian Gray*, published in 1890, Lord Henry Wotton muses, 'I wonder what it was defined man as a rational animal. It was the most premature definition ever given. Man is many things, but he is not rational.' (He says this after Dorian Gray has had a sobbing fit and Basil Hallward, the portraitist, has threatened to destroy the new portrait.)[24]

In debates about the primacy of biology over culture, it is now clear that not only does biology help form consciousness; it helps to make culture as well: our biological predispositions and hereditary endowment forge the social world we inhabit. This will come as a surprise only to those who are in 'biodenial,' as Nadine Weidman puts it, those who dismiss the role that biology plays in pushing behaviour.[25] Irving Gottesman, a biological psychologist at the University of Virginia, was asked in 1998 about the resistance to 'determinism.' He said, 'Well, it's a continuation of general hostility toward anything that can be seen as doing away with free will – anything that is seen as a personal threat to your own self-expression. If you think ... that the drive for self-expression can be compromised by some kind of wiring diagram in your brain, in your neurotransmitter system, that is perceived by some individuals, a small group, as threatening ...'[26]

Indeed. Some readers may be indignant about the argument that we are driven willy-nilly by our bodies in the historic search for pleasure. This book cannot prove that this is so, but at least it can try to make a reasonable case.

CHAPTER TWO

Sex, a Baseline

Is sex like music? There are no new notes, but it's all in the arrangement? Or are there new notes? It's evident that new notes in the history of sexuality do indeed sound, and in our own time some of these new notes are heard with great resonance. But evolution from what? What was sex like before? To gauge the evolution of sensuality, we require a baseline, a description of what sort of sexual behaviour has always been practised. One might think of a baseline as a minimal level of erotic pleasure required for human reproduction.

Part of the assignment is not at all difficult: sex has always offered pleasure. Not only is sex necessary for procreation, for most people it is enjoyable. Thus there is a kind of physiological minimum of pleasure that sex has always given to men and women, despite social restraints, the teachings of the church, or – for women at least – the fear of pregnancy. But where was that minumum set? What was it that most men and women once did in bed that forms a platform for the later spectacular changes?

The baseline corresponds to universal underlying sexual desires the force of which is such that they will be expressed in most times and places – unless the hindrances are extraordinary. Other desires will become expressed as the surrounding society becomes more congenial. The greater the congeniality, the more the expression. Medieval Christian

Europe was most uncongenial, and one barely glimpses the baseline. Today's society is highly congenial, and one sees the whole underlying panoply, the underlying platform of desire, arrayed in its fullest and most colourful effervescence. Historically seen, the changes in sexual behaviour have been spectacular. The purpose of this chapter is not to write a full history of human sexuality but merely to sketch out a status quo ante that lets us judge the surge towards pleasure that takes place after 1900. Of course, there were rivulets on the tide from century to century – an eighteenth-century libertineness among elites, let us say, that contrasts with the enforced piety of the seventeenth century. Yet beneath the elites, for the broad band of average men and women, the rivulets vanish; sexual experience was relatively unchanging from century to century. The big changes have come only in the last hundred years, and in the last forty these have accelerated dramatically. When, therefore, such observers as 'Mr Blue,' a New York maker of pornographic films, assures us that 'Sex has always been around, [it has] always been an element in human life' – he likened it to 'hunger, thirst, and activity'[1] – let us take this with a grain of salt. Declares one popular author, 'I'm amazed how little dalliance has changed since 20 B.C.' She argues that the body of a woman who lived in Roman times and who relished love poetry is 'exactly the same as the body of a woman living in St. Louis right now.'[2] To be sure, the structure of the body is the same, the DNA undiffering. But the physical experiences that the bodies of these two women encounter differ vastly, the kinds of sensations their minds cry out for diverge remarkably.

Playful Sex from Antiquity

In studying the ancient Greeks and Romans we get a sense that ours is not the first society in history to recognize that the whole body can be a vehicle for sexual pleasure – that unrestrained desire leads to 'total body sex.' It is merely the first in a long time. If a taste for total body sex is indeed wired into the basic mechanics of the brain, it would be a surprise if our society, entering the third millennium after Christ, were in fact the first to experience such a thing. How astonishing it would be if all the cultures that have flourished before us – many of them relaxing in the arms of plenty – had not discovered this supposedly fundamental aspect of human desire. Of course many have. This book, owing to the author's own limitations, is mainly about Europe and America after the Middle Ages. Yet it is useful to remind ourselves that previous models for total body sex, and for the mind as the sensual servant of the brain, did exist.

Here is Ovid, a Roman poet who lived several decades before the birth of Christ, advising his mistress on how to behave when together with her husband at a party. Ovid himself was also to be present. Ovid and his lover will communicate with each other, he said, by arching eyebrows, each gesture speaking 'whole silent volumes.' 'When you're thinking about the last time we made love together, touch your rosy cheek with one elegant thumb.' Or she might turn her ring back and forth on her finger when thinking of some special delicacy they performed together in bed.

But it's when Ovid starts instructing her on what not to do that we begin to see the depths of sensuality of the upper classes in ancient Rome: 'Don't let his fingers roam down your dress to touch up those responsive nipples.' (It would be almost two thousand years before references to nipples budding with pleasure start to reappear.)

'So much for what I can see,' said a resigned Ovid. 'But there's plenty goes on under a long evening wrap. The mere thought worries me stiff. Don't start rubbing your thigh against his, don't go playing footsie under the table.'

Describing another lover, he says, 'When at last she stood naked before me, not a stitch of clothing, I couldn't fault her body at any point. Smooth shoulders, delectable arms (I saw, I touched them), nipples inviting caresses, the flat belly outlined beneath that flawless bosom, exquisite curve of a hip, firm youthful thighs.'[3] Ovid appreciated the female body in its full physicality, not just face and genitalia as later would be the case.

A mountain of texts and remaining shards of bowls, mirrors, and statues fill in the picture for us: the ancient Greeks and Romans, generally speaking, worshipped the pleasures of the flesh. Said a French classics professor much later, slightly embarrassed at the texts he had to teach his students, 'Ah! Messieurs, what pigs those Greeks were, but did they have spirit!'[4] The Greek philosopher Plato was not necessarily a sensualist (indeed he seemed suspicious of the pleasures of the body). Yet in his *Symposium*, describing a banquet said to have occurred around 416 BC, he allows the female character Diotima to expound sensually about the pleasures of love. Love, she explains, was a Greek god, the child of Penia (a poor goddess) and Poros (Love's brave, impetuous father). Hence Love had the qualities of both his parents: 'He is by nature neither immortal nor mortal. But now he springs to life when he gets his way; now he dies – all in the very same day. But because he is his father's son he keeps coming back to life ...' If there had been an audience, its members must have been nudging one another and grinning. Diotima was chatting, in this speech, with Socrates – and the book from which it is drawn is, of course, one of the classics of Western philosophy.[5]

Nor were the Romans strangers to this kind of relaxed sexual playfulness. The poet Martial teased his lover about erectile problems:

> When you say – 'Quick: let's get it over' –
> I feel myself a languid lover.
> It's only when you bid me wait
> That I dash from the starting-gate.
> If you are in such haste to go
> You'd better tell me to be slow.[6]

The playfulness of upper-class eroticism in antiquity comes across as well in the surviving art. In a fragment of statuary from the island of Delos in the second century BC, a man enters a woman from behind as she turns her head to kiss him. The sculpture is anything but brutish and crude: the two lovers are locked together in an obvious spasm of ecstasy which the genius of the sculptor has permitted civilizations far removed to feel. In another fragment known as the 'Boston mirror-cover,' from Corinth in fourth-century BC, the woman is bending over, the man is standing behind her. She guides his penis into her vagina with her hand.[7] These must have been typical scenes from the sex lives of the upper classes, else they would have been meaningless to viewers or long destroyed as scandalous pornography.

The erotic art of the Romans embraces even more of the spectrum of human sexuality. One of the frescoes on the walls of a bathhouse just outside the walls of Pompeii in the first century before Christ shows a threesome of two men and a woman. The first man is evidently buggering the second, while the second man has intercourse with the kneeling woman from behind. Following that is another scene, representing a foursome, in which one man, kneeling on the floor, penetrates the man in front, who, in turn, is being fellated by a woman, who, in turn, is receiving cunnilingus from another woman.[8] This is not to say that the average Pompeiian often participated in homoerotic group sex. Yet the sophisticated audience that saw these frescoes would have smiled appreciatively and cracked jokes about them. The entire discussion takes place in a climate of relaxed hedonism that later would have been unthinkable.

There are some limits on the sexuality of the Romans. Oral sex was apparently not condoned among equals, though both men and women could hire prostitutes for its performance.[9] There is little suggestion of the rituals of the consensual sadomasochism of our own time. Also, among Greeks and Romans alike, men evidently had difficulty accepting women as emotional equals in sex.[10] (Ovid is an exception to this, as he relished seeing his partner's orgasm: 'I love the sighs that betray their rapture, that beg me to go slow, to keep it up just a little longer. It's great when my mistress comes, eyes swooning, then collapses, can't take anymore for a long while.')[11] Yet on the whole we encounter among the upper orders of the ancient world an interest in sensuality that suggests society offered few hindrances to the translation of deeply felt sexual desires into action. The Greeks and Romans alike show us the capacity for sensuality inherent in the human condition, in which, in a climate of luxury and permissiveness, the brain drives the mind to pleasure.

A Baseline for Men

But maybe the upper classes of the ancient world two thousand years ago represented only a unique and tiny elite. Perhaps they are typical only of themselves and of nothing more. To talk about a baseline for the human condition, we need to widen our gaze, to look at worlds closer to our own. Let's take Christian Europe after the Middle Ages, a society drenched in piety, constrained by want, and governed by the reproving elders of small towns and villages. Through these layers of hindrance to the expression of underlying sexual desires, what can we glimpse of basic human sexuality? We look at men and women separately, because the fear of pregnancy and anxiety about a sudden and catastrophic loss of one's beauty – for women an important commodity – tended to make sexual issues for women different than for men.

If it is true that the brain drives the mind towards sensuality, one would expect to find most forms of today's sexuality present in the past in embryo, for the brain is unchanged. Some men, surely, must have escaped the brutish restrictiveness of the village and small town in order to free themselves for pleasure. Gay men come immediately to mind. Here we must distinguish between quantity and quality.[12] Quantity means how soon sex begins, how many times per week, and whether it occurs outside the nuptial tie. Quality means what actually happens in bed, what zones of the body are involved. In the quantitative area, not that much has changed for men.

Men have always been sexual adventurers. 'I name, among the trials of my life, the indulgence of the flesh,' said Italian mathematician Jerome Cardano in 1575, a year before his death, as he looked back ruefully upon decades of womanizing, gambling, and other pastimes. 'Finally it came to this, that the very year in which it was believed the end of my life was at hand, brought with it a beginning of living – and that was my forty-third year. That was the moment when ... I made a beginning, turning away from pleasure.'[13] Until his religious conversion at forty-three, Cardano had indulged himself sexually.

There were many who indeed never turned away from pleasure but made it their life's ambition. Gustav Schilling, a young eighteenth-century German writer, described his father as 'the wealthiest cavalier in the county.' '[My father's] first article of belief was, "Love God and your fellow man." His second: People are born for pleasure.' The father made both credos his life plan and retired to his country estate, where he rejected 'the voluntarily assumed shackles of marriage' as inhibiting pleasure, 'the purpose of life.'[14]

For the eighteenth-century Venetian Giacomo Casanova, life itself was just a series of sexual conquests. 'Madame, I am a professional libertine,' he explained to one candidate. Given that he tried to treat women as equals and respect their feelings, it's amazing that he never fell definitively in love, only transitorily. Casanova's problem was the loss of desire after conquest: 'If we succeed [in seducing them], it's certain that we lose our desire for them, for one doesn't desire what one already possesses.'[15]

Casanova stands out against his time because he was a conscious sensualist. 'Cultivating whatever gave pleasure to my senses was always the principal goal of my life,' he wrote in 1797.[16]

So the question is not whether men ardently desired individual women – men and women have always fallen in love – but how ardently men desired sensuality as such. In the scale of life's values, where did sensuality rank? Somewhere near the top, up with running an orderly household and being seen to do one's duty? Or did sensuality fit in farther down, something that was nice if it happened, like eating the roast beef that fell off the wagon but not exactly the purpose of life? This formulation makes opting for sensuality sound like a conscious philosophical choice, like becoming a Unitarian. But the historical reality involved making a series of micro-decisions to seek pleasure, all the while remaining a pious Christian or dedicated husband – subliminal choices, in other words, of which the mind is only dimly aware. In these terms, many men in the past were sensualists, and the concept is part of the male sexual norm.

Thus Samuel Pepys found little contradiction between his Christian faith, his fondness for his wife, and his attempts to pick up female parishioners on Sunday mornings in church. In 1667, Pepys was thirty-four and had been married for twelve years to a beautiful woman with whom he loved to dally mornings in bed. On Sunday, 18 August he attended services at St Dunstan's: 'And [I] stood by a pretty, modest maid, whom I did labour to take by the hand and the body; but she would not, but got further and further from me.' Pepys could see that she had taken a hat pin from her pocket to jab him should he approach again.

So then he spied 'another pretty maid' in a nearby pew. 'And I did go about to take her by the hand, which she suffered a little and then withdrew.' So the sermon ended, and Pepys went home to his wife.[17]

Later that year, on Christmas Eve Day, Pepys went to the Queen's chapel at St James's for a High Mass. Several comely women were present, so he tried something he'd never ventured before: a think-off. 'Here I make myself to do la cosa [orgasm] by mere imagination, mirando a jolie mosa [envisioning intercourse] and with my eyes wide open, which I never did before – and God forgive me for it, it being in the chapel.'[18] On still another occasion Pepys, fixing the image in his mind of a merchant's daughter who was sitting in the upper pew, closed his eyes and masturbated himself in church.[19]

How typical was Pepys? On occasion, he excoriates himself for his wantonness. He went home one day and found that his wife had invited the lovely Mrs Horsely to tea. 'But Lord, to see how my nature could not refrain from temptation, but I must invite them to go to Fox hall ... for an outing, in the hopes of scoring.'[20] He was often rueful about his transgressions, and so he saw himself perhaps as sexually driven. But there is no indication that he regarded himself as untypical of the men in his circle, merely that his astonishingly frank diary has survived whereas many similar diaries perished, burned by the relatives. Yet Pepys's circle of upper-middle-class urban males was a quite restricted one.

If one were to go by the evidence of Pepys, Casanova, and history's other great libertines, one would say that the male baseline included a large component of intense and articulate sexual desire. Yet how typical were these men, in view of the ability of the culture to force the mind to renounce and to turn in horror from the pleasures of the senses? This turning away in horror was far more typical of the experience of the average man before the last third of the nineteenth century than were the Casanovas and Pepyses of this world. The New Year of Christian Gellert, a minor German littérateur, age forty-six, began poorly in 1761: 'I am weak and suffer at night from a disabling excretion, the onset of which I have felt now for several days.' Gellert dwelt upon his sinfulness. These rather vague diary entries continue for months, the nocturnal incidents striking again and again.

On 31 July he noted, 'I slept well, but am awakened by a sexual dream and experienced, just like a year ago, powerful feelings of voluptuousness.' Since his supplications to the Lord for relief had availed not, Gellert decided to consult Dr Hebenstreit, who apparently prescribed quinine water. By Christmas, Gellert was feeling better.[21]

With Gellert, we see the same deep underlying eroticism

that propelled Pepys yet turned into an object of horror in the intense religiosity of German Pietism. But Gellert at least allowed himself to wrestle with daydreams, erections, and nocturnal discharges. For many men, the wrapping in piety was sufficiently tight that sensualism had no chance of victory at all.

Here we have young William Stout, a twenty-six-year-old Quaker shopkeeper living in Lancaster, England. In 1691 he and his sister decided to begin keeping house, in a street where she already had a number of acquaintances. 'But in some time, the familiarity increased so much that I feared that it extended above what it was safe in innocency to allow ... I was very sensible that my neighbour to the street side, whose lodgings with mine were in common up one pair of stairs, took all opportunities in conversation and other insinuations to allure me to her bed, or to introduce herself into mine.' Her husband was abroad in America. Pepys, of course, would have leapt at the opportunity. But how did young Stout respond? He sought recourse to God 'to be preserved innocent, and especially in that prayer of Jesus Christ, viz: "and lead us not into temptation ..."' For several more years Stout continued to live near the woman, 'observing her freedom in discourse, and the entertainment of some young men in her house.'[22] His faith had clearly saved him from debauchery, he thought.

Stout is typical of a theme in the history of male desire that needs no further elaboration because it is so obvious: the struggle with temptation. Autobiography and literature since Augustine are filled with examples of men who wrestled with desire and either won or lost. The point is that male desire, in the form of visiting prostitutes or coveting the wives of others, is probably a historical constant. In drawing a baseline, the only interesting point is whether, and under what circumstances, men have acted on the basis of longing. A few men such as Pepys and Casanova have always responded to these deep urges. Yet in times past, the Pietists, the Counter-Reformation Catholics, and the thin-lipped

Quakers have always been more numerous. It is more likely Stout and Gellert who were sociologically typical in insulating the mind from the urgings of the brain and letting custom and belief stifle the call of desire.

Looking back upon past times, the Parisian food critic Anthelme Brillat-Savarin marvelled in 1826 that physical love had been an object of such uninterest, 'right up to the time of Buffon [mid-eighteenth century].' Brillat-Savarin considered the sexual sense to be just as important as the other special senses such as hearing, taste, touch, and so forth. 'It is astonishing,' he wrote, 'that a sense of such importance could have been misrecognized, and even confused or assimilated to the sense of touch.'[23] Romance and falling in love are separate issues that may or may not include intense physicality. But if Brillat-Savarin was right, for most men who lived before the nineteenth century the sexual baseline did not include acute and arduous desire articulated in the mind as a plan of action. It remained slumbering in the brain.

How about the qualitative side – what men actually did in bed? The question, of course, should be phrased to include women, since the plan of action could only be carried out with a member of the opposite sex. Yet just as men determined much else of what happened in family and political life before the nineteenth century, they determined as well the nature of sexual activity. Here one is astonished by the narrowness of the agenda. For the vast majority of men before the end of the nineteenth century, sexual actions and fantasies were limited to intercourse in the missionary position. There is a great deal of evidence for this bold generalization.

Misinformation on this subject abounds. The *Decameron* of Giovanni Boccaccio, set just outside of Florence in the mid-fourteenth century, laid the basis of the Western tradition of sardonic erotic fiction, featuring wayward friars, lovesick older men, and desirous noblewomen. Behaviour stolen from the *Decameron* has always suggested the erotic and forbidden. Yet if the male baseline is to be sought here, it would be decorous indeed, for Boccaccio's work features very little in the way of non-conventional sex. Boccaccio is discreet about exactly what his creatures are permitted in bed, though occasionally we learn that the couples disported themselves so vigorously that, 'Fra [Brother] Puccio thought he felt the floor of the house shake a little.' The wayward monks seem to favour the missionary position, and if occasionally the woman is on top, it is only because the friar in question is so fat. Readers would not bear away the message that the body is capable of multiple pleasures.[24]

The works of Pietro Aretino several centuries later have similarly become synonyms for wickedness, as at the bedside of one of Casanova's partners. When he, at age twenty-nine, encountered young Marina Morosini ('M.M.') in a convent near Venice in 1754, he discovered that she, worldly young thing of twenty-two, had a copy of Aretino's early-sixteenth-century sonnets. The sonnets were, like the *Decameron*, acidulous send-ups of noble ladies, the clergy, and others who engaged in sexual peccadilloes. Sixteen in number, they had been written to accompany ten copperplate prints of sexual scenes that had been commissioned by one of the popes. The original prints had vanished, but by Casanova's day a good deal of erotic literature was in circulation falsely purporting to represent the lost prints and all of Aretino's numerous postures. Now Casanova proposed to M.M. that in the three hours at their disposition they perform 'some of the postures.'

M.M. replied, 'Some can't possibly be acted out and others are insipid.' Casanova and M.M. agreed to try three, though we aren't told which.[25] The Aretino tradition, in other words, boosts sexual athleticism but no erotic zones save the genitals. It is positionology, not zoneology.

In even libertarian male encounters it was positionology that triumphed over zoneology: the thrill of different bodily positions as opposed to exploring new erotic zones of the body. In the dozens of sexual encounters that Pepys mentions, he seems either to have used the missionary position or to have been standing up, as the situation required. He comments occasionally on deviations from this pattern, but they are few in number. To wit: on Whitsunday, 1666, he goes to the home of his old friend Betty Martin 'and there did what je voudrais avec her, both devante and backward, which is also muy bon plazer.' (Pepys often used this pigdin sex code to describe the details: he penetrated her straight and from behind, both most pleasurable for him.) A year later with another old friend, Mrs Bagwell, he does the act both 'venter and cons,' meaning frontal and back (not anal intercourse). On another occasion he invited Mrs Daniel to step into his coach; they became intimate, and she masturbated him. Finally, Mrs Turner, wife of a colleague at the Navy Office, stayed on at the Pepys home after a small intimate dinner, and she and Pepys touched each other's 'things.' That is the extent of the unconventional in his nine-year saga of sexual adventure.[26]

As for body parts, Pepys was interested solely in his own penis. He never comments on his own nipples: presumably his partners never touched them. And on only one occasion did he comment on experiencing pleasure from playing with a woman's nipples (with Pegg, as they kissed in a closet).[27] From time to time he fondled his partners' breasts. Indeed, breasts in general for the men of his time seem to have been more an object of interest than the erotically much more sensitive nipples. In sexual terms, Pepys was totally and utterly conventional in the context of his age, however randily he may have carried on.

The erotic literature of an era displays its sexual range. Surely here the imagination of a society receives its fullest airing. If a theme isn't present in the sexy fireside tales of an epoch or in its erotic art or pornography, there's a good chance that it simply doesn't exist in that society's sexual repertoire.

Beneath the austerely religious high culture of the Middle Ages there bubbled a lively popular culture, full of broad winks about sexuality. In Old French, this sexual humour was recorded in the *fabliaux* – fables told at the fireside and handed down from generation to generation. They are full of 'randy wandering students, concupiscent clerics, lascivious wives, clever prostitutes, procuresses, and pimps,' as Howard Bloch puts it. Yet in Bloch's analysis, the *fabliaux* are 'orthodox to a fault.' Despite their apparent liberality, they contain virtually no references to homosexuality, anal sex, sadomasochism, or oral sex. The *fabliaux*, filled with detailed descriptions of sexual organs, refer to virtually no sexual posture save the missionary position.[28] So the problem is not modesty; it's the restricted sexual imagination of the era.

We leap forward to seventeenth-century Spain. The Spanish Inquisition has begun and is interrogating wayward priests who fondled their parishioners in the confessional (or worse) about their sexual fantasies. A few of the fantasies were bizarre, a product, in the words of one student, of the 'extreme sexual frustration and repressed longings of the age.' Thus female saints being raped and beautiful virgins with mutilated breasts were the order of the day. Yet the great majority of fantasies of the ordinary priests were perfectly conventional, involving fatherhood, family life, and placing one's head between the breasts of one's handsome young parishioners. Cunnilingus was 'extremely rare.' At the farthest edge of the Spanish sexual imagination was one priest who 'expressed a desire to see Sor Augustina and another nun engage in sex play.'[29]

The pornography of the day emphasizes as well the narrowness of the seventeenth-century erotic imagination. The chief conceit is the size of the penis and the awe with which women look upon such an organ (matched only by their subsequent delight). French eroticist Nicolas Chorier, writing around 1660, allows Tullia and Octavia to have a dialogue about Octavia's recent encounter:

Octavia: 'I soon felt some large warm object between my thighs. He forced me to open up; with a robust effort he shoved that stiff thing against my body and that crack.'

Octavia resists mightily.

Tullia: 'You mean that with one hand you were able to ward off so monstrous a catapult?'

Octavia says that she 'grabbed it and held it aside. But what a mess! I felt myself completely drenched with a shower like fire and, naked as I was, it went right up to my navel.'

Later in the story Tullia relates her own experiences of intercourse. Octavia reassures her, 'The pain is nothing compared to the joys.' The entire humour is focused on the size of the fiancé's penis and the agonies of Octavia's devirgination after her wedding. There are no references to oral sex in the tale.[30]

In the eighteenth century the volume of pornography rises enormously. Of the 457 clandestinely published books that Robert Darnton examined for France in the period 1769 to 1789, 21 per cent treated sex. The big bestseller was a French translation of *Fanny Hill*, John Cleland's 1749 novel.[31]

Indeed *Fanny Hill* illustrates neatly the range of sexual themes in which Cleland believed his readers were interested. As Fanny, fifteen, arrives in London she is seduced by an older lesbian: after a bit of body touching, the focus is completely on the vagina: 'Oh! Let me view the small, dear, tender cleft!' Recruited into prostitution, Fanny soon falls in love with her client Charles. They have several bouts of vaginal sex, references being made to his 'over-fierce attack' and the like. The next candidate, Mr H —, hops into her bed, rapidly covers her body 'with a profusion of kisses,' then scores. Other suitors indulge in scarcely more foreplay, occasionally fondling her breasts. At the climax of the story, she and a lover feel each other all over while standing in a pool of water. In this odyssey, Fanny's most imaginative sexual position is sitting in a chair with her legs up. Throughout, almost all vaginal sex is in the missionary position. There is no oral sex. Several men attempt anal but get no further. The men themselves evidence little interest in being touched. For both men and women, nipple play is a non-theme.[32] The novel typifies the vaginal focus, missionary position, and ram-it-home approach that is characteristic of the baseline of male sexuality.

Virtually all of the plots of eighteenth-century pornographic novels contain the above themes with little variation save the occasional episode of heterosexual anal sex. In none is there much interest in sex as a total body experience.

In a series of thirty pornographic mezzotints from late-eighteenth- and early-nineteenth-century England, the dramatis personae are all engaged in coitus(and to be sure in various positions), but in none of them is there nipple play; the anus is involved in almost none; and oral-genital sex is a non-starter.[33] Despite the apparent wantonness of the sex scenes in the pornographic literature and art of the day, we are still light-years away from total body sex.

In the male baseline, the chief image that aroused desire was the woman's face, the rest of her body being either a mystery or a matter of uninterest. '[It] is a strange slavery that I stand in to beauty, that I value nothing near it,' wrote Pepys in 1664. He had just visited the milliner Doll Stacey and paid an outrageous sum for a pair of gloves trimmed with yellow ribbon. 'But she is so pretty, that, God forgive me, I could not think it too much.'[34] But of course Pepys couldn't see the rest of Doll's body because it was completely covered by clothing. She was a handsome woman, and he fixed his sexual longing upon her face.

What parts of the female body are considered beautiful? asked Agnolo Firenzuola in 1541 in his dialogue *On the Beauty of Women*. Firenzuola had grown up in Florence, knew Aretino in Rome, and now, at forty-five, had returned to Tuscany to live in a rather worldly monastery in Prato. Firenzuola had been around enough to distil the conventional wisdom of the men of his day on the subject of women. He dwells long upon the face and the head: 'the ears then open out from the highest part of the body,' and so on. Then there is a brief paragraph on the breasts, 'like two hills filled with snow and roses.' Then silence! Down to the feet: 'The feet are worthy of much attention and very important for the total beauty of the entire body ...'[35]

This theme is struck again and again in early-modern literature: that what interests men in women is mainly the prettiness of the face. 'Let's talk about looks,' said Pierre de Bourdeilles, called 'Brantôme' after the name of his chateau, in his late-sixteenth-century book, *Worldly Women*. 'There's no lovelier sight on earth than a beautiful woman, either dressed ... or naked between the sheets.' In fact, having sex while dressed was even more exciting, said Brantôme, because of the thrill of not knowing what was underneath: 'The pleasure is redoubled when, of all parts of the body, you can see only the face.' But learning that a beautiful woman has an unattractive body can cut your desire completely, he added. 'Alas, this is the worst! Such beautiful women, such beautiful faces, we see them and admire them, and desire their beautiful bodies for the love of their beautiful faces. And then it happens that, when they get undressed and show themselves naked, we lose our desire: because they're ugly ... so hideous that the face has deceived us completely. And we've [meaning Brantôme himself] made a number of mistakes like this.'[36]

Perhaps it was *faute de mieux* that men were so attached to women's faces: they could see little else. In his *Confessions*, written in 1769, Jean-Jacques Rousseau describes what was visible of Mme Basile, whom he knew at the age of sixteen: 'I devoured with my eyes all that I could see of her without being noticed: the flowers of her gown, the tip of her pretty toe, the section of white firm arm visible between her sleeve and her glove, and whatever one could see between her throat and her kerchief [in her bosom].' Yet the limited nature of the view did not prevent the young man from transpiring with desire: 'As a result of glimpsing what I could, and perhaps even beyond, my eyes grew dim, my chest felt heavy, and my respiration, ever more rapid, became almost uncontrollable, and all I could do was to take my leave without the benefit of audible sighs ...'[37] Thus, it was Mme Basile's face that transported the young student into rapture. He could scarcely see anything else.

It is now 1750. Twenty-five-year-old Casanova has just arrived in Paris. He is at the opera, and one of the other guests in a royal box (where Casanova has been received) asks him, 'Which of the two actresses do you think is more beautiful?'

'That one,' replies Casanova.

'She has ugly legs.'

'One can't see them, Monsieur, and anyway, in assessing the beauty of a woman the first thing I ignore are the legs.'[38]

The overwhelming historical evidence suggests that for men the very minimum of sexual desire – the baseline – focused on the face of the woman, the rest of her anatomy being really a matter of speculation. (And this is a tradition that coasted into the early nineteenth century, English painter Robert Haydon declaring in 1814, 'An eye melting, piercing, shining, full of soul as it beams, is a more lovely object, a more intellectual object, than a great limb or a fine foot. The most interesting part of Nature is the face.')[39]

Historically, there are examples of men of letters praising nudity or the entire female body, yet these have received more attention than they deserve. In Thomas More's *Utopia* (1518), prospective candidates in the marriage market are allowed to inspect each other's bodies naked ('A sad and honest matrone sheweth the woman ... naked to the wooer. And likewise a sage and discreet man exhibiteth the wooer to the woman').[40] But More evidently intends this inspection for medical or hygienic reasons, not to heighten desire. It is, in any event, a fantasy, as are the seventeenth-century poet John Donne's rhapsodies about the naked body: From Donne's 'To His Mistress Going to Bed':

> Full nakedness, all joys are due to thee.
> As souls unbodied, bodies uncloth'd must be
> To taste whole joys.

Yet the editor of Donne's *Elegies* is quick to throw cold water on the idea that these lines might somehow have reflected his experience: the poet's inspiration was largely literary, going back to such Roman sensualists as Ovid. As Donne confided to a correspondent in 1625, 'You knew my uttermost when it was best, and even then I did best when I had least truth for my subjects.'[41] It is Donne's imagination that gives magic to these millennial male fantasies. But in actual practice, the woman's face alone would suffice for sexual arousal, her body being terra incognita.

Even after marriage, essential parts of the woman's body remained unknown territory, at least to hands and eyes. Pepys exhibited an extreme squeamishness about looking at women's private parts. He marvelled, for example, at the story of a pal who had tricked a woman into believing that he was a physician who could treat a vaginal infection. The ruse worked, and as the pal returned with medication, he received 'the sight of her thing below, and did handle it – and he swears the next time that he will do more,' wrote an astonished Pepys. Years later, Pepys finally brought himself to touch 'the thing' of a woman. But not until February 1669, fourteen years after his marriage to Mrs Pepys, did he actually overcome his reluctance to insert his finger in his wife's vagina, and then only in a moment of marital crisis: 'At last [we] ... went to bed betimes, where I did hazer [fuck] her very well, and did this night by chance the first time put my finger in her thing, which did her much pleasure, but I pray God that she does not think that I did know before – or get a trick of liking it.'[42] Just as long as she didn't develop the habit!

In the context of the time, Pepys's squeamishness was not unusual. Brantôme tells of a 'very great prince' who had as his mistress 'a very great princesse.' He was brought to look at and touch her pudendum only after great exhortations. Liking what he saw, however, he made touching and inspecting her vagina a part of her future gratification.[43] Under such circumstances, it would be difficult to talk of total body sex in times past.

Finally, in assessing the baseline of male sexual gratification, there is masturbation.[44] There is no question that men who lived before the mid-nineteenth century masturbated. The only issue is, how often? To what extent was masturbation a part of their daily life, rather than an extraordinary act indulged in deeply secret moments? De facto evidence of the existence of masturbation is the flood of pornography that swept onto the market in the eighteenth century, 'books to be read with only one hand,' as Rousseau said. But personal testimony about masturbation is rare, and we know of the practice mainly from medical condemnations of it, which increased greatly in frequency during the century.

What little we have in the way of personal testimony suggests that masturbation was practised, but not frequently. Pepys's diary offers a frank view of his own sex life, and in the course of the nine years that he diarized, he masturbated only three times aside from the above-mentioned episode in church. Thus Pepys led, from the viewpoint of masturbation, not exactly an over-excited life, but not one totally deprived either. (At present, the average for American men who masturbate is three times a week.)

There is no other historical source comparable to Pepys, yet other authors who specialized in personal revelation do give us some glimpses into their masturbatory life as well. Casanova believed masturbation to be normal in young men, and although he himself did so occasionally, it was with reluctance. In Turin he encountered 'the beautiful Jewess' Lia. Of course he wants to sleep with her. Not tonight, she says, but you can watch me undress. With Casanova hidden in the closet, she disrobes elaborately. 'I was not able to prevent myself from masturbating,' he says, 'an irritation inimical to love.'[45] Rousseau, age nineteen, is totally in love with Mme de Warens of Annecy, who has taken him in as a boarder. 'How many times did I kiss my bedding imagining that it was she who had slept there ... [or kiss] the floor, as I prostrated myself, fantasizing that she had walked upon it.' Once at table, as she was about to put a bite in her mouth, he cried out that there was a hair on it. She spat it out, and he grabbed it and gobbled it down. Thus Rousseau's frame of mind as, in 1729, he began masturbating, 'which is a great stimulant to the lively imagination.' But he did so while fully cognizant of the great health risks he believed himself to be running, and in the future he would do it seldom.[46]

If history's great libertines masturbated rarely, what of the common people? To what extent did masturbation really form part of the common experience for men? We have the most contradictory testimony to sort out: from physicians who believed the locals did it all the time to those who believed their patients to be as pure as the driven snow. In 1760 one French physician alluded to 'this vice, which is only too common in our century.' This contrasts with the affirmation of two doctors in Stuttgart a few decades later that 'the sin of self-abuse has not achieved deep roots here, which speaks well for the mostly blossoming appearance of our boys and girls and is a credit to their parents.'[47] These testimonies cannot possibly be reconciled, and it would be dull to review them in detail.

The last intimate diary we have before coming to the great transformation of the late nineteenth century is that of the English statesman William Gladstone. Even though Gladstone wrestled with the practice as though with the devil himself, it is clear that he masturbated more frequently than did Pepys. And he started earlier than Rousseau. In 1829, at age twenty, Gladstone says that, 'though God has kept the temptation away there has been black sin on my part.' He used this code word for masturbation, suggesting that this indeed was not the first time. A year later he alludes to himself as, 'the sinner within and without, sinner within my rankling passions (passions which I dare not name – shame forbids it and duty does not seem to require it –) and sinner without in the veil of godliness and moderation too which I have cast over them ...' This gives the flavour of the references that continue throughout the diaries: the one sin 'which returns upon me again and again like a flood. God help me ...' In 1837: 'restless cravings towards the quarter I have left,' and so on throughout life.[48] Masturbation was thus part of the baseline of male sexual experience, but it seems to have produced mainly feelings of guilt and remorse rather than constituting a hedonistic encounter with one's body.

The Female Baseline

There is no reason to believe female desire any less ardent than male. The eighteenth-century feminist hero Mary Wollstonecraft was almost certainly wrong when she wrote, 'Men are certainly more under the influence of their appetites than women.'[49] In fact, women desire pleasure with the same intrinsic force as men. Yet historically the external constraints on the expression of women's desire were far greater than those facing men. Hence women in history appear less sexually driven than men, even though their underlying starting point, or baseline, may have been identical. Yet occasionally the glowing coals of female desire do break through to the surface, and we glimpse it across the ages, however briefly. These fleeting sightings represent a reassurance that deep in the spirit, the ardour of female passion glowed as brightly as that of male.

In the fifteenth century, the male Welsh poet Dafydd Llwyd challenged the female poet Gwerful Mechain to a kind of sexual shoot-out: Could she match his challenge?

'Tell me, lovely girl,' he wrote, 'slender are your brows, your look is tender; do [you] have any dish and a long sheath which would contain this [dick]?'

Gwerful replies: 'Here's a hairy pit, until you get tired, Dafydd, to tame your prick; here's a seat for your balls, here you are, if you come as far as the arse ... I'll follow you if I'm not held, brave noble lad with the long cock.'[50]

The glowing coals smoulder into flame in the sonnets of the sixteenth-century French poet Louise Labé, who offers us a female version of the classical male 'kiss poem.' She writes:

> Kiss me once more, kiss me again, and kiss me:
> Give me one of your tastiest kisses,
> Give me one of your most loving ones:
> I'll return you four, hotter than coals.[51]

Hotter than coals. At least some women were willing to articulate such deep-seated desires in poetry. Others wrote them down in memoirs. Looking back in 1793 from her prison cell (where she would shortly be executed), Mme Manon Roland, thirty-nine, recalled the ascetic piety of her girlhood. 'I had read in [our religious texts] that it wasn't allowed us to have any kind of pleasure at all from our bodies, except in marriage.' Then at fourteen she had her first menstruation, and her eyes began to open: 'I was somehow drawn from this most profound sleep in a surprising way. My imagination played no role at all ... I underwent the most extraordinary incandescence of my sensations ... effecting in me a kind of purging, although I had no idea of the cause.' 'What I was experiencing could be called pleasure, thus I was guilty ...'

Roland's guilt at the pleasurable, evidently masturbatory, sensations that her body produced turned into delight once she was married. 'A single night of marriage' overturned all of her philosophical defences against pleasure. Even now, facing death in 1793, she continued to be pleased at how young and desirable she looked.[52]

Mme Françoise de Graffigny, a noblewoman at a provincial court whose letters leave a remarkable account of an early-eighteenth-century emotional life, was something of a hedonist. At age forty-three she exulted in making love in her boyfriend's carriage on the Pont Neuf in Paris.[53] These testimonies are astonishing because there are so few of them directly from women themselves. More numerous are the male lovers who testify how sexually excited their women become. This could be self-serving, yet perhaps the men are telling the truth. Of the Catholic priests put on trial for sex crimes in seventeenth-century Spain, 39 per cent testified that the women responded positively when they, the confessors, came on to them. The marital dissatisfaction of some of these women was heartbreaking. One woman declared that she would 'sometimes rather sleep next to a pregnant pig' than with her husband.[54]

It is no wonder that Casanova, with his charm and his

concern for his partners' satisfaction, was attractive to women. And he reports a number who evidently experienced deep pleasure in his embrace. Anticipating spending a night together with him, a Mme F. says, 'All right, let's try out any game that might please the senses. We'll abandon control over all of our faculties. Devour me. But you must let me do to you whatever I want. And if tonight turns out to be too short, we'll suffer in silence tomorrow, in the certain knowledge that our love will give us yet another night.'[55] In these lines, Mme F. speaks as freely as any man of deep desire. It's clear that her baseline could not have been any shallower than a man's.

A third kind of testimony comes not from men who claim to report female experience but from men, such as Giovanni Boccaccio, who fantasize what it must be like to experience pleasure as a woman.[56] Yet Boccaccio, evidently in his mid-thirties at the time he wrote the *Decameron* (which is set during the plague of 1348 and was written shortly thereafter), had much previous experience with women, including a grand love affair lasting twelve years. The women in his stories are often aflame with desire, one an abbess who captures the gardener and seduces him, another a 'lusty' young lady who takes evident pleasure with a monk. The tales abound with women who 'glow,' who give 'partially suppressed sighs,' and who are always more ready for sex than men. And the women crave variety! Boccaccio wrote: 'As it not seldom happens that one cannot keep ever to the same diet, but would fain at times vary it, so this lady [Madonna Isabella], finding her husband not altogether to her mind, became enamoured of a gallant ...'[57] The problem is that portraying women as crazed with desire is a standard convention of erotic writers who set out to titillate other males. Even though Boccaccio claimed to be writing the *Decameron* for women, he later expressed distaste at the thought that they might read it.[58] So there is a point at which male-generated evidence about women blends into fantasy.

Do we cross this point with the Marquis de Sade late in the

eighteenth century? Or does his extensive experience with seduction make him a reliable gauge of women's desire? His female characters are raging with it to the point of insatiability. In the 'Story of Juliette,' published in 1796, Juliette, her female buddy Clairwil, and the prince are leaving some hideous scene of debauchery. 'Your friend still hasn't had enough,' says the prince to Juliette, pointing to Clairwil, who is entertaining herself by poking at the wounds of the dead who have been left on the field of battle.

'Fuck!' cries Clairwil. 'You don't think we've had enough of this do you? Do you think that one ever really gets enough?"[59]

Sade has held readers spellbound for two centuries now. Surely there was an audience for his view that women could be as rapaciously desirous as men.

Yet women generally speaking were allowed to act on their desire far less often (though some of the women at court constituted an exception). Among women who have left testimony, the vast majority commonly denied all desire, praising instead the path of abstinence. Most of the comments of women about sex are anti-erotic rather than hedonic. There is historic evidence aplenty of women's distaste for sex, of a deep underlying suspicion of eroticism. Few articulated this as well as Mary Wollstonecraft, thirty-three at the time she wrote what was to become the intellectual foundation stone of the feminist movement, *A Vindication of the Rights of Woman* (1792). The book's underlying argument was that, although women are superb as mothers and intellectual companions, sex and passion are a snare for them. Wollstonecraft could not tolerate that women were required to learn about sexual pleasure, for either themselves or others, which she referred to as 'the art of pleasing.' How might one produce virtuous wives? she asked. Don't 'teach her to practise the wanton arts of a mistress ... [demanded] by the sensualist who can no longer relish the artless charms of sincerity or taste the pleasure arising from a tender intimacy.'[60] The sensualist male was the bugbear on the horizon of the virtuous woman.

According to Wollstonecraft, apprenticeship for harlotry began already in boarding school, when girls learned the evil vice of masturbation: 'A number of girls sleep in the same room, and wash together ... I should be very anxious to prevent their acquiring nasty, or immodest habits; and as many girls have learned very nasty tricks from ignorant servants, the mixing them thus indiscriminately together is very improper.' As for adolescent daughters, the last thing they should learn is 'being taught to please.' 'What an example of folly, not to say vice, would [such a mother] be to her innocent daughters!' During the honeymoon, avoid frequent sex: 'The behaviour of many newly married women has often disgusted me. They seem anxious never to let their husbands forget the privilege of marriage; and to find no pleasure in his society unless he is acting the lover.' Then finally, as the husband loses interest, all the seductive charms the woman has acquired along life's highway will be as naught: 'When the husband ceases to be a lover – and the time will inevitably come, her desire of pleasing will then grow languid, or become a spring of bitterness.'[61] Thus the lives of women who interested themselves in sexual pleasure were destined to end in arid disappointment.

Shortly after writing these lines, Mary Wollstonecraft herself became almost unglued with desire for the artist Henry Fuseli – himself apparently something of an SM adept (see below) – as well as for others.[62] Yet it was this book that authorized a strain of sexual primness that would dog the feminist movement for the next several centuries. In *A Vindication* Wollstonecraft was merely voicing in non-religious terms the vein of female mistrust of Eros that has run through the ages.

Some of this mistrust had explicitly religious roots, as in the young Laura Cereta of fifteenth-century Italy, married at fifteen, who lost her husband the following year. After this brief taste of marital sex, she spent the rest of her days devoting herself to the study of 'religious texts.'[63] After the Englishwoman Margery Kempe heard one night 'a sound of melody so sweet and delectable that she thought she had been in Paradise,' she decided to renounce the flesh. 'And after this time she had never desired to commune fleshly with her husband, for the debt of matrimony was so abominable to her that she would rather, she thought, have eaten or drunk the ooze and the muck in the gutter than consent to any fleshly communing, save only for obedience.'[64] One notes the phrase, 'the debt of matrimony,' the subtext of which is, sensuality is something women must do, not something they enjoy.

We follow the trajectory of Lady Elizabeth Delaval, a seventeenth-century English noblewoman, as she matures:

At fourteen, in 1663: 'I have done little or no good. I have done much evil.'

At fifteen: 'I who am but vile dust and ashes ...'

At sixteen: 'Sin like a crust of leprosy has spread me all over, Lord ...'

At twenty-two: 'O grant that my study may be evermore to contemn all such imaginary pleasures of the body, and so to elevate my mind that ... I may bear all afflictions ...'

One could say that this is merely the rhetoric of sin and guilt in a century fearful of hellfire. Yet the point is that for Elizabeth Delaval there would apparently be no apprenticeship in the art of pleasing, no discovery of her own capacities for pleasure, no surrender to the sensual impulses beating out from somewhere deep in her brain or soul – because she does allude vaguely to physical longing as a young man courts her ('for I have hitherto kept myself from giving him any other love than what a sister may have for a brother, yet I know not how long I may so well defend my heart ...').[65]

The dubiety, however, that most women expressed about Eros before the nineteenth century was not rooted so much in religion as in experience. If they saw the pleasures of the flesh as dangerous to them, it was not for ascetic reasons but because they had been disappointed by sex, mainly in the form of unwanted pregnancies or unfaithful husbands. 'Whoever wants to put an end to all laughter should get married in

France,' wrote Liselotte of the Palatinate in 1699 to her sister back in Frankfurt. Liselotte, a German princess married to the Duke of Orléans, was bitterly unhappy at court. On another occasion she said, 'Getting married in this country is a risky business, one soon followed by remorse.' At fifty, she considered herself past the point of experiencing pleasure. 'In this world I no longer expect happiness of any kind. I'm too old to enjoy anything.'[66]

Liselotte had suffered terribly from the prince's cruelty and infidelity. The Marchioness of Newcastle, by contrast, had great affection and respect for her husband, her 'Lord,' as she put it. 'He was the only person I ever was in love with,' she wrote in 1656. 'But it was not amorous love.' What kind of love was it? Evidently not carnal, for 'I am chaste both by nature and education insomuch as I do abhor an unchaste thought.'[67] Such comments from women were common enough in the god-fearing seventeenth century.

But this vein endures long after the fires of religious ardour have burned out. In the reputedly pleasure-loving eighteenth century, among the great majority of women who talk of such things, the tenor of the discussion remains anti-erotic, anti-sensual. We are not talking about Bible-thumping female prisses. Lady Mary, the daughter of Lord Kingston, despite being urbane, witty, and well-educated, was nonetheless at the receiving end of generations of women's folklore about men and the suffering they cause. 'Our aunts and grandmothers always tell us men are a sort of animals, that if ever they are constant 'tis only where they are ill us'd.' In her circle, lifelong misery was the usual scenario: people marry, retire to the country, and become bored with each other: 'The gentleman falls in love with his dogs and horses, and out of love with everything else.'[68]

But Lady Mary was resolved to do it differently, to combine the affection of friendship with the stability of marriage. When she eloped with Edward Wortley Montagu in 1712 at age twenty-one, it was in an apparent marriage of love. Yet she had warned him in advance, 'If you expect passion I am

utterly unacquainted with any. It may be a fault of my tem-
per. 'Tis a stupidity I could never justify, but I do not know I
was in my life ever touched with any.' Nor did things get any
better. 'Love,' she later explained to him, 'signifies a passion
rather founded on fancy than reason.' She preferred 'friendship, I mean a mixture of tenderness and esteem.' By 1739 the
marriage had collapsed, and she went to live in France and
Italy, where she had several affairs. Yet her rhetoric remained
resolutely unsensual. She could hardly believe that a woman
of forty – a friend of hers whose lover was said to have leaped
out the window upon being discovered by the husband – was
capable of adulterous passion. As she told her daughter
in 1753, slightly tongue-in-cheek, 'My true vocation was a
monastery.'[69]

These testimonials are much more typical of the buried
world of female sensuality than are those of Mme de Graffigny
or Mme Roland. There is no doubt that the great majority of
women who lived before 1850 – and who were able to put
pen to paper – scorned their capacity for physical pleasure
and associated 'sensuality' with lustful overweight men. 'He
is a gross, fat, paralytic glutton,' wrote young noblewoman
Fanny Burney in 1779 of a village clergyman; 'such a sensualist that I love not his sight.'[70] In assessing the female baseline
of pleasure, it is clear that, outside of the court aristocracy,
women historically were much less ardent than men.

That women of the aristocracy were so different means
that we are talking here about actual practice rather than
about biology.

In Touch with Desire: Women Aristocrats

The European court aristocracy played by different rules than
the common people and lesser nobility. 'A vast luxury bordello' was one description of court life in France around
1600.[71] It was common for courtiers in Paris to boast that they
could achieve six orgasms a night, and when one failed to
fulfil his promises, the lady responded, 'You can't get it up

any more? Then get out of my bed. I haven't loaned it to you like some kind of hotel where you can take it easy and relax. So fuck off.'[72] So deliriously did the upper orders revel in pleasure that they believed it was reserved for them alone, the peasants by contrast content with defecating in an open clearing.[73]

Within the court aristocracy we do find women, unlike Liselotte, who relish desire. We would expect this. Released from the constraints of sustenance and shelter that held back women in the lesser orders, released from the narrow primness of community opinion, these *grandes dames* were virtually as free as the aristocratic males to act on the basis of desire.

Yet there are a couple of caveats. Aristocratic women had the same vulnerability as other women to pregnancy and to such catastrophic disfigurements as smallpox. Also, however wanton they are portrayed as being, the women at court rarely held a candle to the sexual depredations of their male counterparts. Finally, we are talking about women at opulent courts, where hedonism often struck the dominant note, rather than about noble women or wealthy women in general. The world we have lost was filled with nobility of various kinds: by some estimates up to 10 per cent of the total population of places like Hungary and France. Yet only at court – and not out there in village and small-town society – did conditions conspire to let noblewomen behave freely.

Many of the women of the court aristocracy manifested a sovereign control over their sexual pleasure unfamiliar to women of the lower orders. Brantôme, who is our eye on sixteenth-century court life – and a man not unsympathetic to female pleasure – spoke of women who shun furtive couplings. 'They want to communicate with their lovers, not as with pieces of rock or marble, but after selecting them well, being properly and gently served and loved by them.' These are women who take pleasure with their lovers, 'not masked, or in silence, or mute, or in the night and shadow, but who in the lovely light of day let themselves be seen, and touched, and explored, and embraced.' Yet, said Brantôme, these were women who knew how to excite their men in bed 'with great sex talk, using lascivious phrases that drive men wild.'[74] Brantôme described women 'drunk with pleasure' who wanted to have sex all night.

In mid-eighteenth-century Paris, the women of the aristocracy perfected the so-called butterfly style (*papillotage*), flitting from one lover to the next. *Le papillotage*, said one anonymous observer in 1769, 'is the refinement of elegance and sensuousness [*volupté*], the quintessence of parties and love affairs.' Under its influence, romance was said to be 'as changeable as fashion.' 'In Paris, women find a new lover once a month, and men a mistress once weekly.'[75]

These, then, were the ladies of the court aristocracy in Old Regime Paris. Said the commentator of 1769, 'Most of the women display their coquetterie as one might display a flag. Their conversation is reduced to double entendres. Adultery is seen as a stroke of fortune, and modesty becomes an embarrassment. Husbands rarely make love to their wives, and [husband and wife] really split into two couples and two households in the same dwelling.'[76] Through the reproving tone we view upper-class women making their own decisions about pleasure.

At the French court we begin to get a glimpse of total body sex for the first time in history, so much were the reins removed from traditional female chastity and modesty. Few men historically have exulted over any female body parts save the face and the ankles (the only parts visible). Yet men at the French court admired good-looking female legs, and the women tried to please them. 'I've known lots of beautiful gentlewomen and girls, who have been just as avid [as the men] to keep their beautiful legs precious and clean and nice,' said Brantôme. 'And they are right, because legs are sexier than one may think.' 'As long as we're on the subject of getting pleasure from pretty legs,' Brantôme continued, 'it wasn't just the king (as I've heard tell) but all the gallants of the court who got marvellous pleasure from contemplating and admiring the legs of those beautiful women, so terrifically displayed that the temptation was irresistible to go up to the second floor [for sex] ...'[77] Interest in legs is already a dim indication that the entire body is coming into sexual play.

Yet by the end of the Old Regime, in the days of Marie Antoinette, the evidence is even more interesting. One pornographer, writing in 1790, assigns to her the ability 'to fuck in the ass, the cunt, the armpits, the tits, the mouth, the hair, and the supple loins.'[78] That such stories of court life start to appear in the pornographic imagination is curious. It shows that for this privileged few, to whom literally nothing was denied, a taste for sex involving all of the body was at least being imagined.

Similar reports of aristocratic debauchery appear for most of the other courts of Europe, from London to the Vatican (before the Counter-Reformation), from Berlin to Vienna. But there was one major extension of the principle of libertineness outside the court aristocracy: the system of 'cavalier servitude' – as Byron called it – of the upper classes of such Italian merchant cities as Florence and Venice. Virtually at the same time that a young woman married there, she also took a lover, the *cicisbeo*, or *cavalière servente*. Though she would conceive her children with her husband, the servant-cavalier would make love to her, escort her socially, and generally play the practical role of husband, including giving her an allowance. (Her husband might, in turn, be a servant-cavalier to some other woman.) Speaking of his Italian experiences around the years 1818 to 1820, Byron said, 'Their system has its rules ... so as to be reduced to a kind of discipline, or game at hearts, which admits few deviations unless you wish to lose it. They [the women] are extremely tenacious, and jealous as furies, not permitting their lovers even to marry if they can help it, and keeping them always close to them in public as in private whenever they can. In short they transfer marriage to adultery.' This was not exactly a system in which women were free to roam at will, yet, as at the great courts, in Florence and Venice female desire rears its head. 'The reason is that they marry for their parents and love for themselves,' Byron explained.[79]

When Donatien, Count de Sade, visited Florence in 1775 he found the *cicisbeo* system functioning smoothly. 'Even if conjugal fidelity is not respected in Florence, the fidelity promised to the *cicisbeo* lasts considerably longer. He is a friend, a kind of second husband, typically a relative chosen by the woman herself from the first day of matrimony onwards and from whom she never separates ... The husband never gets in the way or creates jealous scenes.'[80]

Had these upper-class Italian women merely exchanged one form of servitude for another, the husband for the permanent lover? Not exactly. The stability rules collapsed when a handsome foreigner rode into town. Said a rather envious Sade: 'If a distinguished foreigner arrives in Florence, above all some Englishman announces that he's going to stay for a while, all the arrangements are poised to rupture. It seems that each of the women competes for the honor of devirginating him. And in these cases, the [*cicisbeo*] arrangements sometimes break down.'[81]

'It seems that women had a weakness for foreigners, especially for the English,' notes one historian of the *cicisbeo* system.[82] These women were not passive objects. It was they who decided (but also often their parents and husbands) whom they would take as a servant cavalier[83] and whether to see a dashing foreigner on the side if they so chose.

This freedom of female choice left Mary Wortley Montagu, then living in an Italian village, scandalized. She thought the moral fabric of the land disintegrating. As she wrote to a female confidante in England in 1751, 'The Italian [women] go far beyond their patterns, the Parisian ladies, in the extent of their liberty. I am not so much surprised at the women's conduct as I am amazed at the change in the men's sentiments [since the 1730s, which Lady Mary imagined to be some golden age of stability]. Jealousy, which was once a point of honour amongst them, is exploded to that degree it is the most infamous and ridiculous of all characters, and you cannot more affront a gentleman than to suppose him capable of it.' These women are constantly divorcing, she noted, 'several of the finest and greatest ladies [in Genoa] having two husbands alive. The constant pretext is impotency, to which the man often pleads guilty ...'[84]

In the context of Western society before 1850, these aristocratic women at court and north Italian women of the upper classes were pioneers.[85] They acted on the basis of desire. For them, the constraints that bound other women to chastity, fidelity, and monogamy were lifted, and their bodies had the opportunity to dictate an agenda of pleasure to the mind, just as for the men of their circle. This suggests that the female baseline of pleasure – the minimum amount of sex pleasure consistent with the function of reproduction – is not all that different from the male, merely that far fewer women than men were permitted to seek pleasure actively.

CHAPTER THREE

A Baseline for Gays and Lesbians

In September 1923, Julien Green, a young Parisian who had just finished an undergraduate degree at the University of Virginia and was now back home, wrote to his former student friend Malcolm, with whom he had fallen somewhat in love, 'I am horribly sensual. I have done everything that the human brain can imagine and the flesh can undertake. Don't think that I can't resist temptation. I can do so very well. In fact,' said Green, who was a devout Catholic, 'I am much more strongly drawn to good rather than to evil. I have chosen evil because I think that evil is more interesting and more beautiful.'[1] Struggling with his homoerotic feelings, Green considered them evil. Yet he chose the pathway of desire.

Why would the history of desire be different for gays and lesbians than for straights? Of course it's not, except for being more deeply secret. Just as the erotic history of heterosexuals is driven by deep neural programs that are doubtless genetically determined, much evidence suggests that homosexuality springs also from a biological predisposition. Pleasure chooses gays, rather than the reverse. Thus, homosexuality has always existed, and gays and lesbians must have a historic baseline – a minimum repertoire to make the whole thing worthwhile – in the same way that heterosexuals do. 'Sex still goes first, and hands eyes mouth brain follow,' poetized Edward Carpenter in 1883, an English labour militant who publicly proclaimed his gayness. 'From the midst of belly and thighs radiate the knowledge of self, religion, and immortality.'[2] For homosexuals no less than for heterosexuals, desire is one of the master variables that helps drive everything else.

There are many similarities between the histories of heterosexuals and homosexuals. Both have a point of departure in the Middle Ages that permits only limited expression of erotic feeling; both undergo a great breakout in the last third of the nineteenth century; both experience a rapid acceleration in erotic amplitude after 1960.

But there is one big difference. Unlike heterosexuality, in which at least the missionary position has always been socially acceptable, *all* forms of homosexuality have always been rigorously forbidden. There have always been strict religious and secular ordinances against buggery and against women's physical intimacy with each other. One is reminded that Catherina Linck in eighteenth-century Germany was beheaded because she penetrated another woman with a leather penis.[3]

Thus, when the scope of erotic expression in the gay community widens, it must be owing to circumstances other than diminished repression – because the level of repression until our own time has remained high and unchanged. (There are, of course, historic nuances in society's toleration of homosexuality, yet nowhere in the West has anal intercourse ever been accepted with benevolent neutrality.) The history of homosexuality cautions us, therefore, against attributing too much importance to the church or the courts in times of changing sexuality, and points to other factors that might regulate erotic expression such as the opportunity for privacy, improved personal hygiene and more agreeable body odours, or fewer distracting physical sensations, such as itching or hunger.

Inborn Orientation or Social Construction?

Around 1900, French novelist André Gide had been in love with a woman without wanting her sexually. 'I was too swept

away to be perfectly clear to myself that I did not desire her.'
Then Gide realized that he was gay. 'What can you do?' a
friend asked him. 'Change your desires?'

'It's that I can't change them,' Gide replied. 'This is the
dilemma for which ... so many others saw no solution except
a pistol shot.' (The dialogue, doubtless imaginary, was reconstructed in Gide's 1911 novel, *Corydon*.)[4]

For André Gide, as for so many other homosexual men and
women, sexual orientation was inborn and unalterable. Homosexuals were gay or lesbian as a matter of constitution,
genetics, earliest childhood awareness, and deepest inclination. Contrary to the social-construction view, they were not
perfectly bisexual, awaiting only happenstance events in
order to make a more or less arbitrary choice.[5] 'If anything
tends to disprove the idea that personality and behaviour are
purely the results of choice,' wrote gay historian Rictor Norton
many years later, 'it is homosexuality.'[6]

Indeed, late-nineteenth-century English writer John
Addington Symonds insisted that his homosexuality was congenital and that he would always 'love beauty above virtue,
& think that nowhere is beauty more eminent than in young
men.' He believed himself, as his biographer Phyllis
Grosskurth puts it, 'to be obeying the inexorable law of his
own nature.'[7] Turn-of-the-century German psychiatrist Paul
Näcke, who himself was openly gay, believed that it was
unrealistic to contemplate changing one's sexual orientation:
'I consider the real and lasting conversion of a homosexual
into a heterosexual and vice versa virtually impossible, because we are dealing with the deepest possible character
traits *ab ovo* [from conception].'[8]

The only real interruption in this stream of 'essentialist,'
or inborn, sentiment among gay people occurred under the
influence of psychoanalysis after the Second World War. In
1951, Donald Webster Cory, in the first analysis of gay life in
post-Second World War America, proceeded to speculate about
bisexuality and how mothers – *à la* Sigmund Freud – turned
basically ambidextrous young males towards same-sex

choices.[9] Yet even 'Cory,' a pseudonym of Edward Sagarin, a sociologist at City College of New York, asked in rage, 'How ... can a world condemn an individual for being what he was made to be?' Cory declared, 'We homosexuals are utterly incapable of being other than what we are.'[10]

Few within the gay community after the 1960s could possibly have believed their sexuality was not nature-given, and the very ubiquity of biological views among insiders makes it all the more puzzling that social-constructionist views persist within the ivory tower even today. The notion that homosexuality is constructed by outside, environmental influences represents the triumph of a kind of perfervid academic ratiocination over the claims of biology.

This question of inborn versus societal shaping is important for us because, if homosexuality does not rise from some deep interior wellspring of desire, the taking-the-lid-off model this book proposes for heterosexuality would not apply to gays and lesbians. 'Take the lid off and nothing happens: it's society that creates gays,' they might respond. What is required, say the social constructionists, are doctors who invent such terms as 'homosexual' in order to give people clarity about what they are, to make them realize that they now have an identity.[11]

According to Näcke, writing in 1909, 'True homosexuals demonstrate an abnormal course of development in childhood ... Very early on, the boy feels himself excluded by most of his comrades, and unconsciously drawn to a certain older man, or even a number of such men. So the others view him as an outsider.'[12] Indeed, today awareness of being homosexual begins early in life. According to one study of 180 gay youths, the average age at which awareness of same-sex attractions dawns is 8 years; the first gay sexual encounter occurs at 14.1 years; recognition of oneself as gay or bisexual happens on the average at 16.9 years.[13] Given a melioration of social taboos, the gay experience dawns soon in childhood and puberty. It is inborn, not socially induced.

The bottom line is that few men are really bisexual; most

do not drift restlessly back and forth from one sexual orientation to another. Bisexuality is a phase of transition, not a state.
It is not a transition from one state to another but from an
assumption of heterosexuality to a recognition of the innate
state of homosexuality. Dean Hamer, a scientist at the National Institutes of Health in Bethesda, Maryland, who initiated the search for the 'gay gene' in the 1990s, said, 'The
strongest evidence for the stability of sexual orientation is the
consistent failure of attempts to change gay men to straight.'[14]
One recalls the fruitless – and demeaning – outcomes of past
decades of 'aversive' therapy and eager psychoanalysis. In
Rictor Norton's view, the dubious concept of 'bisexuality'
merely marked the past struggles of married men to be dis-
creetly gay. For him, bisexuality 'involves coming to grips
with an essentially homosexual identity in a heterosexual
society.'[15]

Historically, many lesbians as well had the sense that their
sexual orientation was absolutely inborn. Natalie Barney, a
prominent Paris lesbian in the belle époque, said in her autobiography that, 'I considered myself without shame: albinos
aren't reproached for having pink eyes and whitish hair; why
should they hold it against me for being a lesbian? It's a
question of Nature. My queerness isn't a vice, isn't deliberate,
and harms no one.'[16] As English novelist Radclyffe ('John')
Hall reassured a young Russian émigrée in France named
Souline who was about to become her lover in 1934, 'I have
never felt an impulse towards a man in all my life, this
because I am a congenital invert [homosexual].' John added,
apparently because Souline had muttered apprehensions
about perversion, 'Do try, for my sake and for your own, to
look upon inversion as a part of nature.'[17] Of the twenty-five
older lesbian women whom Claudie Lesselier interviewed in
Paris in the 1980s, many affirmed the 'naturalness' of their
lesbianism, its 'obviousness.' 'It was for me so self-evident,'
said one.[18] They clearly believed they were born with their
sexual orientation rather than having casually selected it from
a range of options.

A final piece of evidence: of the 2,525 American lesbian women who responded to a questionnaire circulated by *The Advocate* magazine in 1995, only 15 per cent said they believed that 'choice' had anything to do with their sexual orientation. And more than half thought they were born with it.[19]

A number of lesbian women prefer 'butch,' or mannish, roles, and, as Del Martin and Phyllis Lyon reported in their survey of American lesbian life in the 1970s, lesbians often perceive these roles from the first dawning of same-sex consciousness: 'It is those women who feel that they are "born butch" who tend to ape all the least desirable characteristics of men.'[20] (They mean swaggering around and seeming to be unfeeling in bed.) Research today suggests that many more adult gays and lesbians recall from childhood 'gender nonconforming behavior' ('sissy' boys, girls uninterested in 'feminine' things) than do heterosexuals.[21] So it is possible that even specific roles, such as the tough 'dyke' or the prancing 'fairy,' have an inborn quality to them.

Physicians in the past – the much-maligned 'sexologists' of the late nineteenth century, some of whom believed that homosexuality was evidence of 'degeneration' – were equally convinced that sexual orientation was largely an inborn affair, not acquired through life's experiences. The first authority to take this position seems to have been Johann Ludwig Casper, a forensic medicine specialist in Berlin, who wrote in 1852 – actually tossing off the observation in passing – 'The man-to-man sexual inclination is inborn among many of these unfortunates, I suspect among the minority, while many other men turn to it later in life because of oversaturation in Venus's customary service.'[22]

For many years, Vienna psychiatrist Richard von Krafft-Ebing held the view that homosexuality was a sign of degeneration.[23] Then late in the century he changed his mind. In 1901, a year before his death in 1902, he declared that homosexuality was 'not an illness but rather an anomaly.' He commented in an article, published in a gay-identified journal, that science had finally approached the viewpoint of homo-sexuals themselves, that their 'singular sexual orientation,' though minoritarian, nonetheless represents for them 'an adequate, natural and thus legitimate' mode of sexuality.[24]

In these years English sexologist Havelock Ellis argued for the 'sexual instinct' as 'inborn.' In twenty-nine of the thirty-three cases he had examined, same-sex feelings began early in life, suggesting that, 'We must regard sexual inversion as largely a congenital phenomenon.'[25] In 1905 Amsterdam psychiatrist L.S. Römer observed, on the basis of a sample of data that he had gathered in the Netherlands and that Magnus Hirschfeld had augmented from Berlin, that homosexuality seemed to have a genetics of its own: in at least 35 per cent of the gay males in his file, there was a family history of homo-sexuality. He believed that no other factors were capable of 'causing' homosexuality if an inborn predisposition was not present.[26]

Similarly, a good deal of scientific research today also suggests that sexual orientation is an inborn or genetic phenomenon. While to date no 'gay gene' has been found, it is likely that sexual preference is determined by a number of separate genes acting in unison. Gayness, so goes one theory, is produced genetically as a by-product of nature's efforts to provide for a 'diversity in phenotypes [the entire physical make-up of a person] within each generation so that at least one phenotype will be well adapted for whatever conditions occur.' Economist Edward Miller's somewhat controversial theory is that differing balances of masculinizing and femi-nizing hormones in the brain produce these various pheno-types.[27] Whether that is true – and many masculine gays and feminine lesbians would stoutly argue that it is not – need not be resolved here.

Yet the evidence that homosexuality has a genetics of its own, accompanied by physical differences in brain and body structure, is now overwhelming. The first piece of evidence was Franz Kallmann's study of forty one-egg (monozygotic) and forty-five two-egg (dizygotic) twin pairs, in which at least one member of the pair was gay, drawn from the mental hospitals, prisons, and 'clandestine homosexual world' of New York State in the 1940s. Kallmann was a German-Jewish refugee who is considered the virtual founder of twin-pair studies. He thought that genetic influences would be especially apparent in the differences between one-egg pairs (who have common genes) and two-egg pairs (who have nothing more in common genetically than any brothers and sisters). Astonishingly, in the forty one-egg pairs, both members of each twin pair were gay. The second twin in the two-egg pairs, by contrast, demonstrated no greater tendency to homosexuality than was found (Kallmann believed) in the population as a whole. He noted that, 'The majority of one-egg pairs not only are fully *concordant* as to the overt practice [of homosexuality] ... but they even tend to be *very similar* in both the part taken in their individual sex activities and the visible extent of feminized appearance and behavior displayed by some of them.'[28]

Latter-day twin studies confirm the general drift of Kallmann's work, though the concordances are not so dramatic. In a large study of adult Australian twins, investigators found modest concordances in monozygotic twins for homosexuality: 20 per cent for gays, 24 per cent for lesbians. (One bears in mind that about 2 per cent of the adult population as a whole is homosexual.) 'Childhood gender nonconformity was significantly heritable for both men and women,' the Australian researchers also noted.[29] This study represented the lowest concordance in such research (Kallmann's being the highest). Numerous other twin studies in homosexuality come in around 50 or 60 per cent;[30] for example, Whitam and researchers found a concordance for homosexuality of 66 per cent in the 38 pairs of monozygotic twins they studied, 30 per cent for the dizygotic.[31]

In non-genetic research, many investigators of birth order have noted that later-born children have a greater chance of becoming homosexual than first-born children. In the past, psychological explanations of the phenomenon prevailed:

later-borns got more mothering and thus were made gay by smother love. But no. It turns out that later-borns in fact get less mothering than first-borns. Or could it be that later-born males, who generally speaking have lower levels of testosterone, turn out gay because they are less drenched in maleness in utero? Many explanations of the 'later-born equals gay' phenomenon have been ventured, with no firm conclusions at this writing.[32] Nonetheless, such a significant birth-order phenomenon, occurring in many different societies at different periods, means we are not dealing with social construction.

Homosexuals stand a 39 per cent greater chance of being left-handed than do straights (34 per cent greater for gays, 91 per cent greater for lesbians) – significant because handedness seems to have a neurodevelopmental basis, determined in the womb or very early childhood.[33] What causes handedness isn't understood yet, but the underlying neural process is somehow linked to sexual orientation.

At a street fair in San Francisco in 1999, one group of researchers asked 720 randomly encountered adults about sexual orientation, measuring as well the length of their fingers. (Finger length is influenced in the womb by fetal androgens.) It turned out that lesbians had significantly longer fingers (measured as a ratio of the index finger to the fourth digit) than did non-lesbian women. This didn't apply to homosexual men.[34]

In terms of neuroanatomy, meaning the actual structure of the brain, gay and straight men show some interesting differences. In gay men, one of the four cell groups (INAH 3) in the anterior part of the hypothalamus is 50 per cent smaller than in non-gays; it is also generally smaller in women than in men. This was the first real discovery of a brain-structure difference in something that previously was assumed to be socially constructed; the finding appeared in 1991 in one of the world's premier scientific journals, *Science*.[35]

A final hint of the essential biological stability of homosexuality is the apparently unchanging nature of its prevalence in the population. The first serious statistics on the rate of homosexuality per 100 population come from Magnus Hirschfeld's surveys in Germany about 1900. Studying around thirty micro-milieux (by interrogating people who knew the sexual orientation of small groups of co-workers, fellow soldiers, fellow patients, and the like), Hirschfeld estimated the overall rate of male homosexuality in the population as 1.99 per cent. (Among groups studied by questionnaire, Hirschfeld and others obtained higher rates – on the order of 4 to 6 per cent – probably because the non-response rate was so high: gays may have returned questionnaires at a higher rate than straights.)[36] Hirschfeld's overall rate of 2 per cent coincides neatly with current estimates from American and British populations, which also come in at around 2 per cent.[37] (Kinsey's figure of 10 per cent was much too high because, being gay himself, he preferentially sampled homosexuals.)

These accounts of gays' and lesbians' own self-perceptions, of historical medical opinion, and of current biological research make the assumption plausible that the sexual behaviour of gays and lesbians is as brain-driven as that of heterosexuals seems to be. Homosexuals therefore might have undergone the same historic changes in sexuality as heterosexuals: a long traditional period characterized by a limited range of sexual expression, a breakout towards the end of the nineteenth century in which all zones of the body begin to come into play, and an acceleration towards total body sex at the end of the twentieth century and the beginning of the twenty-first. The remainder of this chapter looks at what constituted homosexual sex before this breakout – during the traditional period.

The Ancient Scene

The historic baseline for male homosexuals was, not to put too fine a point on it, buggery. This surfaces clearly in ancient Greece and Rome, and provides a continuous narrative thread for the next millennium and a half. One bears in mind that the frequency of anal sex, however, is naturally exaggerated by the use of criminal records as sources. It was buggery, not handholding, that was illegal, so in court documents we're clearly going to be reading about anal sex. Nonetheless, a variety of other sources as well confirm the predominance of anal sex to the exclusion of the other main forms of sexual contact.

Because the subject of sodomy once caused such discomfort, even in enlightened academic circles, scholars have tended to portray Greek homosexuality through rose-coloured glasses, emphasizing that the Greeks loved primarily beauty, and that their ideal of beauty just happened to be male, especially that of adolescent boys. Classical scholar Paul Brandt, who wrote in the 1920s under the pseudonym 'Hans Licht' and is considered the founder of sexual studies in antiquity, emphasized that upper-class males in ancient Greece spent morning to evening together with adolescent boys, who were said to be working out in the gym in Athens three-quarters of the time. 'For all of these physical exercises, the boys were naked.' So, one thing just led to another and Licht, with a bit of special pleading here, argued that pederastic relations were absolutely the most natural thing in the world. Licht identified a strong homoerotic – indeed, pederastic – strain in Greek culture from the Homeric epics at the beginning until the final fall of Hellenic civilization. Greek pederasty, in his view, was based on aesthetic and religious (rather than hedonic) principles, and aimed to reinforce concepts of civic and personal virtue. '[Pederasty] was not antipathetical to marriage but complemented it as important principle of pedagogy. Thus one can speak of a pronounced bisexuality among the Greeks.'[38]

Indeed, Plato's *Symposium*, the locus classicus of views about the uplifting features of man-boy love in ancient Athens, argues that it was normal for older married men to fall in love with boys – adolescents are meant here. The boy was supposed to enjoy penetration, though Plato certainly does not use such a rude term. The master had everything to teach, the boy to learn. Once the boy reached maturity, the affair was over. Plato allows Aristophanes, for example, to say of the origins of sexual identity, 'People who are split from a male [at creation] are male-oriented. While they are boys, because they are chips off the male block, they love men and enjoy lying with men and being embraced by men; those are the best of boys and lads, because they are the most manly in their nature.'[39]

Greek literature is relatively silent about what happens sexually in relations between men and men, and men and boys. But John Clarke's careful analysis of pictorial evidence from shards of vases and the like makes clear what they are doing together: they are having anal intercourse, 'the man as phallic penetrator and boy as passive orifice.' A large agate gemstone now in the Royal Coin Cabinet at Leiden shows 'a man lying prone [who] raises his body up ... and turns his head around in profile ... to gaze at the man who is penetrating him.' Also visible in the representation is the large erect penis of the man on the bottom.[40] Licht glancingly concedes the existence of sodomy in man-love by citing such phrases from a Greek source as 'Hey boys, turn around.'[41] Oral sex, by contrast, seems to have been little practised between Greek males.[42]

Under the Romans, the male homosexual scene changes a bit. Anal sex remains in the centre of the picture, but man-boy relations become confined to slaves as the passive partners. (See the Roman poet Martial, who counted 'among the poet's needs ... a young and well-grown serving lad.')[43] What is striking about Roman society is the positive value it places on man-man sex. After an exacting analysis of the surviving imagery – almost all of it showing anal penetration – John Clarke concludes that a virtual 'homosexual subculture' existed among the upper classes in cities like Rome, so common was it for men to buy slaves for their sexual delectation.[44] Fellatio, as among the Greeks, remained taboo.[45]

Yet it is unlikely that the sexual choices of these men were as indiscriminate as modern authors suggest. For Clarke, 'the elite male would have his pretty boy to make love to. He would probably also have his female love toys – all under the same roof with his wife.'[46] Classical scholar John Boswell postulates 'the absolute indifference of most Latin authors to the question of gender,' and comments on 'the bisexuality of the time.'[47] Yet the sources of such affirmations tend to be the cynical poets, and observers of the twenty-second century would get just as screwy an idea of the sexuality of our own society in relying upon the comic monologues of Chris Rock as evidence.

Of lesbians in ancient times we know much less, although the woman-woman love patterns of the Greeks were to supply the vocabulary of lesbian love for all the ages to come. The celebrated poet Sappho was born in 612 BC in Eresos on the isle of Lesbos and gathered a circle of young females about her whom she trained in all the musical arts. The poet Horace found her a 'masculine' figure. She felt highly passionate attractions to other women: exactly how these were played out was left unspecified in her poetry, though she speaks in the language of desire.[48] In one fragment Sappho wrote,

> You came and I was craving you.
> My wits were kindled with desire
> And you set them aflame.

On another occasion, she reminded a departing lover,

> And sweetly on soft beds
> You rapidly slaked
> Your passion for young women.[49]

The inhabitants of Lesbos figure in what is virtually the sole description of lesbian sexual activity from antiquity. It is a lively one. In the dialogues of second-century Greek poet Lucien, a courtesan, Leona, tells a male friend of being forced to make love with a rich lady of Lesbos and her friend. She describes being kissed and having her breasts touched. But after noting that the lady had said to her, 'You're going to see that I can make love in a much sweeter way [than a man],' Leona provides no further details.[50]

Yet this conversation is a more explicit account of lesbian sexuality than any description for virtually the next two thousand years. That it was penned by a man does not necessarily mean that it was not true. It reflects the playfulness and wide-ranging sensuality – which gays shared as well – of the classical period. All that would shortly come to an end.

Gays and Lesbians in Christian Europe

The real baseline for gay and lesbian sex is not what the ancients were doing. They were almost as de-repressed as the early twenty-first century. The minimum in terms of erotic activity is represented by the long Christian centuries between the fall of the Roman Empire and the great changes of the 1800s. Normally, one would not regard such a huge span as a uniform time block. But so little changed in terms of gay sexual activity over these years that we can treat this large period as defining the pre-modern profile of gay sexuality. What components belong to it? What have gays 'always' done?

From the early days of Christian Europe to the mid-nineteenth century, buggery was the main component of gay sexual practices.[51] Indeed, its long use over the centuries gave gays a – today undeserved – reputation as 'buggers.' Focus on the anus may strike one as strange, given the complete taboo in the past against heterosexual anal intercourse. Yet for gays, anal penetration is the functional equivalent of the missionary position, and social conditions that limit the expression of sexual activity to all people will limit it as well for gays.

The evidence is considerable. After a careful review of primary sources from Germany and northern Italy, historian Bernd-Ulrich Hergemöller suggests that the core content of the vague accusation of 'sodomy' was anal penetration. Bishop

Burchard of Worms, in the eleventh century, advised his par-
ish priests to ask about 'sodomy' in the confessional in the
following terms: 'Have you committed a sexual offence of the
kind the Sodomites do, that is, have you introduced your
penis into the backside or anus of a man, and thus in a
sodomitical manner had sex?' As the Dominican monk Johann
von Schwenkenfeld began the search for heretics in 1332, he
cast the sexual net wide and sought out 'all kinds of sins of
the Sodomites,' including heterosexual anal sex as well as
tongue kissing in church. But there was no doubt, says
Hergemöller, that '*Sodomiticus*,' written large in his instructions, applied to man-man sex.[52]

Court proceedings for sodomy offer some insight into what
gays were actually doing. A study of such cases in fourteenth-
and fifteenth-century Venice determined that some of the
accused stopped at intercrural sex (a leg between the other
person's thighs); others progressed to anal; others still proceeded directly to anal sex. In this terrible Venetian fear of
'sodomy,' the emphasis was certainly on the evilness of the
anus. Similarly, in the huge amount of homosexual activity
that went on in Florence in these years, anal penetration
seems to have dominated the interaction: fellatio was mentioned in only 12 per cent of the confessions.[53]

By the late seventeenth or early eighteenth centuries, a
large and very active gay subculture had established itself in
London, centred in the 'molly' houses (the contemporary
term for gay). In his 1684 play, *Sodom; or, The Quintessence of
Buggery*, the Earl of Rochester has the King declaim,[54]

> Since I have bugger'd human arse, I find
> Pintle to cunt is not so much inclined.
> What though the lechery be dry, 'tis smart;
> A Turkish arse I love with all my heart.
> ... the brawny muscles of its side
> Tickling the nerve, their rowling eyes do glance,
> And all mankind with vast delight intrance.
> May as the Gods his name immortal be
> That first received the gift of buggery!

English homosexual men apparently shared these views. A careful study of London's gay milieu in the first decades of the eighteenth century found little evidence of fellatio among the 'mollies.' Instead, 'Anal intercourse was the preferred route, without refinements.'[55] Finally, a tabulation of eighty-eight reports of police spies to the authorities in Paris in the years 1723–4 found that sodomy prevailed; fellatio and kissing were mentioned in only 22 per cent. The author of the study was 'amazed at the apparent absence of the mouth as an erogenous zone.'[56]

Why gays historically have avoided the mouth as an erogenous zone is an interesting question. The parallelism to straights, who also avoided oral sex, is striking. But it may not be that people shunned oral relations as such, but rather odour. The Roman poet Martial says to Zoilus, 'The bathwater's fouled when your buttocks you swill. Just put in your head; 'twill be dirtier still.'[57] These were societies in which, with the exception of a few members of the upper classes, the vast majority did not wash. They feared contact with water as causing 'colds.' As a result, people stank, especially about the anus and perineum, and the missionary position for straights and anal penetration from behind for gays may have been popular precisely because these positions minimized exposure to the stench of one's partner.

Odour certainly played a role in the decision of the sixteen-year-old Rousseau to repel the advances of a gay priest in Turin, where Rousseau was receiving religious instruction. 'One evening he wanted to sleep with me; I refused on the grounds that my bed was too small. He urged me to come into his. I refused again because the poor fellow was so filthy and stank so strongly of chewed tobacco that it gave me a stomach ache.'[58] Elisabeth Charlotte of Orléans ('Liselotte') was complaining to her sister back in Germany late in the seventeenth century of the Duke d'Ussy in the Paris court, who had given his wife a fatal venereal infection: 'I cannot understand how she could have loved him. He is horribly ugly, stinks like a goat ... drinks with his lackeys and does even worse things with them because he has unquestionably acquired this vice [sodomy].'[59] Thus we have the prospect of oral sex with someone who stinks like a goat ...

A second component of the baseline for gay males is awareness of oneself as being, in fact, gay. In the case of heterosexuals this would seem too obvious even to point out ('Yes, we're heteros!') were it not for one reading of gay history that argues that an understanding of sexual identity is an invention of the late nineteenth century: only after the doctors stamp same-sex relations as pathological do gays somehow learn who they are. Rather, it seems to be true from the very beginning in Christian Europe that gays had a common sense of same-sex desire, that they were readily aware of one another, and that they sought sexual contacts in common meeting places. (Whether society had an understanding of gays as a separate identity, rather than just as criminal practitioners of illicit forms of sex, is an entirely different matter.) Yet equally true is that cities seem necessary for the development of a proper gay subculture, where, in Norton's terms, 'there is an opportunity for revealing sexual organs, as in urinals and baths ... of seeing many people in a short period of time in a small area ... and where there is an opportunity for loitering without calling attention to oneself (and for making an easy escape if necessary).'[60] William Monter puts the minimum size of cities filling such preconditions at about 100,000 for northern Europe and 60,000 for Italy.[61]

'People run after young boys here, falling in love with this one or that one, just as a young virgin gets pursued in Germany,' wrote Liselotte to her sister back home in 1699 about the French court. She hoped that the Counts of Nassau, who had intermarried into the French nobility, 'won't learn anything nasty here. I'd be very thankful to our good honest Germans if they don't fall into these ghastly practices that are so on the rise here.' The English whom she saw were even worse, 'all of them horribly debauched, especially with other men; it's said to be even worse there than here in France and in Italy.'[62] From the viewpoint of the scandalized Liselotte, Sodom had been recreated, but in the eyes of the gay and lesbian courtiers, they moved in a homosexual subculture at the French (and English and Italian) courts – quite comparable to that of the post-1960s.

In Paris, by 1748 there were at least eight gay taverns 'where groups of fifteen to thirty people gathered in the evening with the shutters closed.' The participants ate, danced, sang, and seduced, committing 'acts' – as the police spies put it – not only on the premises but on the road home.[63] Cruising grounds in the French capital were the gardens of the Tuileries, the Luxembourg Palace and the Palais-Royal, and quite especially the Champs-Élysées, by which was meant not the later avenue with that famous name but the parkland on both sides of the avenue that runs between Rond-Point and the Place de la Concorde.[64] One mid-nineteenth-century observer, Paul Lacroix, described this area, including the Allée des Veuves, as a kind of 'meat-rack,' to use a modern expression for a place where gays can meet under trees or behind bushes to have sex. Men were said to come there every evening from all over Paris, 'and after the invasion of these occupiers, normal strollers no longer hazarded wandering beneath the complaisant trees that extended their secular shadow over this vast space where sodomy came into its own.' There was apparently a password that permitted 'new arrivals to be freely admitted for the free exercise of their customary pastime.' One evening in 1831, novelist Victor Hugo, deep in thought, strolled by the Allée des Veuves, reciting his own poetry loudly to himself and was turned back by one of the men 'guarding' the area from outsiders.[65]

In London a 'molly' subculture of equal amplitude flourished from the late seventeenth century on, beginning possibly with the introduction of the first public urinals in 1692 near Lincoln's Inn (and cited as a 'molly market').[66] Early in the new century the Earl of Sunderland set up a sodomitical brandy house – apparently the first 'molly house' – near Jermyn Street, where in 1709 nine gay men were arrested. By the mid-1720s there was a network of such houses, which we know about because they were raided. In the decades ahead, however, the molly houses declined in the face of organized gay prostitution and public cruising grounds. By the mid-eighteenth century, London possessed a huge homosexual underworld, whose members, of course, were all conscious of being 'mollies' and 'madge culls,' a slang expression for the female pudendum.[67]

Amsterdam knew its meeting places for gays in the eighteenth century in bars, inns, and public toilets. The latter, made out of wood and placed under bridges, were ideal 'tea rooms' (as they would later be called) because individuals descending the stairs in the wooden clogs of the working classes would make a lot of noise and warn the group below.[68] By the mid-eighteenth century even the middle-sized Dutch cities had subcultures of institutions where gays could meet and, in some of the inns of Amsterdam, The Hague, and Utrecht, even have sex.[69]

Finally, there is the extraordinary case of Italy. The cities of northern Italy had been identified with homosexuality since time out of mind. In German, a homosexual was known as a 'Florenzer,' and many seventeenth-century French people thought of homosexuality as 'the Italian vice.'[70] An English visitor to Padua in 1609 stormed that, 'Sodomy is as rife here as in Rome, Naples, Florence ... Parma not being exempted, nor yet the smallest village of Italy: A monstrous filthiness, and yet to them a pleasant pastime, making songs, and singing sonnets of the beauty and pleasure of their bardassi, or buggered boys.'[71]

A lot of this was true: in cities like Venice and Florence the majority of young men were obliged to undergo a kind of *rite de passage* in which they were buggered by a small number of older men, some of the latter married, and some not. The true dimensions of this story were unknown until the publication in 1996 of Michael Rocke's *Forbidden Friendships*, an account of homosexuality in Florence in the fifteenth and sixteenth centuries. According to Rocke, 'In the later fifteenth century, the majority of local males at least once during their lifetimes were officially incriminated for engaging in homosexual relations.' On the basis of the number of men who came to the attention of a special court, the Office of the Night, between 1459 and 1502 – some 350 annually – Rocke estimates that by age thirty, at least one half of the young men of Florence had been formally implicated in sodomy and that by age forty 'at least two of every three men had been incriminated.' Typically, adolescent males under eighteen (but not children) would be sodomized by men in their late twenties. The active partners tended not to be married: 24 per cent married, versus 51 per cent of all Florentine men. After eighteen, the adolescents' passive role was over, and most went on to marry. Rocke says that adult men did not have sex with each other.[72] (This seems rather unlikely: perhaps they did, and were not prosecuted by the Office of the Night.)

How do we explain the quasi-universality of sodomy among the young men of Florence? For Rocke, we're dealing with a low-marriage society, and this 'abundance of virile young ... bachelors denied legitimate sexual outlets tended to foster an environment in which unauthorized sexual activity of all sorts flourished.' In other words, all men are basically bisexual, and given the right circumstances, they will as easily choose homosexuality as heterosexuality.

This explanation doesn't really wash. We may be dealing with a situation of establishing hierarchy among men regardless of sexual orientation. In Florence, there was evidently a group of older men, unable to marry for various reasons, who were able to seize control of socialization rituals and to impose a rite of passage similar to that of American prisons today, where sodomy is commonly used by the inmates to establish a pecking order: the stronger sodomize the weaker, and so on down the chain.[73] Outside, these convicts are rarely gay. Indeed, Rocke concedes that, 'In many ways, pederasty was an expression of the power adult men wielded over boys.' A number of the boys suffered anal injuries, but some liked it. This is consistent with a biological model in which some males, born homosexual, would indeed like it, and remain single as adults in a gay subculture, as we have seen in other cities. Rocke, however, denies that such a subculture existed: the huge volume of homosexual activity effaced the lines between gay and straight, he says. 'There was only a single male sexual culture with a prominent homoerotic character.'[74]

These issues are extremely important because they point either towards, or away from, a biological origin of homosexuality. On the basis of Florence, gay historian Randolph Trumbach concludes, 'In traditional European society all adult males had desired both women and adolescent males.'[75] If Florence turns out to be typical of many north Italian cities – or of Europe in the main – one would concede to gayness a large cultural component that may indeed have been socially constructed: if men as a whole are basically bisexual, many will go gay when induced to do so. It may be, on the other hand, that Florence constituted a curious exception. The pattern of a rigid dividing line between gay and straight observed elsewhere would suggest that, in general, people sort themselves out on the basis of biological, brain-driven desire, rather than on the basis of happenstance opportunities for interchangeable 'outlets.'

Finally, is effeminacy part of the historic gay profile? 'Nances,' 'queens,' and 'fairies' have always been associated with the gay world, but is the effeminate homosexual just part of the wallpaper or fundamental to the orientation? Within 'queer' scholarship, as it is now called, the consensus says that effeminate homosexuals arose only in the eighteenth century as part of a so-called 'third sex,' feminized men situated somewhere between traditional males and women. Trumbach is the main advocate of this view, asserting that a 'gender revolution' around 1700 created three genders: men, women, and sodomites. The masculinized lesbian arose, he says, around the same time. Until that time, men had desired women and other men – or rather, boys – equally; but with the gender revolution, masculine and effeminate men find an attraction to each other. Once inside the molly houses, the effeminate homosexuals could dress up in drag and call each other 'Miss Thing,' and generally behave like classic queens.[76]

There are two problems with the argument of a gender revolution producing a third, effeminate sex around 1700, aside from the intrinsic implausibility of the idea that every sexual variant becomes a separate 'gender.' One is that, long before 1700, there were references to effeminate male homosexuals. Hans Licht pointed out that the Greeks knew 'half-men, who through female gestures, make-up and other feminine toilet practices drew contempt upon themselves.' People mocked them: 'They don't want to be men, and yet they weren't born as women, and they aren't men either since they let themselves be used as women.' In the Greek comedies, such 'sissies' were given female names, and Aristophanes' audiences howled over a nance named Kleonyme ('Kleonymos' would have been the proper masculine ending.)[77]

More than one medieval cleric thundered against effeminate homosexuals who constituted the passive, receiving partners in the gay duo. Versified one divine: 'Because this one thing, the backside, isn't just yours alone to offer, no, Lentulus you sissy: Everybody's got one!'[78] In the gay subculture of seventeenth-century Lisbon, effeminate gay men cruised in inns and danced together at public festivals in drag. Some of them took on feminine nicknames such as 'Miss Turk' and 'Miss Galicia.'[79]

A second objection to the idea that another, effeminate gender was created around 1700 is that the most careful student of gay life in London at the time of the supposed gender revolution, Rictor Norton, denies specifically any element of effeminacy in the world of the mollies. For him, they were manly working-class males, even if they did tease one another with feminine nicknames in a gay slang called the Female Dialect: 'Where have you been you saucy Queen?' Norton sees effeminacy mainly as a form of 'self-advertisement,' an announcement that one is available 'in the same way that a coquette establishes contact.' By contrast, men in the molly culture radiated a 'vigorous and lusty bonhomie ... and evinced more vitality than effeteness.' There was no butch-femme role playing in the mollies' world.[80] As for the mollies forming a 'third gender,' not in the slightest.

On balance, effeminacy seems scarcely to form part of a constant gay sexual trait. Though it is present throughout history, its occurrence in the centuries of Christian Europe was too sporadic to represent an inborn kind of theme. Effeminacy becomes much commoner in the late nineteenth and early twentieth centuries, yet as a kind of 'overlay,' a societally induced coloration of the basic sexual picture that may be present in some times and places but not in others.

The baseline of male homosexuality thus seems structured much like that of heterosexuality in its limitation to a few erotic themes and its preservation of the elemental force of desire in the face of repression. For heterosexuals, the entire society, of course, was their 'subculture'; yet homosexual men have always been able to recognize one another at a glance, and they too were conscious of their special communality.

A Lesbian Baseline

Why would lesbian sexuality be less ardent than any other variety? There's no reason to think that it would be. In the French Revolution, the Parisian actress with the stage name Mlle de Raucourt fainted after she learned that the Paris prostitutes had plans to downgrade her and her lesbian circle to the status of prostitutes. Her companions revived her by stimulating her genitals. 'My first impulse,' she said afterwards, 'was to put my hand on my cunt to assure myself of my existence.'[81]

Lesbians seem to have been just as passionate as anybody else, yet much less is known about their sexuality in Christian Europe, mainly because lesbian women have always been extremely discreet about what they do in bed. Also, the authorities found lesbian offences so shocking that they often refrained from mentioning what was entailed.[82] Thus it is virtually impossible to answer some key questions in comparing lesbians, gay men, and straights. What, for lesbians, was the equivalent of the missionary position (for heterosexuals), or anal sex (for homosexual men)? Is there a lesbian tradition of using appliances such as dildoes, or this is an imputation of male fantasy?[83] Finally, is there a historic continuity in lesbian culture that values such symbols as the colour purple or special rings?[84]

We know a few things. First of all, anal sex is definitely not part of the lesbian baseline. It is simply never mentioned. The 'classic form of female sodomy,' according to one scholar, is tribadism, or rubbing pelvises together. We glimpse it in the sex life of Benedetta, a lesbian nun and member of the Theatine Order in Pescia in Italy in the early seventeenth century, who kissed the breasts of her lover, then engaged in mutual masturbation and genital rubbing. More than that was just not on.[85]

Such few, spare accounts never mention the anus. Or if so, then in horror: Mlle de Raucourt, in her battle against the prostitutes, urged cross-dressing lesbians to make common cause with the male gay community of Paris, 'even if it meant subjecting themselves to anal intercourse.'[86] This suggested, of course, that for Paris lesbians, normally the anus was strictly off limits. Nowhere in the growing literature on the history of lesbian sexuality does one encounter the notion, before the beginning of the twentieth century, that lesbians experimented with anal penetration.

What they did instead would have remained largely a mystery were it not for the publication in 1992 and 1998 of the extraordinary two-volume set of diaries of Anne Lister, a lesbian gentlewoman in the English countryside in the 1820s and 1830s. Believing that she was writing for herself alone, Lister conveys the quality of her intimate life in a way that is without historical precedent and that would not again be matched until the flood of self-revelations of the 1980s and beyond.

She describes her love affairs with women, including kissing, orgasms, and fantasies. It is often unclear exactly what she and her lovers were doing in bed, but there are hints that they may have engaged in oral sex and mutual masturbation: 'Goodish touching and pressing last night – she much and long on the *amoroso* and I had as much kiss as possible with drawers on.' (The *amoroso* is evidently a reference to Walker's [her partner's] orgasm; that things would get even better for Lister with panties off means either that they were having oral sex, or that the thick panties of the day interfered with mutual rubbing and masturbation.) There are also references to tribadism or 'grubbling' as Anne called it: 'She was at first tired and sleepy but by and by roused up and during a long grubbling said often we had never done it so well before. I was hot to washing-tub wetness ...' (So much for the official historians of lesbianism who claim that the whole thing is about friendship and mutual career support.)[87]

Anne Lister's diary is the founding document of the history of lesbian sexuality. Although it is unexplicit on the subject of oral sex (anal was not a theme), it limns a fully sexualized woman, as Anne Lister and her partners exchange deep kisses (Lister almost bit Walker's lip through one night);[88] they grasp each other's bodies from top to bottom and rub passionately together. Anne's relationships reflect the same rather narrow erotic range of gays and heterosexuals in the period of Christian Europe. Yet there can be no question of the quality of ardour for lesbians being somehow set lower than for gays and straights: these early-nineteenth-century English country gentlewomen were all over each other.

What about their identity as lesbians? In the countryside around Halifax where Anne lived, were there lesbian bars and inns corresponding to those of gay men in the big cities? Of course not. Yet Anne is continually surprised at encountering so many lesbian women in the rural West Riding. After meeting Miss Pickford and learning her secret (while not divulging her own same-sex tastes), Anne muses, 'Are there more Miss Pickfords in the world than I have ever before thought of?'[89] Anne meets her potential partners through family contacts and social get-togethers of the gentry; some also at church. Just as it would not surprise us to learn there were many gay men in the West Riding, lesbian women also abounded.

In other sources as well, it is obvious that lesbian women share consciously as a common denominator their desire for other women. The well-organized Paris lesbians of the late eighteenth century, with Mlle de Raucourt at their epicentre, have already been mentioned. They were, in fact, split into competing clubs.[90] The convents of the day, filled with young women idling away their time until marriage, knew plenty of lesbian relations. Casanova describes how in 1754 the abbess 'M.M.' initiates the fourteen-year-old Caterina Capretta 'into the mysteries of Sappho.'[91] There was said to have been a social circle of 'tribades' in Dublin in the 1730s, ruled over by Lady Frances Brudenell, the widowed Duchess of Newburgh. The actress Mary Yates presided in the 1780s and earlier over a lesbian club in London.[92] We know virtually nothing about how these women felt and thought about their sexuality, but they could not have been so different from Anne Lister, who told Miss Pickford, apropos two women sleeping together, that 'Many would censure unqualifiedly but I did not. If it had been done from books and not from nature, the thing would have been different ... But as it was, nature was the guide.'[93]

Which brings us to the point about butch and femme lesbians, the exact counterpart of manly and effeminate gays. Did nature make them part of the basic scene? Butches are mannish lesbians, femmes, of course, feminine ones, and the two often pair up. Some observers feel that the butch-femme dyad is a creation of late-nineteenth-century urban life, others that it has been present from the start.[94]

Even today, when butch-femme relationships tend to be frowned on as resurrecting patriarchal images, many lesbian women feel strongly that they are – and always have been – one or the other. Lesbian journalist Susie Bright – co-founder in 1984 of a 'lesbian entertainment' magazine called *On Our Backs* – threatened to 'get out of the *lesbian* magazine business and into the *butch-femme* magazine business – there really should be a magazine for people who are attracted to butches, and another for people who are attracted to femmes.' Then she wouldn't have to endure letters from someone saying, 'Oh, everybody in your magazine's too hard and cold and masculine for me.' Other readers, by contrast, would write in, 'If you show one more woman with lipstick, I am going to throw your magazine into the trash.' So Bright, tongue-in-cheek, said, 'Let's just make it really *simple* for the whole world': If you want to look at this or that kind of person, here's the magazine for you.[95]

Butch and femme, in other words, may be natural categories.

Anne Lister was very butch. On 7 May 1821, she fantasizes about having intercourse with another woman, 'taking her into a shed ... and being connected with her. Supposing myself in men's clothes and having a penis ...' People told her 'how much I am like a man,' and at one point she even started growing a moustache. (Her lover M— called her 'Fred.') On one occasion, after supervising a gang of fifteen men in the field she wrote, 'All this ordering and work and exercise seemed to excite my manly feelings. I saw a pretty young girl go up the lane and desire rather came over me.'[96]

One of the reasons Anne and Miss Pickford didn't get together sexually was that Miss Pickford was even more mannish, and would actually cross-dress and flirt with women under the name of 'Captain Cowper.' Did Anne see herself as embodying some kind of 'third sex'? She certainly did conceive of her world in such categories, but she did not need the late-nineteenth-century sexologists, with their 'third sex' thinking, to tell her how to behave.[97]

There are many historical records of cross-dressing women 'passing' as male. Some often considered themselves 'lesbian' and played the butch role with their mates just as Anne Lister did. Mme Catherine de la Guette, in seventeenth-century

France, had always thought of herself as having a 'warrior' temperament; her father trained her in the military arts and, to defend her estate in the civil wars known as the Fronde, she cross-dressed as a soldier, fighting on horseback alongside her men. 'I've always been more of a mind for war,' she said, 'than for peacefully putting the chicken in the pot and spinning with the distaff.' There were numerous such women in the tumult of mid-seventeenth-century France, all of them, of course, not necessarily lesbian. As for Mme de la Guette, we know only that she was attracted to handsome young women and that at first she resisted her conjugal duties of intercourse, though otherwise she drops a veil of silence over her sexual tastes.[98]

In the late-nineteenth-century United States, Lucy Ann Slater had cross-dressed for years as 'Joe' Lobdell, living with women in 'Lesbian love,' as her psychiatrist put it. (Quite independently of this fact, in 1880 she was admitted to a psychiatric hospital at age fifty-six with some kind of disease resulting in progressive dementia.) She did not consider herself a man, merely that she had same-sex tastes and an enlarged clitoris.[99]

Mme de la Guette, Lucy Ann Slater, and Anne Lister were all typical of a minority strain in lesbian sexual attraction that echoes across the ages. Whether the origin of butch-style behaviour is biological or some cultural variant that mannish women invent for themselves is unclear. But it seems always to have been present in lesbianism and represents part of the historic tradition.

From this baseline a dramatic change in gay and lesbian sexuality would burst forth in the late nineteenth century.

CHAPTER FOUR

Hindrances

The low priority attached to sexual pleasure by people who lived in distant times is inexplicable unless one considers the hindrances that existed in those days. Hindrances to pleasure – such physical distractions as chronic itching or chronic pain, the lack of privacy in family life, an antisensual culture, and fear of pregnancy in women – all inhibited the mind's ability to act on whatever hedonic urging it received from the brain. The antisexual messages from the village community, from the church, from life itself screamed so loudly that the neural signals were deafened. In a profoundly antisexual culture, biology does not transmit itself into action. It would occur to few men today to go out and have sex with the first woman they see passing on the street, even though broadcasting in this random fashion would give their seed an evolutionary advantage in the gene pool, because our society has declared itself against this kind of importunity. Similarly, it occurred to few husbands in the seventeenth century to demand oral sex from their wives – however gratifying that might have been for their peripheral sensory receptors – because everything they had learned since childhood spoke against such sin. (And because the wives doubtless thought that their husbands smelled repulsive.) The hindrances drowned out the voice of desire.

After the mid-nineteenth century, these hindrances start to be removed, and the great surge towards pleasure begins. For the previous thousand years, however, from the Dark Ages to the Industrial Revolution, there were really few changes in dirt, misery, and disease, and in the obstacles to pleasure that village and small-town life threw up. Of course this characterization may raise eyebrows among specialists who are accustomed to teasing out differences between the thirteenth and eighteenth centuries! Yet in the domains we treat here, the differences were few.

Physical Distractions from Sensuality

Super-sex is inconceivable if one is constantly grimacing, scratching, and writhing to escape intolerable itching. Itching is an example of a physical distraction from sensual pleasure, and it was once extremely common, the result of daily infestations among the common people of scabies, lice, and fleas, tiny vermin that bit, stung, or burrowed their way into the skin, leaving a legacy of cutaneous misery. Complained an Upper-Bavarian folk song,

> No matter how deep in bed I nest,
> Those devlish fleas will give no rest.
> They make the night a living hell
> And romp in covers thick as well.
> It never stops: scratch here, scratch there.
> And scratch your ass and all that's bare.
> Biting, biting, biting never ends.[1]

Itching was once an everyday experience for most people. And of the various bugs that cause chronic itching, worst was the ectoparasite responsible for scabies, or the itch. Itching in scabies is especially severe because the impregnated female itch mite tunnels beneath the skin and deposits her eggs along the burrow. As the larvae hatch, they congregate to hair follicles and cause an acute itching that is distracting indeed for the sufferer. Peasant women would dig the tiny white larvae out of their skin with needles. The disease is associated with rural and working-class life, because peasants, servants, and factory workers tended to sleep three or four to a bed – and the itch mite is transmitted in direct skin-to-skin contact.

How common was scabies? Very common. Ulrich Bräker, a poor peasant in Switzerland's Toggenburg district, mentions casually of his childhood in the 1740s, 'Now we hired another female hand. That was alright with Dad because she worked hard, but Mom and Grandma couldn't stand her because she sucked up to him and tattled to him about everything. Also, she had scabies, and gave it to everyone in the house.'[2] Towards the end of the nineteenth century, scabies was the single most frequent diagnosis in Munich's main hospital, the Hospital Left-of-the Isar: in a 10 per cent sample of patients for the year 1894, the thirty-seven patients with scabies constituted the largest single diagnostic category.[3] These were people almost driven mad by the itching and by the secondary infections that followed.

Other itching disorders were scattered more generously throughout the social hierarchy. Casanova made his first contact with fleas – which, unlike the itch mite, can live on clothing and bedding – at age nine at a pension in Padua where he was lodging in order to attend school. His first night was hideous, the fleas biting him all over, rats leaping back and forth across his bed.[4] Of course, fleas were not universal. Casanova, a minor aristocrat, had grown up in a well-kept household. Yet these people in Padua were not living in desperate poverty, and still they were infested from top to bottom.

Lice were another source of chronic itching. On a January evening in 1669, Samuel Pepys had an unpleasant surprise. 'So to my wife's chamber, and there supped and got her to cut my hair and look [at] my shirt, for I have itched mightily these six or seven days; and when all came to all, she finds that I am louzy, having found in my head and body above 20 lice, little and great ...' Pepys was puzzled, since for the preceding twenty years he had been lice-free, 'so how they came, I know not.'[5] (Yet Pepys's world was not exactly innocent of lice, for on a previous occasion, when he sent to his wigmaker for a periwig he found it 'full of nits,' lice being the wigmaker's 'old fault.'[6]

The households of the literate, such as Casanova and Pepys, were relatively free of vermin, but we know that lice and fleas infested the common people because almost every time the wealthy stayed in an inn or hotel before the nineteenth century they came away scratching themselves. As French essayist Michel de Montaigne travelled in Italy in 1581, at San Lorenzo he was obliged to sleep fully clothed on top of a table, 'because of the fleas, something that I have otherwise encountered only in Florence.'[7] After the Scottish writer and physician Tobias Smollett had dined at an inn in the little town of Noli near Genoa in 1765, he retired for the night. 'But I had not been in bed five minutes, when I felt something crawling on different parts of my body, and taking a light to examine, perceived above a dozen large bugs.' He leapt out of bed, wrapped himself in his overcoat, and spent the night atop a chest.[8]

How little Italy had changed by the 1830s, when English politician William Gladstone travelled in Sicily: 'We fared pretty well on our last night's mattresses: everyone in Sicily should be particularly watchful of the fleas which spring upon the feet and ankles from the floors and may be inadvertently carried into bed.' Perhaps, he said, 'it is ... a question worth considering whether (on account of sleep) a person who suffers much from vermin should come to Sicily at all.'[9] Thus we have the Italians, the nation of lovers, scratching themselves constantly.

But it was not just those nasty Mediterraneans. Many Englishmen must also have been scratching themselves after travelling at home. In 1782 pastor James Woodforde, a country parson in a small town in Norfolk, came down to London and stayed at the Bell Savage inn. It was a mistake. 'I was bit terribly by the bugs last night, but did not wake me,' he reported in his diary. He must have forgotten this experience because four years later he stayed at the Bell Savage again.

'Very much pestered and bit by the bugs in the night,' he noted.[10]

The reports of bug-bitten travellers are fairly uniform. The point is that the lower classes – meaning the vast majority of people – in the countries through which our reporters were travelling lived amid vermin; people were constantly bitten by them and must have been continually itching and scratching themselves. For the full deployment of sensuality, a minimum of physical comfort or physical serenity is required. And amid the constant burrowing, creeping, and biting of itch mites, fleas, and lice this must have been difficult to attain.

Another distraction from the sexual enjoyment of the whole body is chronic pain. It is not that chronic pain has somehow disappeared from our own society. Every year 600,000 Americans experience pain from arthritis for the first time; 25 million have regular migraine headaches; and 7 million wrestle with low back pain. 'Fully 80 percent of all physician consults are pain related,' says one government source.[11] Yet the experience of disablement from chronic pain is a subjective one, and every society makes its decisions about what constitutes unacceptable pain. In the world before analgesia and anesthesia, that threshold was set very high. In that world, many people regularly experienced the kind of pain that we would consider intolerable.

Take the sort of pain that affects sexual functioning, that is intense, and for which relief exists today: the pain of kidney and bladder stone. Little stones form in the kidneys, slide painfully down the ureters, then lie in the bladder swelling with additional urate crystals until they are either voided in agonizing pain – or not, in which case the sufferer dies of uremia. Michel de Montaigne suffered for many years from bladder stone. 'You are seen to sweat in anguish,' he wrote, 'to turn pale and red, to tremble and vomit blood, to suffer strange contractions and convulsions, at times to let great tears drop from your eyes, to discharge black, thick, and dreadful urine, or to have it checked by some sharp, rough

stone that cruelly pricks and tears the neck of your [bladder].'
In the meantime, said Montaigne, you are trying to hold
conversations with bystanders or ride about on your horse
(for many years he had been an army officer).[12]

Both Samuel Pepys and Elizabeth, first Duchess of
Northumberland, also complained in their diaries of stones.
The pain of stone did make a difference in people's sex lives.
Jean-Jacques Rousseau's encounter with bladder stone in 1756
at age forty-four certainly suspended his sexual pleasures for
a while. Here he is in bed with pain: 'Aside from the fact that
one certainly doesn't feel like making love when in pain, my
imagination was inspired by the countryside, lying beneath
the trees. But [in reality] I languish and die in a room beneath
the beams of the ceiling.'[13]

Thus a society beset by high-order chronic pain: 'We are
born to grow old, to grow weak, and to be sick in despite of
all medicine,' said Montaigne in 1586. 'We must suffer quietly
the laws of our condition.'[14] Yes, indeed. But this is a recipe
for asceticism, not hedonism.

Memento Mori

Today, people try not to dwell overly upon death and usually
do not discuss it at the dinner table or reflect about it in their
busy days. In the world we have lost things were different.
Death was omnipresent, an awareness of it seldom far from
consciousness. People who live amid fear of death do not
fling themselves about in gay abandon. They do not shout
'Carpe diem! Live for the day!' and party on. Rather, they
seek refuge in religion, and in religious reflections of the most
puritanical and antihedonistic sort.

In those days, death could strike at any time of life, not just
in old age as is characteristic of our society. Here we are in the
German village of Wollbach. It is the 1720s. Jacob Lorentz, a
twenty-three-year-old labourer, has just married a young
woman exactly his age named Veronika Wirslin. They pro-
ceed to have seven children, yet his career as paterfamilias is

cut off fifteen years later as he dies. The seven children were steadily scythed away. One – Johannes – died eight days after birth; a second Johannes died at sixteen; three daughters were all dead before ten; one child we lose sight of; and one final child, Anna, survived to old age.

Yet this was not the end of the story for their mother, Veronika. After Jacob himself died in 1737, she remarried two years later, to a man whose wife had just died. This new husband then died shortly thereafter, and Veronika went on, in 1745, to give birth to an illegitimate daughter, who died at fourteen.[15] There was nothing unusual about Wollbach. Nor was the Lorentz family particularly star-crossed.

Even in the relatively healthy United States, the average life expectancy at birth in 1850 for men was 38.3, for women 40.5 (the statistics are for Massachusetts). These figures are so low because they are dragged down by high infant mortality: one child in seven would not survive the first year of life. Yet even if you made it to age 20 – prime dating age – you would probably not make it past sixty, an age that we now associate with full sexual vigour.[16] (Today in the United States, by contrast, the average life expectancy at birth is 74.1 for men, 79.5 for women.)[17] In Christian Europe, with its stifling sexual restrictions, epidemics of plague, smallpox, cholera (after the 1830s), and typhus swept back and forth across the adult population. Tuberculosis was an endemic disease, meaning constantly present, and pneumonia probably the single commonest cause of death. All of these diseases could strike literally any time of the day or night: it was not unusual for entire families to die within days or weeks of one another. Memento mori, indeed.

Some people are, of course, constitutionally jolly, but in the remote past the sadness born of continual mourning seems to have been more representative of the average person's mood. Glückel, a middle-class Jewish woman who lived in the German town of Hameln in the mid-seventeenth century, was probably more typical than the jolly monk Rabelais. She had lost her sister, a nephew, and a brother-in-law before she

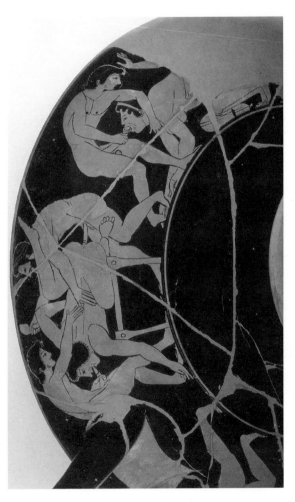

Total body sex in classical antiquity: The relaxed sexual playfulness of the ancient Greeks and Romans is evident in their art. The orgy scenes depicted in this Greek bowl from the 5th century BC reveal an erotic range that virtually disappears from western culture until the latter half of the 19th century. Red figure cup, circa 510–500 BCE, attributed to Pedieus Painter (6 BCE). (Photo: Chuzeville. Réunion des Musées Nationaux / Art Resource, NY /Louvre, Paris, France)

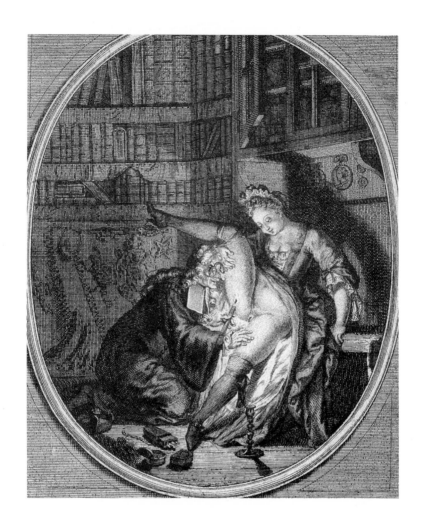

Traditional sexual baselines: Although the volume of pornographic art and literature rose dramatically during the 18th
century, the sexual imagination remained focused on vaginal
intercourse. Illustration from J. Grand-Carteret, *Die Erotik in der
Französischen Karikatur* (Wien/Liepzig, 1909).

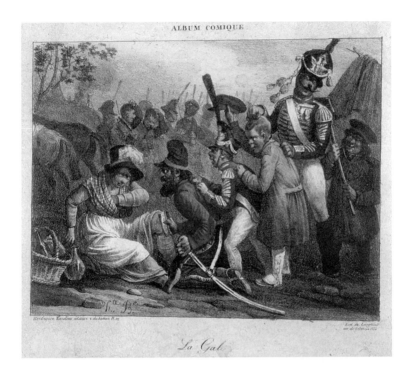

La Gale

Distractions from sensuality: Scabies. Super-sex is inconceivable for people who are constantly scratching and writhing to escape the intolerable itching of scabies, like the sufferers in this early 19th century French cartoon. *La gale*, coloured lithograph by Langlumé. Illustration in Hippolyte Bellangé, *Album comique de pathologie pittoresque* (Paris: Tardieu, 1823). (National Library of Medicine, USA)

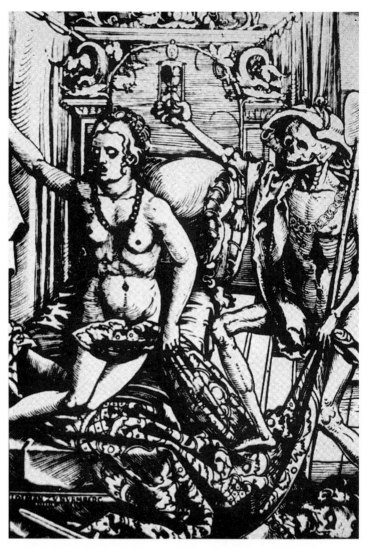

Distractions from sensuality: *Memento mori* and an antihedonistic culture. Constant mindfulness of death and belief in the sinfulness of physical desire were powerful hindrances to sensuality in medieval and early modern Europe. Both themes are apparent in Niklas Meldemann's 1522 engraving *Lust und Tod* (Lust and Death).

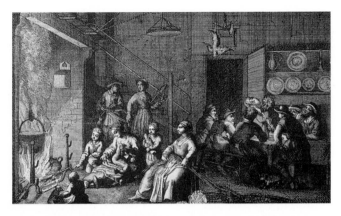

Community controls begin at home: Domestic privacy was non-existent in traditional society, with whole families – and in peasant families, sometimes the livestock as well – crowded into a single room. *Ménage champêtre,* 17th century French engraving in *Histoire du people francais* (Paris: Nouvelle Librairie de France, 1951).

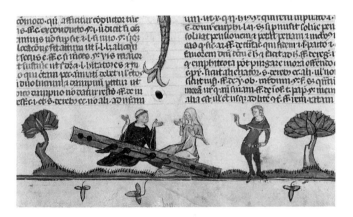

Community controls enforced by local authorities: In traditional European towns and villages, public penalties and humiliations were frequently inflicted upon people who violated community sexual standards. Illustration in the border of the Smithfield Decretals, an illuminated copy of the decrees of Pope Gregory IX, ca. 1300 – ca. 1325. (Courtesy of the Heritage Image Partnerships)

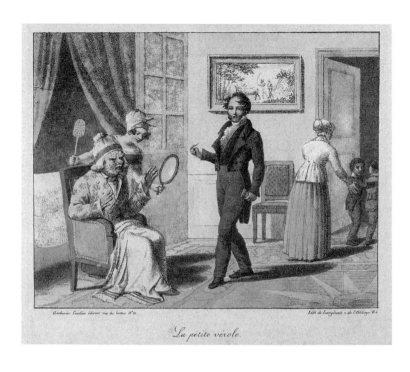

La petite vérole.

The vulnerability of beauty: Before the advent of vaccination, 20 to 30 per cent of the population in some European countries suffered facial scarring from smallpox infections. For women, whose faces were their fortune, disfiguration by smallpox was a social catastrophe. *La petite vérole*, coloured lithgraph by Langlumé. Illustration in Hippolyte Bellangé, *Album comique de pathologie pittoresque* (Paris: Tardieu, 1823). (Courtesy of the Wellcome Library, London, U.K.)

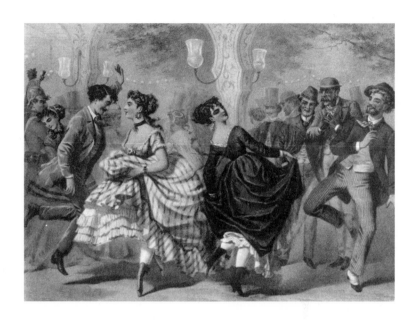

The great breakout: As people moved from countryside to city during the 19th century they exchanged the stifling restrictions of the rural village for the anonymity and sexual freedom of urban life. At the Parisian dance hall Mabille, men and women could meet and mingle without interference from disapproving elders. *Bal Mabille* (1839). (J. Boudet Collection)

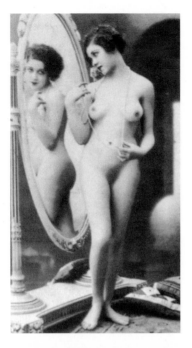

The great breakout: In the privacy of the city young women like Zola's courtesan Nana could explore the sensuality of their bodies in front of the bedroom mirror. (Collection Romi)

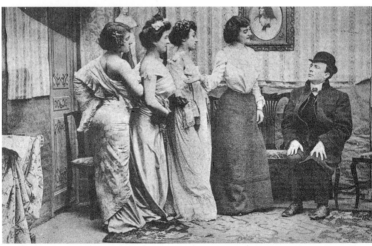

The great breakout: City life offered new opportunities and choices for every sexual taste – as celebrated here in 'Le Choix,' a 1905 postcard from a French bordello. (Collection Romi)

started to bear, and then lost her own children. After her husband and a married daughter died, she writes that she cannot enjoy life: 'No,' she said. 'My sins are too heavy to bear. I am a sinner. Every day, every hour, every minute, every second – full of sins ... For these I weep and mine eyes runneth down with water [Lamentations 1:16].'[18]

But it was certainly not only the Jewish families whose religious beliefs reminded them that they were sinners living in a vale of tears. The rhetoric of both Protestant and Catholic churches emphasized life's grim nature, asceticism, and redemption through suffering. The Bible is very clear, Psalm 90 having admonished humankind for thousands of years that, 'Thou carriest them away as with a flood; they are as a sleep: in the morning they are like grass which groweth up; in the evening it is cut down, and withereth.'

In the gospel of St Luke, a rich man reflects that it's now finally time to enjoy himself: I've laid up goods for many years. I should take my ease, 'eat, drink and be merry.'

But God says to him, 'Thou fool, this night thy soul shall be required of thee: then whose shall those things be, which thou hast provided?'[19] A more explicitly antihedonistic text could not be imagined.

Medieval writers did not necessarily celebrate illness. Yet it is true, as Carolyn Bynum tells us, 'that sickness and suffering were sometimes seen by medieval people as conditions "to be endured" rather than "cured."' One nun, in the monastery of Töss, wrote a poem in which Christ said to her: 'The sicker you are, the dearer you are to me.'[20] The late-medieval preacher Johann Spangenberg compared this mortal coil to an inn run by the devil: 'Here in this world we are in Satan's kingdom, where the innkeeper is a rogue, a thief, a robber, and a murderer. And because we have to eat, drink, rest, and sleep in this inn, so must we finally pay. Yet the innkeeper gives no other fare than pestilence, fever, and other illnesses. There's also nothing to drink except vanity, poison, and death.'[21]

Other preachers in the Middle Ages likened this doleful

world to the sea: 'One. Because of the disquiet that is in both the world and the sea. Two, just as the sea never runs out, so are the sins of the world. Three, just as the sea is bitter, so is everything that belongs to the world mixed with bitterness.' Yet with the ship of penance, it was said, we reach the heavenly city and eternal life.[22] The bitterness of the world? The ship of penance? Where in this discourse is there place for sensuality?

The medieval church viewed 'concupiscence' – or Adam and Eve's blunder of letting the sex organs escape the control of volition – as the source of most human depravity since the Fall. Permitting pleasure to sweep across the sexual scene was comparable to mankind's original disobedience towards God. The church, in a sense, recognized the basic argument of the present book: that humankind's historic sin had been letting the genitals respond to the brain rather than to the mind. Indeed, one scholar speaks of the 'shameful disobedience of the genital organs.'[23]

Without a doubt, the antisexual views of the medieval church influenced the way real people viewed their sexuality. Christine de Pizan, a female writer of the early fifteenth century (and in some ways a feminist because of her scorn of the church's misogyny), praised women who renounced the pleasures of the flesh. In her *Book of the City of Ladies* (1405) she lauds 'Zenobia, Queen of the Palmyrenes': 'This maiden despised all physical love and refused to marry for a long time, for she was a woman who wished to keep her virginity for life.' In the various misadventures that fortune placed in her path, Zenobia remained 'supremely chaste. Not only did she avoid other men, but she also slept with her husband only to have children, and demonstrated this clearly by not sleeping with her husband when she was pregnant.' That was the tale told by 'Lady Reason.' Later in the book 'Lady Rectitude' is permitted to second these sentiments, apostrophizing the reader, 'How many valiant and chaste ladies does Holy Scripture mention who chose death rather than transgress against the chastity and purity of their bodies.' At the end, the author urges women, 'Oh my ladies, flee, flee the foolish love [that men] urge on you! Flee it, for God's sake, flee!'[24]

With the Reformation of the sixteenth century, the medieval church split between the Protestant denominations and the renewed Catholic faith of the Counter-Reformation that shortly came forth. It would be difficult to decide which was more purse-lipped about physical pleasure and hedonism. Every Sunday morning and often during the week as well, the Lutheran pastors drummed into their parishioners the message of how quickly joy is lost. Howled one sixteenth-century Lutheran divine from the pulpit, 'Ay ay! The grass soon withers. Today you're the master, tomorrow a stinking fish ... Everything passes, like yesterday; everything is dark, like the blackest night; everything runs away, like the river; everything is transitory, like a dream, as inconstant as the green grass and the lovely weather.'[25] One can imagine in what mood the parishioners might emerge after a sermon like this. Ready for total body sex? Hardly.

People were mindful of these lessons and did not merely shake them from their heads as they left church. One law professor in Hildesheim built himself a lovely house, in which he arranged for a special room whose walls were covered with biblical sayings and pictures. He called the room 'Life and Death,' spent much time there preparing himself for death, and wished there to die. It was common for people to have coffins made out of oak prepared long in advance, where apples would be stored until the event arrived. And if the coffin was not actually built, having oaken 'coffin wood' on hand was almost universal.[26] Thus memento mori rang through one's life.

A constant mindfulness of death, the yearning for a better life in the hereafter, and the view of the body as a prison: all conspired to deflect people's attention from sensuality; all were internalized prescriptions to hinder the mind from choosing the path of hedonism.

Community Controls

Yet it would be incorrect to make the asceticism of traditional society entirely the fault of 'the church.' The world we have lost was an antihedonic society, as the Marquis de Sade clearly realized in his 1801 novel, 'The Story of Juliette.' Young Juliette is admitted to a convent, where she encounters the abbess Mme Delbène, who is a complete voluptuary. Juliette can't believe that Mme Delbène is no longer interested in her 'reputation' or in society's limit for acceptable behaviour. Delbène says, 'What are they, these limits? Let's just try to envisage them with sang-froid. They are social conventions almost always promulgated without the consent of the members of society, detested by our hearts ... absurd conventions that are real only in the eyes of the idiots who want to submit to them.'[27]

Absurd, perhaps, but nonetheless real. The neighbourhood communities in these small towns and villages watched vigilantly for pleasure seeking and snuffed it out wherever possible save at feast times, on the logic that hedonism militated against social stability; and if one value in these little burghs was elevated above all others, it was stability.

The control of pleasure seeking entailed surveillance. The village community had mechanisms in place for watching people and ensuring that they did not have deviant sex, or that their dinner tables were not groaning with juicy roasts, or that they were not clothing themselves above their station.

Surveillance began at home. The forum par excellence for denying people the privacy needed for hedonism was the family and household. In these small communities, where people made a living from farming and handicrafts, rarely did the nuclear family live alone. Live-in servants were common, as were stray relatives and travellers who stopped for the night. And all were crowded into one little room, often – in peasant life – together with some of the livestock. In such a setting one could basically forget about pleasure as a means of personal gratification.

'You often see three or four beds in the hole in the wall they call the "room,"' said the local doctor of the Breton town of Lamballe in 1787. 'There, the sick sleep alongside the healthy, often two in the same bed.' If the sick sweated heavily or soiled themselves, there was no question of changing the linen. The entire family slept in the same putrid dungeon.[28] In the German village of Frankenheim in the Rhön region there were 2.6 people per bed, a region where commonly 'there are more than two people for most beds.' Some households had seven people per bed, and a family of ten people might have two beds. 'The moral consequences of this over-crowding ... might well be imagined,' sniffed the local doctor.[29]

Was all this merely owing to the consequences of rural poverty? Not really. It was much more custom and convention that dictated this lack of privacy. Prosperous peasants in the Querfurt district of northern Germany 'content themselves with a single room which is used as a family room, for eating et cetera, and may also serve as a dining room for the hired hands.' The family also slept in this single room, throwing down straw on the bedsteads and covering it with a single comforter, where they would all spend the night together.[30]

Thus the parents had sex in front of the children, not sashaying about the room dressed in pink nighties and looking at themselves in the mirror, but burrowed under the covers. 'It's not just that the cottager sleeps with his children in the same small room, but in the same bed even after the children are grown,' said one observer of Ravensberg County in Westphalia in 1793. 'They are witnesses to marital intimacies that cannot be kept sufficiently secret ...'[31] Under these circumstances, could there be any question of total body sex in Ravensberg County?

Then there was asceticism enforced at the level of town and village. Luxury and pleasure seeking were seen as disruptive of the hierarchy, so that in places with sumptuary laws or strong customs, the lower classes were not permitted to dress as splendidly as the upper classes. It was not that fine clothes would put revolutionary ideas into the heads of the workers; rather, these sartorial badges of rank reminded everyone of stability and order. In Pervy, a wealthy farm village in central France, custom forbade the wives of farmers to wear ribbons in their bonnets as 'an accessory of inappropriate luxury.' The logic, in the words of Pervy's folklorist, was that 'any sign of luxury was feared because of the threat of new ideas by association.'[32] Similarly, the elders of Vaud Canton in Switzerland prescribed dress appropriate for each class in order to 'fight against vanity.' 'Such jewels and ornaments of the body' could only result in 'scandal, pride, and lasciviousness.' Overcoats – done only in black – were reserved for the higher classes and were to be worn in all seasons. The lower orders, whatever the weather, wore a shirt plus a vest.[33]

Things were no different in Germany. As Lady Mary Wortley Montagu travelled through Nuremberg in 1716, she wrote to a friend, 'They have sumptuary laws in this town which distinguish their rank by their dress and prevents that excess which ruins so many other cities ... I wish these laws were in force in other parts of the world.' Much better, said Lady Mary, never to have known pleasure than 'to fall into a folly which betrays [young people] to that want of money which is the source of a thousand basenesses.'[34] Such laws were in force in many parts of Europe, though not in England, as a way of sending people an antipleasure message.

Then there was the surveillance of Sunday churchgoing, in a society where the church was the centre of the community. In the days of Lutheran orthodoxy in seventeenth- and eighteenth-century Sweden and Finland, church attendance was mandatory. The newspaper was read out from the pulpit. 'At the church the harvest prospects were discussed, servants were hired, many a love match was started, and there also preparations were made, with very practical reasons, for marriage.'[35] It would have been inconceivable for young people to carry on hedonically in a way that offended the sensibilities of these steely-eyed elders.

In many parts of the world we have lost, public penalties

and humiliations were inflicted upon young people who had sex before marriage. One example among many: as late as 1800 in Sigmaringen, Germany, young women who had pre-marital sex (and who became pregnant) would be cast into the stocks in the town square, forced to wear mocking crowns of straw, or tied to the 'post of shame.'[36]

Even the timing of intercourse among married people would be subject to community regulation, not with spies peering into the bedroom window, but through a generally accepted sense of what behaviour was acceptable and when. There were proverbs about what *months* not to sleep with your wife.[37] An analysis of the seasonality of conception in seventeenth-century English villages shows that June was the month for marital sex, October the month to avoid. Fair enough, given the burst of April marriages and the exhaustion of early-autumn field labour, but just imagine connubial spontaneity under this regimen.[38]

And wifely spontaneity? On the Channel island of Guernsey, then belonging to France, women who took the sexual initiative in bed with their husbands might be grabbed by the neighbours and paraded about on a donkey.[39]

No, in these past eras, the local community mandated the rules of intimate life, and they were the rules of Christian Europe.

Obstacles to Pleasure for Women in Particular

There were some obstacles to pleasure that affected women in particular. These help explain why, generally speaking, before the mid-nineteenth century the sex act was more pleasurable for men than for women, although some physicians believed otherwise.[40] Among those circumstances were that in peasant and artisan families custom made a woman subservient to her husband, obliged to do his bidding in bed and out. Also, women's beauty – one of the few chips they personally had to bring to the table – was subject to sudden devastation through such maladies as smallpox. Finally, since women were subject to mutilation and death in childbirth, in this pre-birth-control society, where any act of intercourse might mean a conception, sex was a source of potential danger rather than pleasure. All these circumstances acted on women in a strongly anti-erotic manner.

The brutality and indifference of peasant men towards their wives seems almost inconceivable to today's reader. We can scarcely imagine that a brutish lack of feeling was once the norm for the great majority of the population in small towns and villages. Yet the authorities of the day – the small-town doctors and schoolteachers who knew their communities well – leave no doubt that this was so. Here is Abel Hugo, commenting in 1835 on women's lives in the Finistère department of Brittany. 'Among these Lower Bretons, the women are the first servants in their households; they plough the land, look after the house, eat after their husbands, who never speak to them other than with curtness, meanness, and even with a kind of contempt. If the horse and the wife fall sick at the same time, the Lower Breton will rush to the blacksmith to look after the animal, and leave to nature the task of curing his wife.'[41] In the Creuse department in central France, Hugo found that, as elsewhere, the women did exhausting work, 'yet without the little recompenses that the men receive at the bar on Sundays or holidays. There are few women who drink wine. If they accompany their husbands or relatives to the bar, it is to wait respectfully for them outside and not to share a brew. The subordination and submissiveness of the women towards men are extreme.'[42]

This litany of female obedience to men continues for other parts of France. Of the commune of Saint-Romain-en-Galles near Lyon it was said, 'The women have a certain respect for their husbands, calling them only "the lord, the lord master, the chief" [notre homme, notre maître, notre gros]. They never use the "tu" form with men. Women serve the men at table and eat only behind them standing up. It's only with difficulty that you can get women to sit down on the day of their wedding at the banquet table.'[43] Near Mantes, closer to Paris, the lot of married women was so lacking in pleasure that young women wore mourning clothes as wedding gowns. 'This garment of sadness conveys to the girl that the joys of youth and of life are brief, that happiness has no morrow, and that in this world you no longer need a party dress but a mourning dress.'[44] Marriage as the end of happiness! Could any antipleasure message have been more forceful?

One's beauty was as fleeting as one's happiness. For men, perhaps, it mattered less, since men have never needed to be beautiful to marry well. But for women beauty mattered. 'I know that beauty is perishable,' Fanny Burney's husband wrote to her in 1816, apropos the need to marry for something other than beauty. 'An accident, a difficult labour etc can transform it into ugliness.'[45]

Their beauty was highly important to women, possibly more so than today, for it gave them the message that their bodies were for finding partners above all else, not for pleasure. This antisensual message was exacerbated by the stress women lived under, knowing full well that this beauty was extremely vulnerable, a social tool that could be lost at any time.

Beauty was vulnerable to smallpox, a viral infection that left the skin pitted. The French novelist Honoré de Balzac described smallpox as 'the battle of Waterloo for women': once they'd had it, their allies vanished.[46] In the eighteenth century, smallpox caused 10 to 15 percent of all deaths in some European countries.[47] Twice as many again survived but with scarred faces. For women in the middle classes and aristocracy in particular (peasant men married more for strength than for beauty), these faces were destiny.

Women themselves believed their disfigurement from smallpox to be catastrophic. Lady Mary Wortley Montagu declared herself indifferent to sensuality, but perhaps it was because she herself had been similarly mutilated by the disease. She composed this poem ('Machaon' refers to her doctor):

Machaon too, the great Machaon, known
By his red cloak and his superior frown;
And why, he cry'd, this grief and this despair?
You shall again be well, again be fair;
Believe my oath; (with that an oath he swore)
False was his oath; my beauty is no more![48]

Of course working-class women had smallpox too, though the above testimonies are from the aristocracy. Prostitutes, for example, felt compelled to mention it in their ads in order to prepare the john in advance for the shock. Julie, who worked the streets of central Paris, said of herself in a 1791 advertisement, 'open to everything [*extrêmement coquine*]; has never been indifferent to pleasure; the prettiest eyes in the world; smallpox has changed her a bit, but she's lost none of her vigour.'[49] Smallpox, then, was something that women thought about constantly.

A final anti-erotic turn-off for women was the fear that they might become pregnant in any given sexual encounter. 'Why do we find this natural sadness among all peoples after the act of intercourse,' asked French writer Charles-Augustin Sainte-Beuve in 1851. 'It's because an inner voice says, "You've given life to a human being, and thus it's you yourself who are closer to death."'[50] Given that maternal mortality in times past was about 10 per cent on a lifetime basis, a woman stood a one-in-ten chance of dying from sex.[51] Before the late nineteenth century, you as a woman in a village would have to know only ten or so other women to realize that one of you would perish as a consequence of the sex act. Thus American family historian Carl Degler, commenting on the lack of birth control in the nineteenth century, has called the risk of conception 'a dark shadow over every act of intercourse.'[52]

Women's helplessness was exacerbated by completely false information about the timing of ovulation. Over the centuries the view of the second-century Greek physician Soranus of Ephesus had prevailed that the fertile period was just before and after menstruation.[53] Exactly wrong! Even prudent women were walking into a lava pit.

What subjective evidence is there that women found the risk of pregnancy anti-erotic? Early-eighteenth-century French obstetrician Guillaume de la Motte had patients who feared conception so greatly that they would vomit after intercourse.[54] According to Jacques Gélis, a French historian of obstetrics, 'Young women, horrified at the tale of lethal deliveries, refused to marry from fear of pregnancy and the complications of delivery. Women rejected the approach of their husbands after a long and painful delivery from which they emerged miraculously yet mutilated in their bodies.'[55] Truly, it is difficult to imagine that these women, terrified of mutilation and dying in the act of birth, experienced much joy in the act of sex.[56]

Since the dawn of humankind, the fear of pregnancy had acted as a brake on female sexuality. The playing field between men and women was not equal, for only women could get pregnant and suffer the risk of dying in a difficult delivery or from a postpartum infection. Perhaps it is this fear, more than any other mentioned in this chapter, that made women appear as cautious, pious creatures in contrast to the men who swashbuckled across the stage of history. Thus for centuries the view prevailed that women had a lesser appetite for pleasure than men.

As we have seen, the brain drives the mind in the search for pleasure. Yet if external hindrances such as physical discomfort, poor hygiene, pain, fear of death and disability, and so on, present themselves as insurmountable, these neural instructions will not be acted on. The mind will decide, 'I have to walk twelve miles through snow to feed my family. I have no time for total body sex.' The narrative of the history of desire therefore begins late in the nineteenth century, as these various hindrances are lifted and the mind is set free to follow the urgings of the brain towards sensuality.

CHAPTER FIVE

Why Not the Romantics?

The year was 1830. The young French poet Alfred de Musset, age nineteen, was attending 'a grand dinner party after a masked ball. My friends about me were richly costumed, on every side young men and women sparkling with beauty and joy.' The wine began to rise in his veins. 'People spontaneously embraced everyone who smiled at them. I felt myself the brother of everyone present.'

He planned to meet with his girlfriend, a widow, later that night. But before the evening was through he had caught her holding hands and rubbing feet with, and caressing, another young man at the dinner table. The hero of this thinly disguised autobiographical novel by one of France's great romantic poets muses bitterly about this bubbling lovey-dovey: 'C'était la maladie du siècle.' It was the sickness of our century.[1]

What was the sickness of the century? Why does our story of the onward march of pleasure not start here? Why do the romantics, exponents of the great explosion of feeling that swept Europe between the middle of the eighteenth century and the middle of the nineteenth, not mark the beginning of the surfacing of desire? Like Musset, they were not immune to sensuality. They were certainly not prudish and were willing to bury their grief in the bosoms of sex workers from time to time. They inhabited a world that permitted men and women, or at least widows, to freely cohabit. Why may we not assert that the revolution in physical sensuality that has given rise so directly to our own times began in 1770 rather than in 1870?

The illness of the century, Musset said, was in 'not realizing that life consisted of other things than loving.' Too much on one heart touching another. Musset later does become, in his personal life, something of a sensualist, but his critique of his time was that the love fantasies that men and women entertained for each other caused them to be carried away by rank emotionalism.

Yet all this talk about feeling also effaced the reality of desire. In the novel, Musset's worldly wise friend Desgenais says, 'There is a big secret, my friend, a key to the whole picture. If you think about it a bit, you realize that debauchery is natural. Someday they'll prove that it's natural.' Desgenais meant that men naturally yearned to 'push aside the pleasures of thought in favour of physical embraces.'[2] Disguising this natural desire with romantic pretty-talk constituted, for Musset, a century-long error (one that the turn-of-the-century futurists would finally put right). At this point no one was talking of women and desire.

The reason our story does not begin at mid-eighteenth century, rather than mid-nineteenth, is that the romantics, immersed as they were in the entwining of souls, retained all the scruples of traditional society about the physicality of sex. The naked soul, laid bare in the tear-smeared entries of a diary, appealed greatly to the romantic temperament. The writhing together of naked bodies did not. (As Fanny Burney confided to her diary in 1768 at age sixteen, 'I must confess my *every* thought, must open my whole Heart!')[3] In her world such values as friendship and togetherness came to matter much more than physical passion. Having now become Mme d'Arblay, she told correspondents, 'You all must know that to me a crust of bread with a little roof for shelter and a fire for warmth, near you, would bring me to peace, to happiness – to all that my Heart holds dear ... I cannot picture such a fate with dry eyes.' Her husband would be there somewhere in the background too.[4] But as for physical relations, in this whole torrent of heartfelt letters and journals she virtually never mentioned them, save to note that she had been offended by a suitor's physicality as he put his arm about her waist.[5]

The De-corporealization of Feeling

The key to understanding the romantics is their very absence of physicality: They exalted feeling, as manifest in such non-physical forms of sensuality as literature, art, and above all, music. As the young German romantic poet Friedrich Hebbel asked himself in 1835, 'Why can't I listen to music any longer than a quarter of an hour? I say to myself, the soul has its depths, and once these are stirred up, it only remains to torture them or kill them off. The pain lies in that which endures, the joy in the momentary.'[6] For this young writer, the exquisiteness of the new sensibility lay in the aesthetics of music, not in actually reaching out and physically touching another person – or being touched.

The romantics vibrated with abstract feeling. In 1815, the English romantic painter Benjamin Robert Haydon, age twenty-nine, saw the tragic actress Eliza O'Neill play Isabelle in Thomas Southerne's seventeenth-century tragedy *The Fatal Marriage*. 'Really there was no bearing it. I sat with the tears trickling over my cheeks like a woman ... I sobbed with remembrances. It touched a chord of my own sensitive heart that the World will never be acquainted with.' Months later, he confided to his diary, 'My feelings are keen and cutting, nervous, alive, and trembling.'[7]

By the following year Haydon said of his 'passions,' 'They are now more intense, more burning, more furious than ever.' What touched off this effusion was the sight, earlier that day, of a woman, 'a little, lively, plump, ambling creature,' strolling along the Strand in London. 'I passed, but her image had sunk into my soul.' Was it that he found her attractive and wanted to have sex with her? No. 'I saw her air and sweetness bright to my inmost sense.' He wandered along the Strand all day in an effort to find her again, not necessarily to ask her out on a date but because 'this creature's figure had clenched my Soul with a red hot clutch, which stopped breath and almost bereft me of sense.'[8] This is the etherealization of desire.

Behind all this romantic gush lay an abstract longing for the world of nature, as distinct from the baroque and rococo artifice of previous centuries. The romantics – from the landscape paintings of William Turner to Beethoven's symphony no. 6, *The Pastoral* – preferred natural forms to contrived. In 1774, Fanny Burney exulted at how well the South Seas tribal chief Omai, just arrived in England on board Captain Cook's *Adventure*, had turned out 'with no tutor but Nature.' '[Omai] appears in a new world like a man who had all his life studied the graces ... I think this shows how much more Nature can do without art, than art with all her refinement, unassisted by Nature.'[9] In 1786, the twenty-year-old Munich physician Franz von Baader, fresh out of medical school, enthused in his diary about 'Nature ... which in jollier, better moments fills my spirit with heavenly desire, an enchanting notion that brightens, warms and gladdens my soul ...' Baader, later a famous philosopher, would devote himself at length to the study of 'heavenly desires,' little to carnal.[10]

Where, in this world of nature, did sex belong?

Romantic Women

In sexual attitudes, women with a passion for romanticism differed little from traditional women. The evidence these women have left behind is very meagre, yet some insights break through the tumble of diary entries and heart-throbbing letters of the time. Julie de Lespinasse was a Parisian society woman whom one wag called 'the biggest bundle of emotions in the eighteenth century.'[11] She had already been passionately but chastely involved with a number of men, including 'Encyclopedist' Jean d'Alembert, by the time she met the great love of her life, François, Count of Guibord, in 1772. She was forty. Their exchanges were intense. How much, she told him in October 1774, she had liked a previous letter of his: 'This need to live life at the limit [*vivre fort*] is, I think, one of the characteristics of the damned,' a characteristic that she said she shared with her lover. 'If ever I should become calm again, as people put it, it's then that I would think of myself as crucified upon the wheel [a device for torturing prisoners]. This kind of talk [of passion] is only at the disposition of those of us who believe themselves endowed with a sixth sense, the soul. Yes, my friend, I am as fortunate, or as unfortunate, as you in having the same dictionary as you.'[12] What kind of passion did Mlle Lespinasse have in mind?

Although she had given herself physically to the Count, a dictionary of sensual intimacy is just about the last thing one finds in her impassioned letters to him. She refers to her own body as 'ma machine,' as in 'my poor machine,' a standard eighteenth-century usage but still not one that conjures up great physical rapture. Throughout, she endured a constant series of psychosomatic and opium-induced illnesses as a result of conflicts over the Count's other mistress and over his bride-to-be. For someone who believed her soul to have the same physiological status as seeing, hearing, and tasting, it is unsurprising that she experienced romance as pain. 'My friend, I wanted to write to you all day yesterday, but I just didn't have the strength. I was in such a state of suffering that the power to speak and to move had vanished. I can no longer eat. The words food and pain have become synonyms for me.' Later: 'I haven't breathed since last Wednesday.' By October 1774 she had started taking hemlock. 'If I could take it in the same manner as Socrates, I would do so with pleasure! It would cure me of this slow and incurable disease that one calls life.'

By 1775 she believes herself to be ruled solely by her 'soul.' 'Yes, I know, my soul is made entirely for excesses: loving feebly is impossible for me.' Nowhere in this catalogue of physical sufferings that she dispatched to Count Guibord was there any reference to possible physical pleasure that she might have experienced with him, although she declared that she loved him deeply and threatened suicide after he married. Nowhere were there hints of any special little activities they might undertake in bed, of preparing her toilette to appeal, or of any charming little physical graces that he might possess. Instead, she identified with Clarissa, the long-suffering heroine of Samuel Richardson's 1748 novel of that title, the French translation of which had appeared in 1751. But you, you beast, she addressed the Count later in 1775, 'are not worthy of the suffering you inflict!'[13] So there it was, love among the romantics as soul torture rather than physical passion. She died, apparently of opium intoxication, the following year.

By the post-Napoleonic period, this preoccupation with the soul had produced romance-groupies, forerunners of the rock-groupies of a later era. Parisian novelist Arsène Houssaye recalled of the 1830s flocks of young women chasing after the fashionable novelists of the day such as Honoré de Balzac or Alexandre Dumas: 'You could recognize them by their diaphanous looks, their moist, searching eyes, their disarrayed hair. Passion had made them all pale, passion for poetry, or for the ideal man, or for love.'[14] In later years, said Houssaye, it would be 'sexual desire' [*volupté*] that drove such women. But not in the romantic 1830s.

The married Countess Marie d'Agoult, known to the reading public as novelist Daniel Stern, met the budding twenty-year-old Hungarian composer and pianist Franz Liszt in 1830. It was one of the century's great love affairs, but of interest is the timid pace at which the meeting of the two hearts is accompanied by the meeting of bodies.

Liszt, of course, was immersed as well in the literature of romanticism, Byron's epic poem *Childe Harold* being among his favourites. Liszt would come to play for the Countess, and, both unhappy in their personal lives, they would have soulful discussions. 'In the voice of the young enchanter, in his vibrant words, there opened before me a whole infinity,

sometimes luminous, sometimes shadowed, constantly changing, into which my mind plunged with no recourse. In my
intimacy with Franz there was no question of coquetry or of
gallantry, as is appropriate between people of different sexes
in my particular circle.' They met every day, always agreeing
to meet again the following day.

Her family went on vacation, and she asked Franz to come
and join them. There was, one afternoon, a moment of awk-
wardness, their eyes locked, then he fell at her feet, embracing her knees. Mutual love was declared. Only at this point
did their hands touch! A week later Franz and Marie left
France together for Italy. Only as they are sitting in the coach,
leaving for a destination unknown to her, does he embrace
her, throwing his arms around her. 'Grand Dieu!' she cries.[15]

In the course of their long relationship, Marie d'Agoult
would indeed discover Eros and begin writing novels under
the pen name of a male. The point, however, is that physical
intimacy played virtually no role in the genesis of their relationship. It was not mainly about bodies meeting but souls.

These stories represent a mere post-holing amid the vast
field of women's sexual experience in the romantic years.
Perhaps there were women in the period 1750 to 1850 who
had riotously diverse sexual encounters before marriage, filled
with lustiness and physical abandon. But the present author
has seen no references to anything like this, and doubts that
such experiences were common. For women, the lustiness
comes later.

Romantic Men

Jean-Jacques Rousseau stands as the founding figure of the
romantic movement, and, more than any other document, it
was Rousseau's *Confessions*, published posthumously in 1789,
that conferred an image of the romantics as panting with
desire. Yet even though the adolescent Rousseau did indeed pant with desire, at the summit of his courtship years
Rousseau was mainly interested in a union of souls, and

indeed with the great love of his life he had no physical contact at all.

Rousseau later remembered himself, as an eighteen-year-old around 1730, being 'restless, distracted, dreamy: I sobbed, I sighed, I desired a kind of happiness I was unable to describe yet the privation of which I resented ... My boiling blood filled my head incessantly with thoughts of girls and women.' His desire for a woman mounted steadily and was gratified shortly thereafter by an older woman nicknamed 'Maman,' who conferred upon the young man much tenderness but only a minimum of carnal pleasure. In 1737 that relationship gave way to a brief affair with Mme de Larnage, entraining 'a sensuality whose pleasure was so fiery and an intimacy so sweet in our rapports' that it would remain in his head for decades afterwards. Yet it wasn't true love, Rousseau said, and he moved on.

In 1745 Rousseau began a long relationship with the twenty-three-year-old Thérèse Levasseur that lasted until his death in 1794, producing a number of children, all of whom were given up to the foundling hospital. Yet Rousseau claimed that he never really loved her, that he had no more desire for her than for Maman, and that he maintained coital relations with her merely to release himself physically.

The great love of Rousseau's life was Mme d'Houdetot, whom he met in 1757 when he was forty-four and she, 'not at all pretty and her faced marked with smallpox,' about thirty. Living in an arranged marriage, she had never loved her husband. Her already existing lover told her she should meet Rousseau. The relationship between Mme d'Houdetot and Rousseau was rather asymmetrical: 'We were both drunk with love, she for her lover, and me for her.' There were scenes in the clearing at midnight. 'When I think of the intoxicating tears that I deposited on her knees!' A single kiss from her put 'my machine into an inconceivable disarray': his head spun, he felt he was about to go blind, his knees trembled and would scarcely hold him upright.

And that was it. They never made love. 'Such was the sole

amorous moment in the life of this man with the most com-
bustible temperament [himself] – and perhaps the greatest
timidity – that Nature has ever produced.' After Mme
d'Houdetot, Rousseau renounced love forever.[16]

Rousseau's historic importance lies in suggesting that personal happiness is within reach, rather than in establishing
the primacy of the physical. As Mme Roland awaited the
guillotine in her cell in the Bastille during the French Revolution, she recalled that when she was twenty-one her tutor
had given her a copy of Rousseau's *La Nouvelle Heloïse*, published in 1761. 'This was really the first thing that got me
thinking.' 'Rousseau showed me what domestic contentment
I could aspire to, the exquisite delicacies that I would be
capable of sampling.'[17] But of course they were delicacies of
the heart rather than of the flesh.

Yet Rousseau, with his breezy confessions of masturbation
and orgasmic urgency, gives a misleading impression of the
openness of the romantic male towards sexuality. In Théophile
Gautier's 1835 novel, *Mademoiselle de Maupin*, which positively flutters with romantic sensibilities, the hero has become addicted to sex. He declares, 'I have become so weakened
by sexual desire [*volupté*], this poison has become so profoundly insinuated into my bones ...'[18] Thus, for Gautier, sex
was an addictive poison.

So much did Genevan writer Henri-Frédéric Amiel fear
this poison that at age nineteen he would wash his body at
bedtime with vinegar to avoid having a wet dream. As he
confided to his diary in 1840, 'I passed a terrible night; I had
forgotten to wash my abdomen with vinegar, as I usually do;
the heat of the bed affected my senses, and I had an emission.
It's entirely physical, because I had no bad dreams [sic], and
for a long time now I've warded off all bad thoughts. I'm
terrified as I recall the words of the doctor: "Each ejaculation
is a dagger's thrust into your eyes": Expiate, that's the secret.'
In fact, Amiel feared he was going blind as a result of repeated wet dreams, and consulted his aunt because of 'the
immense gravity of the situation.'[19]

The English painter Haydon also struggled to resist masturbation and expressed self-loathing after sexual adventures. Marriage turns out to be his haven: 'I hate vice, – but I love passion faithfully directed, and adore that beautiful sex which excites it.'[20] Thus a man like Haydon represents the age-old standard of male sexual desire with a romantic overlay of feeling. But there is nothing new in his sexuality, in either quantitative terms – meaning how much sex (indeed, he used abstinence as a means of marital birth control), or qualitative terms – meaning what parts of the body are involved (he enjoyed kissing but not with the tongue).

For students of sexuality and romanticism, the great conundrum is Lord Byron. George Gordon, Lord Byron, has passed into history as an icon for tempestuous, violent sensuality, his numerous conquests coining an image of the romantic heroes as physically impassioned lovers, unlike every generation of males that went before. This image is certainly false for the romantics in general, and somewhat off the mark for Byron, because his major sexual interest seems to have been other men. Because homosexuality was so strongly taboo in the past, it has been little appreciated that Byron was gay, at best bisexual. His letters to his friends boast of his female conquests, but then gayness was not gladly advertised in the early nineteenth century. Indeed, an inadvertent outing may have been the occasion of his sudden and unexplained exile from England in 1809.[21]

Even as a youth Byron boasted of his heterosexual conquests while allowing a certain homoerotic fondness. In 1807, at nineteen, he tells the Earl of Clare that 'my attentions have been divided amongst so many fair damsels' that his correspondence has suffered. Yet two years later he says that he intends to offer a treatise on 'Sodomy simplified or Paederasty proved to be praiseworthy from ancient authors and modern practice.'[22]

In brief, Byron represents an unleashing of the physical passions that is not really typical of his romantic contemporaries.[23] Given his homosexuality, he may have been following different cues than the romantic heterosexuals. (The narrative of homosexual history differs somewhat from heterosexual, emerging early in time with explosive force simply because it was so persecuted and repressed.) Yet hetero- or homosexual, Byron loses his sexual energy early in life, a much more fitting romantic apotheosis. At thirty-six, writing to a friend from Genoa in 1823, he declared that his ardour seemed to be flagging: '[Indeed I had indulged] in some portion of dissipation, but it was to *sow my wild oats* so as not to prolong *those* vices beyond a certain period ... In this I think I have succeeded whatever may be said upon the subject.' Given the dictum that one vice drives out another, Byron now anticipated, he said, an attack of avarice.[24]

In the 1870s and after, a new sensuality would turn its back on the romantics. George Moore, a young English writer in his early twenties, is visiting Paris for the first time. Suddenly a light goes on for him. 'Shelley's teaching had been, while accepting the body, to dream of the soul as a star ... But now I saw suddenly, with delightful clearness and with intoxicating conviction, that by looking without shame and accepting with love the flesh, I might raise it to as high a place ... as even the soul had been set in.' 'Here,' said Moore of Paris in the 1870s, 'was a new creed proclaiming the divinity of the body.'[25]

The age-old hindrances to physical pleasure for its own sake were at last coming away.

CHAPTER SIX

The Great Breakout

In July 1912 English writer D.H. Lawrence had just stolen away with his German girlfriend, Frieda von Richthofen, who was then married to another Englishman, to 'the little top floor of the Bavarian peasant-house in Isartal.' It was a secluded chalet next to a stream. From the balcony, Lawrence looked down on Frieda. 'She swims finely, and looks fearfully voluptuous, rolling in the pale green water,' he told a friend. She was swimming naked.[1]

'What a life!' said Frieda. 'We had lost all ordinary sense of time and place.' She and Lawrence concentrated on the physicality of their existence. He told her, 'Take all you want of me, everything, I am yours.' Frieda reflected, 'I took and gave equally, without thought.' 'I knew he loved the essence of me as he loved the blueness of the gentians.' They spent much of the day naked, and lived on black bread, fresh eggs, and strawberries.[2]

There is a frisson of sensuality in these accounts that would not have been present a hundred years previously, the tremor of a new sexual era. It is not just that Lawrence, then an obscure English littérateur from the provinces, had stolen another man's wife and run off to Valhalla with her (although that was unusual enough in the context of the day). Of interest is his description to a friend back home of his erectile pleasure at the sight of his girlfriend's sleek body tumbling in the water. Frieda, in turn, describes surrendering her body totally to him. A page has been turned. The great breakout from the trammels of the sexuality of Christian Europe had begun.

'Sexual life occupies such a large place in the life of our society, indeed in the life of our nation,' wrote Armand Dubarry in the preface to his 1896 novel about homosexuality in Paris. 'It occupies such a large place in our thoughts, our acts, and exercises such an influence upon all of us, that not dealing with this power that controls us ... is the height of absurdity and imprudence.'[3] By the turn of the twentieth century, an entire moral order was slipping away. The former hindrances to pleasure now lay in ruins, and in their stead rose a newly assertive sensuality.

Virginia Woolf rather whimsically put the change around 1910. 'I will hazard a second assertion, which is more disputable perhaps,' she told the members of a literary club in Cambridge in 1924. The first assertion had been that all present were doubtless skilled judges of character. The second: 'On or about December 1910 human character changed.'[4] She meant that human relations were becoming more subjective, less formal. She herself was too reserved to speak directly of sex to club members, yet she in her own life – and the others in the Bloomsbury circle (named after the district of London where they all lived) – had recently begun to feel in very personal and subjective ways that a new sexual era was dawning.

Woolf remembered it had been around 1904 that they had started talking about sex in her home at 46 Gordon Square. (This she did not tell to the literary club.) 'Suddenly the door opened and the long and sinister figure of Mr. Lytton Strachey stood on the threshold. He pointed his finger at a stain on [Virginia's sister] Vanessa's white dress.

'"Semen?" he said.'

All present burst out laughing. Virginia thought to herself, 'Can one really say it?'

This was the beginning of the sexualizing of Bloomsbury. 'With that one word all barriers of reticence and reserve went down. A flood of the sacred fluid seemed to overwhelm us. Sex permeated our conversation. The word bugger was never far from our lips. [Many of the males in the group, including the writer Strachey, were homosexuals.] We discussed copulation with the same excitement and openness that we had discussed the nature of good. It is strange to think how reticent, how reserved we had been and for how long.'[5]

Virginia Woolf's account faithfully reflected her own experience, but it fell short in two ways as an analysis of middle-class England or of Western society. It placed the great sexual breakout in the Edwardian period, the decade before the First World War. Also, it suggested that the change lay mainly in the willingness to discuss sex rather than in sexual behaviour. In fact, the historic upheavals in the sexual agenda had begun, generally speaking, around mid-century, towards 1860 or 1870, as the pace of social change began to accelerate dramatically. French social historian Alain Corbin dates the making of modern sexuality in fact to this decade: 'The contemporary history of sexuality begins around 1860,' he writes of France. 'A gnawing kind of hunger overthrows the traditional culture, and the erotic imagination becomes transformed. Sheltered in the sphere of private life, the middle classes begin to suffer from their previous morality.'[6]

The change affected not so much the quantitative aspect of sex life as the qualitative: not so much at what age people begin to have sex, or whether they are adulterous, or how many times a week they do it, but rather what, exactly, they do in bed. This qualitative aspect began to shift late in the nineteenth century as society started to edge towards total body sex.

The quantitative aspect of sexuality is capable of changing too, of course. Late in the eighteenth century, working-class people and peasants began to free themselves increasingly of peonage by becoming economically independent in the early days of the Industrial Revolution.[7] This resulted in a virtual sexual revolution as men and women who could earn their own keep began to have sex before marriage. One result was a huge explosion of out-of-wedlock births that continued for approximately the next hundred years, until the advent of safer abortions and cheaper contraceptives. But that explosion of premarital sexual activity seems to have involved few qualitative changes: by all accounts, among working-class people the missionary position was as firmly ensconced in the saddle, as it were, at the end of the nineteenth century as at the end of the eighteenth.

Rather, the surge towards qualitative change involved new parts of the body and different styles of making love, parts that had previously been erotically silent over the long eons of time. This is of interest because the body as a whole is sexually responsive, and the brain seems keen to register erotic signals from head to foot. And once the process of brain-driven sexuality begins, it never stops, or at least it has continued uninterrupted until our own time. These qualitative changes were initiated within the middle classes and spread downwards from there. But qualitative or quantitative, both kinds of changes in sexuality entailed lifting the previous hindrances.

Lifting the Hindrances

'When human relationships change,' said Virginia Woolf, 'there is at the same time a change in religion, conduct, politics, and literature.'[8] The transformation of sexuality was made possible by the removal of the historic hindrances upon the free expression of desire. Between the 1860s and the 1920s the world altered in an almost unrecognizable manner, perhaps even more strikingly than it did towards the end of the twentieth century, with the celebrated changes that led to so much astonishment around the year 2000 about 'how far we've come.' Although the pace of change in our own time is undeniable, in the course of the nineteenth century the residence of the average person changed from countryside to city and the place of work from home to factory or counting-house. In the United States, the average life expectancy for males at birth rose from the 38.3 years we previously saw for 1850 to 59.3 in 1929 (and for females from 40.5 years to 62.6).[9] More than twenty extra years of life! Computers, email, and fast planes are important. But the changes of the nineteenth century transformed fundamentally the nature of the human condition. They were equally portentous for the history of sensuality.

Privacy, for example, is essential for sensuality. One cannot shiver with delight at explorations of new body areas if the farmhands are gawking astonished through the cottage window. And there is a special kind of privacy that goes with urbanization. As people move from countryside to city they exchange the stifling control of community life for the anonymity of the metropolis. The population of Paris increased almost fivefold in the years 1801 to 1896. In 1801, one Englishman in seven lived in a city; by 1891, one in two. In the United States there were no cities larger than 100,000 in 1800; by 1890 there were twenty-eight.[10]

During the Second Empire one French writer describes how the eyes of the men and women at the Parisian dancehall Mabille hunt for each other:

> The blue-grey smoke of cigarettes
> Curls from the lessening ends that glow;
> The men are thinking of the bets,
> The women of the debts they owe.
>
> Then their eyes meet, and in their eyes
> The accustomed smile comes up to call,
> A look half-miserably wise,
> Half-heedlessly ironical.[11]

Of course the eyes of men and women have always sought each other. But in the garden of the Mabille, after many turns of the chahut-dance and glasses of wine, the men and women might leave together. This would not happen in the village.

The cities have always meant a freer life, unobserved encounters, the cosiness of privacy. As the Parisian man about town André de Fouquières later said, 'Even the most modest bourgeois of the nineteenth century insisted that his home be divided into two watertight zones, one for "company," which was gussied up, the other for himself, where every kind of negligence was accepted.'[12] The French phrase *chacun chez soi*, or 'people have a right to privacy,' came into common usage in these years. Even in the working-class households of Paris, for the first time in history, 'the bedroom becomes the exclusive place for sex,' in historian Alain Corbin's words.[13]

Magnus Hirschfeld, a pioneer of gay rights in Germany, said in 1904 that homosexuals fled to Berlin to escape the social surveillance of the small town: 'That's just what excites them ... a city of a million, where the individual isn't subject to the control of the neighbourhood as in the smaller towns ... There, people can easily be watched – and are eagerly watched over to see when, where, and with whom you have been eating and drinking, going for a stroll or going to bed. But in Berlin the people in apartment block A have no idea who lives in block B ...'[14] (A similar logic applied to gay men in Paris: of those arrested for sodomy between 1860 and 1870, 59 per cent were born in the provinces, and 9 per cent were foreigners.)[15]

In the city, people could do as they wished, for the locks were tight and the doors thick. In his 1880 novel, *Nana*, Emile Zola explained that one of the heroine's pleasures 'was to undress in front of her wardrobe mirror ... Naked, she looked at herself for a long time. She had a passion for her own body, a love affair with the satin of her skin and the supple lines of her hips that made her serious and attentive, absorbed in love of herself.'[16] Perhaps Paris had ten thousand Nanas, young courtesans like the figure in Zola's novel who squeezed their breasts and kissed their arms in front of the mirror, perhaps only a few. The point is that such intimate self-absorption could be accomplished only in an apartment that guaranteed absolute privacy, and from which few sounds escaped.

One didn't find rooms such as Nana's on the second floor

of the butcher shop looking out over the village square. Such secrecy, privacy, and anonymity could only be guaranteed in 'the chaos of the living city,' in Baudelaire's phrase. For the middle classes to get serious about pleasure, they would first have to acquire an urban platform for it.

Yet the city meant more than privacy for the middle classes and for young women like Nana – Parisian slang for 'babe' – whom the paterfamilias kept. The metropolis symbolized sexual adventure and release. New erotic horizons beckoned for all who moved there. In trying to explain why so many young men and women were fleeing agriculture from the French province of Touraine for Paris, economist Henri Baudrillart told his readers not to seek the cause in such conventional explanations as rural poverty (there were plenty of jobs back home) or the filthiness of rural dwellings (no worse than elsewhere). 'The main cause, in this pleasure-loving country, we shan't find elsewhere than in the attractions of the city. People go there to seek ... a freer life.'[17]

And please: no circumlocutions when it comes to talk of a freer life. The great majority of young people sought the sexual independence of the city, which, in that pre-contraceptive society meant an inevitable reflux of the disappointed to places like the Maternity Hospital of Poitiers. Said its medical director in 1857 of the many enthusiastic young people who years before had set their caps for the big time, 'A deplorable tendency leads young men today to leave the plough to find better pay or easier work, demoralizing them with tastes and penchants they can't always satisfy. We see the same tendency to escape maternal surveillance end up even more deplorably for the young women, causing their even more profound demoralization and the loss of their honour.'[18] According to Iwan Bloch, a militant for gay rights in Germany before the First World War, city life actually heightened sexual desire. 'The sexual impulse is, in every possible way, influenced, increased, elaborated, and complicated, by the civilization of the present day. Especially the life of the great cities, where the essence of modern civilization is found in its most concentrated form, serves as a sexual stimulant in the highest degree ...' All these gastronomic and alcoholic excesses, said Bloch, created the idea that 'after work comes pleasure and not repose.'[19] For these authors, then, there was absolutely no doubt that urban life was overthrowing the hindrance of community control to sexual expression.

Pain and chronic discomfort represented a second hindrance overcome in the years 1860 to 1920. One recalls the great physical distraction of scabies that had plagued humankind over the centuries. In 1911, a pharmacist named Marcussen at the City Hospital of Copenhagen developed a sulphur ointment for the intolerable itching of scabies, a clear yellow solution obtained by heating a kilogram of sublimated sulphur together with a 50 per cent solution of potassium hydroxide. People loved the ointment for its 'soothing properties.' 'In a typical case,' said one authority, 'within an hour the itching ceases.'[20]

A new era in pain relief began in November 1853, when Alexander Wood, an Edinburgh physician casting about for a method of introducing morphine into painful nerves, recalled that Mr Ferguson, of Giltspur Street in London, had recently manufactured 'an elegant little syringe.' Wood procured the instrument, resolving to try it out at the first opportunity. He did not have long to wait. An elderly female patient of his had been unable to sleep for four or five days because of 'a most violent attack of cervico-brachial neuralgia' (arm pain). Wood introduced the needle of the syringe, which contained a solution of morphine mixed with sherry ('because it would not rust the instrument as a water solution of opium would do'), into her shoulder joint. 'In about five minutes the patient's eyes became injected, and looked just like the eyes of a drunken person, and she complained that her head was in a confused state. She soon afterwards fell asleep.' When Wood called on her the following morning, he was alarmed to see her sleeping still. After shaking her awake, he realized he had probably given her too much. Nonetheless, 'This treatment quite cured the old lady of the neuralgic pains, which never returned.'

Wood's treatment became widely adopted in Edinburgh in the following years. Young women there often complained of lower abdominal pains, 'and females suffering from them have very often been treated, by mistake, for uterine disease when there was nothing of the kind,' Wood said. Often doctors had forced speculums into their virginal patients' vaginas. 'Caustic has been employed, and the most severe treatment adopted, when the little instrument I will soon describe to you,' he told a British medical audience in 1858, 'would have almost immediately relieved the pain.'[21]

To be sure, opiates had always existed in medicine, yet the acids of the stomach neutralize much of their action before they can reach the bloodstream. Morphine, an alkaloid of opium, had been described early in the nineteenth century. Yet only with Wood's discovery of the syringe did the effective delivery of a powerful medication for pain become possible.

In the years that followed, other less addictive forms of pain relief came onto the market as well. Yet in the world of analgesia there was nothing comparable to the Bayer Company's introduction of Aspirin in 1899. In 1897 Bayer chemist Felix Hoffmann had synthesized acetylsalicylic acid, as it is known generically, and after Aspirin hit the market it became an instant worldwide best-seller. There was no competitor available until Tylenol (acetaminophen) was approved by the U.S. Food and Drug Administration in 1952. Today, Tylenol dominates the $2.5 billion yearly American pain-relief market with over 40 per cent of total sales, followed by Ibuprofen, Naproxen, and others. Bayer Aspirin's share of sales has shrunk to 5 per cent.[22] Yet the gate opened by Aspirin has made a profound difference in the pharmacology of everyday life.

Chronic pain is still very common, yet these remedies at least hold out the promise of coping with it, making pain not incompatible with the experience of pleasure in other domains of life. None of these options existed before the middle of the nineteenth century, when pain could be countered only with fortitude.

The antisensual dimensions of religious faith have more or less been hoisted out of the picture, as well, first by the determination of people simply to ignore them, later by a decision on the part of both Protestant and Catholic churches to become more accepting of pleasure. 'What does an eternity of damnation matter to whoever finds in an instant the infinity of a climax,' wrote French poet Charles Baudelaire sometime around the mid-nineteenth century.[23] By 1875 in Sweden, the young August Strindberg – later a famous playwright – had become a ladies' man, intent upon repeated conquests. Why was I like this? he asked. As he later reflected: 'The emptiness left behind after I exiled religion from my life was becoming filled again: the need to adore appeared in a new form. God had been toppled and women took his place.'[24] For Strindberg, there were no longer any obstacles to acting on the basis of desire (which, of course, he later bitterly regretted because of relationship complications).

Like a lit fuse, the pleasure that began to ignite in popular life blew away traditional religious antihedonism. As Natalie Barney, hedonistic, lesbian, and very Parisian, later put it, looking back on the sensual emptiness of the couple's life in the traditional family, 'The considering of physical relations as a sin, tolerated solely from the viewpoint of reproduction, demands such a desolating courage that only a religious wife, who had never experienced pleasure nor proffered complaints, could tolerate it.'[25] Such thinking was as far from the circle of her chic Parisian friends of the 1920s as night from day. Once you had savoured desire there was no looking back.

Ultimately, religious dogma changed to accommodate the push towards pleasure. After the turn of the century, the Protestant churches began to embrace sensuality as a part of the humanity that God has given, and the American Catholic church became tacitly accepting of pleasures such as premarital sex that previously would have merited the fires of purgatory. Such turn-of-the-century medical writers as William Hammond, Denslow Lewis, and Robert Latou Dickinson advocated the enjoyment of sex as part of one's Christian faith. In the view of the feminist birth-control advocate Margaret Sanger in the 1920s – also a devout Christian – women's sexual desires had a redemptive religious power.[26] Today, 93 per cent of Americans say they have a religious faith, and 40 per cent attend church at least once a week.[27] Yet most of these people enjoy the sensual bounty that postmodern life holds out to them.

In antihedonism, the differences between the traditional Protestant and Catholic faiths were always marginal, the Lutheran divines of the seventeenth century thundering against this world as a veil of tears no less fervently than their Catholic counterparts.

Similarly, in the modern religious acceptance of hedonism the differences between the faiths are minimal. In a 1948 Gallup Poll, 57 per cent of Protestants declared the just-released Kinsey Report on male sexuality to be 'a good thing,' as compared to 49 per cent of Catholics, a marginal difference.[28] Members of both faiths, in other words, believed it suitable to have detailed information on sexual behaviour.

Finally, one of the major hindrances to sexual pleasure for women – the fear of conception – was steadily eroded by more convenient and reliable contraception. How exactly couples prevent pregnancy belongs to their most intimate secrets. Yet we know that in the last third of the nineteenth century couples began to practise some form of birth control, simply because the birth rate began to drop sharply. One recalls that in traditional society, the average woman might have six live births, with stillbirths and abortions added on. In England and Wales, this began to change in the 1880s, as the fertility rate (measured by a demographic index called 'Ig') fell by 44 per cent from 1881 to 1921; in Germany the rate fell by 31 per cent from 1875 to 1910. Figures for other West European countries are similar, the big exception being France where the decline began earlier and more powerfully.[29] When the birth rate declines, various factors may be at work, such as less marital intercourse, higher abortion rates, or greater fetal loss as a result of malnutrition. Yet these would scarcely be inducements to sensuality. The only factor that would permit women a greater sense of serenity about intercourse – removing the fear that any sex act might result in conception – is improved contraception.

There is a good deal of evidence that better contraception came to the aid of middle-class women, both married and unmarried, late in the century. In 1885, H.A. Allbutt, a physician from Leeds, published a pamphlet, *The Wife's Handbook*, describing the diaphragm, tampons, and the cervical cap, and recommending the condom. Its circulation was in the hundreds of thousands, and it became translated into a number of other languages.[30] As one physician told a national commission in Britain convened just before the First World War to consider the causes of this (to many) alarming decline in the birth rate, 'One frequently hears that a woman refuses to have any children for a time, or even to have any children at all, and even unknown to her husband, she will either introduce into the passage some chemical agent which will destroy the spermatozoa, or she will sometimes wear a cap over the neck of the womb, which takes the place, in the female, of the "letters" that men wear ...'[31] These letters, or condoms, were known to be effective. When Peter Ackerley, a child unwanted by all, was born in 1895 at the family home in Melcombe Place in London, his Aunt Bunny later told him, somewhat viciously, of the circumstances of his conception: 'Your father happened to run out of french letters that day.'[32]

Surveys support these anecdotes. In Katharine Bement Davis's survey of 1,000 women in the early 1920s, 74 per cent of those polled responded that they used contraceptives (11 per cent also relied on abortion).[33] What techniques were American women using in those years? In the four decades between 1880 and 1920, New York gynecologist Robert Latou Dickinson quizzed many of his thirtyish, married, middle-class patients about their sex lives. Of the 229 couples exercising 'deliberate control' over fertility, one in five used abstinence, one-third used female-initiated techniques (such as douches and occlusive pessaries), a further third used male-initiated techniques (condom, withdrawal), and one-eighth were doubly sure, both the man and the woman undertaking some preventive measure.[34] These chemicals, caps, and condoms may not have been as effective as the later birth-control pill, but they were a considerable sight better than what had existed previously – namely coitus interruptus, with unsafe drug abortion as a backup[35] – and the availability of these techniques helped remove what had been for many women a very specific and concrete impediment to sexual pleasure: the fear of conceiving.

Men and women have the same capacity for pleasure. Yet for women, the historic hindrances to the expression of pleasure, such as the constant fear of pregnancy and of death in childbirth, were incomparably more rigorous. When in the late nineteenth century these hindrances began to fall away, women experienced a sexual revolution of their own, more dramatic than the great breakout in men's lives precisely because the degree of erotic fulfilment to which women were accustomed was lower. For women, pleasure becomes an option, within marriage and without. Alain Corbin writes of 'the eroticizing of the wives.'[36] This is the beginning of women's sexual revolution.

But in the years after 1860 both men and women started to experience remarkable changes in their sexual lives. The steady removal of previous barriers – medical, social, and cultural – encouraged millions of people to pursue sensuality. In the last third of the nineteenth century, chronic physical discomfort diminished; the realm of personal privacy expanded; and the ability of an intrusive community to surveil personal pleasures collapsed. A platform was thus created for the pursuit of hedonism. What is the evidence that the mind did, finally, respond to the brain's hedonic urges?

New Body Zones

The last third of the nineteenth century sees a slow and hesitant tapping towards the concept of total body sexuality: an appreciation of every surface of the body for its sexual potential instead of an exclusive focus upon the face and genitals. This is qualitative sexuality: changes not just in the frequency of intercourse or the position but in the very zones of the body that are involved. Evidence on this point is difficult to come by since even today public-opinion polls about sexuality do not ask the right questions: Do you like having your nipples played with? Do you respond to your partner's muscularity? Do you find your partner's buttocks sexually appealing? (And questions about anal and oral sex are often posed with such vagueness and discretion that one gets little sense of what the partners are actually doing.) Yet there is evidence. And it suggests that parts of the body that were previously taboo or ignored are starting to come to life.

Deep kissing, 'the basic building block of intimacy,'[37] is probably the touchstone of total body sex: people whose tongues are not entwined will likely not display a strong interest in any part of their partner's body save the genitals. Today, deep kissing marks the true beginning of a young person's sexual initiation, as for the first time the overwhelming power of Eros floods into a welcoming but completely inexperienced mind.

Deep tongue kissing had formed a fundamental part of the sexuality of the ancients, with their ludic attitude towards the body and its zones. 'There's pleasure too keen for comfort,' wrote Ovid. 'Why did our tongues ever meet? ... Such kisses could only be learnt in bed. Some *maestro* [who taught her tongue kissing] has been well paid.'[38]

With the passing of the Romans and the advent of the Catholic Middle Ages, deep kissing virtually disappears from discussion. A few self-declared libertines such as Casanova admit to it, as for example in 1753 he passes a first night of passion with the young nun M.M., 'having spent hours without doing anything more than continually swallowing her saliva mixed together with mine.' On another occasion Mme F. tells him why she has fallen in love with him: 'After the first kiss I was no longer mistress of myself. I didn't know that a kiss could have such great consequences.'[39] These must have been, in the Casanova style, deep kisses.

But Casanova represented an erotic underworld. From the Middle Ages until the end of the nineteenth century there are remarkably few references to deep kissing in either folklore or literature. Indeed, several late-nineteenth-century treatises on Eros, kissing, and the like, do not even refer to tongue kissing, so profoundly had the subject been repressed in the erotic imagination. A turn-of-the-century treatise on *The Kiss and Its History* by Danish philologist Christopher Nyrop makes it sound as though kissing is really about noise making, loud smacking that certainly does not involve tongue thrusting. 'A person should not be too wet around the mouth,' declared the ancient Norsemen, and nice German girls of yore were said to scorn 'a kiss with sauce.' Indeed, said Nyrop, in peasant society the whole subject of kissing was viewed with some suspicion, because it could lead to romantic entanglement. Nyrop cited references across the ages to 'sweet' kisses, and 'burning' kisses, and even biting ones, but no references to deep or tongue kisses.[40]

Of course, one cannot say that deep kissing is necessarily more erotic than simple lip kissing, because each epoch gets the Eros it deserves. Yet deep tongue kissing does implicate the body more fully. Henry Finck's 1887 account of 'love kissing' is filled with passionate burnings and rapturous smackings, but not a single word is given over to the tongue. Here is Finck on how to kiss: 'A lover should not hold his bride by the ears in kissing her,' he warns. 'A more graceful way ... is to put your right arm round her neck, your fingers under her chin, raise the chin, and then gently but firmly press your lips on hers.' She will learn that 'it doesn't hurt' after a few repetitions and will become 'as gentle as a lamb.'[41] That represented the summation of nineteenth-century kissing lore.

Yet late in the nineteenth century, references to open-mouthed kissing do begin to appear in droves, and by the First World War the tongue kiss has clearly become the standard form of kissing among young people. For Americans who came of age in the 1920s and 1930s, tongue kissing was manifestly part of the repertoire: Alfred Kinsey found that 69 per cent of the white males with a college education whom he quizzed had done 'much' of it premaritally, 46 per cent of the females.[42]

Other zones come to life as well aside from the mucosa of the mouth. We note, for example, the nipples. For men, the historical silence about their own nipples is deafening. There simply are no references to heterosexual men enjoying play with their own nipples. Even master sensualist Casanova was uninterested in his nipples. As he meets the ravishing young nun Caterina ('C.C.') in Venice in 1753, they embrace passionately. He tries to guide her hands to his crotch, 'where she would find evidence that I merited her grace.' Yet 'she refuses to remove her hands from my chest, where she could not have found anything of interest.'[43] Evidently Casanova had no desire to let the eager Caterina stimulate his nipples.

Iwan Bloch's comprehensive history of Western sexuality mentions as 'erogenic areas' of the body 'the lips ... the region of the anus, the female genital organs, and the nipples of the female breast.'[44] He is silent on the male nipples.

Yet in the real world, as opposed to the tower of scholarship, there is evidence that early in the twentieth century men's interest in nipple play does begin to break through. In the mid-1920s Gilbert Hamilton quizzed a sample of 100 middle-class New York males about their sex lives: 'What, if anything, does your wife do, either before or during the sex act, to increase your pleasure?' Three of the men responded, 'stimulating [my] breasts.'[45] This theme becomes more important later.

Women by contrast seem always to have appreciated play with their own nipples, their pleasure perhaps more readily prompted by neurophysiology: sucking on the female nipples causes the pituitary gland to release the hormone oxytocin, which in turn affects the smooth muscle of the uterus and vagina. (In men there has been speculation that nipple-play releases opioids and the like,[46] yet this is unproven.)

References are scattered throughout history to women's enjoyment of breast play. In Boccaccio's mid-fourteenth-century tale *The Decameron*, on the second day, as the survivors of the plague hide away, Alessandro learns that 'the abbott' is a woman. The abbott had begun by playing with Alessandro's chest, obtaining no response. Then 'the abbott' throws off her own chemise 'and taking Alessandro's hand, lays it on her bosom, saying, "Alessandro, dismiss thy foolish thought, feel here, and learn what I conceal."' Alessandro proceeds to feel 'two little teats, round, firm and delicate, as if they had been of ivory.' This woman, previously unknown to Alessandro, responds to his touch. After a bit, 'they embraced, and to their no small mutual satisfaction solaced themselves for the rest of the night.'[47]

In the scholarly world until recently, it has been the convention to think of women's breasts as displayed openly before the nineteenth century, then steadily becoming covered under the repressive influence of the supposedly rising bourgeoisie. Yet according to scholar Hans-Peter Duerr, whose massive work stands as the last word on the subject, the real story was the reverse. Contrary to what most cultural historians have maintained, 'There is no evidence that within the last millennium anywhere in Europe women have gone about with their breasts exposed.' It has only been since the 1860s, Duerr says, that women have begun showing massive cleavage, indeed some hint of the presence of nipples. Duerr's work stands as a demonstration of the extent to which previous scholars have missed the real history of the body because they were so intent upon incriminating 'capitalism.'[48]

We know that American youth who came of age between the world wars paid some attention to tongueing their female partners' nipples premaritally because Kinsey asked about it: 45 per cent of his male subjects remembered having done it 'much' or 'some.'[49] Kinsey was so uninterested in the male nipples that he didn't even ask whether the women had gone after them or not.

Thus in the panoply of total body sex, for the nipples there are only dim stirrings.

Oral Sex

Oral sex, in a way, seems so obvious, that one would expect every generation to discover it for itself. And over the centuries there are indeed scattered references to the pleasure that oral sex brings both men and women.

Yet the ancients evidenced little interest in mouth-genital contact. Despite their merry approach to lovemaking on the whole, the Greeks and Romans seemed to view oral sex as a kind of degrading act one could request only of a prostitute or slave. In the Middle Ages, oral sex seems to vanish from view, so few are the references to it. To be sure, the aristocracy constitutes a libertine exception, and Brantôme assures us that the ladies at court find it enchanting. He tells of the Spanish gallant who said: 'I kiss your hands and feet, senora.' The lady replies, 'Senor, the best part is in the middle.' Brantôme follows vaguely, 'In doing this, some ladies say that their husbands and suitors derive a good deal of delicatesse and pleasure and are spurred on anew.'[50]

Yet aside from among the aristocracy, oral sex apparently was little practised. Among the 405 Spanish clerics who in the seventeenth century were prosecuted for soliciting sex from their parishioners, only 3 displayed any interest in fellatio. Cunnilingus appeared in the imaginings of only one priest. Concludes historian Stephen Haliczer, 'Cunnilingus ... was extremely rare among the priests and penitents in the Inquisition records and undoubtedly rare in the sexual practices of Spanish society as a whole ...'[51] On the basis of data about prostitutes in early-eighteenth-century London, historian Randolph Trumbach surmises that, in their repertoire of services, fellatio was likely to have been unusual.[52]

The common people seem to have been familiar with the concept, and incorporated it in folksayings, yet the evidence that they actually performed it is thin to non-existent. In Finland, apropos the withdrawal technique of birth control, people said, 'You thresh with the ass, you sow with the mouth.'[53] The population around Sorrento in Italy referred to a woman who fellated her husband as 'una bucchinara,' derived from trumpeter.[54] The reference is not complimentary (and implies the extent to which the entire community was aware of a couple's sexual practices).

Elsewhere as well, having one's genitals 'sucked' counted as an allegory for nastiness, not a description of real behaviour. In an anti-aristocratic diatribe of the French Revolution, the whore 'who yesterday in plain view of marquises and counts had [her] hot clitoris rubbed by prelates and her vagina sucked by barons' now has no customers.[55]

Between the last part of the nineteenth century and the first of the twentieth, references to oral sex begin to multiply. Some intimate letters of the Count de la Rochefoucault, written in 1859 to a certain Mrs Chicester while he was attaché to the French embassy in Rome, have survived. He describes in graphic detail the kindnesses he would like to bestow upon her body, yet most interesting is his sense of her body as a whole as an object for his tongue: 'In you everything appears different and pure, the purity which reigns in your every feature, the excess of refinement which exists in your whole body, your hands, your feet, your legs, your cunt, your bottom, the hairs of your private parts, all is appetising.'[56] The effusion is an early expression, from a social class often in advance, of behaviour that was to democratize itself within a few years.

At the end of the century oral sex was on the minds of many young men. In 1909 novelist James Joyce, twenty-seven, wrote to his bride Nora Barnacle that he could not wait until he felt 'your hot lips sucking off my cock while my head is wedged in between your fat thighs, my hands clutching the round cushions of your bum and my tongue licking ravenously up your red cunt.'[57] Austrian novelist Robert Musil looked back, much later in life, to the moonlit nights in autumn that he as a nineteen-year-old had passed around 1899 on the shores of the Wörthersee, one of Austria's beautiful little lakes. The mood was erotic. 'Sexuality loves the unappetizing,' he mused, 'or whatever is not exactly appetizing. The odour of the vagina, a suspicious odour in any event, becomes heaven.'[58]

By 1919 American novelist Theodore Dreiser, age forty-eight and living in Greenwich Village in New York, was no longer a young man; his girlfriend, Helen Richardson, was only twenty. On Friday, 7 November, Dreiser commented favourably on 'Helen's Sweetie ways ... Her interest in all things seductive. Licks my P & A [prick and ass] – Can't let my roger alone.' Four days later: 'She looks like an angel or a classic figure and yet is sensuality to the core. We indulge in a long suck and then I put her on her knees. A wild finish. Return to my work.'[59]

In the Roaring Twenties, Dreiser was fully in step with his time. Oral sex was becoming a constant part of the sexuality package in middle-class America just as it was in Europe. Kinsey found that a quarter of college-educated married men performed it 'some' or 'much.' (A fifth of college-educated wives fellated their husbands.)[60] An analysis of American pornographic films in the 1920s found them full of fellatio and cunnilingus. One stag film, *Wonders of the Unseen World* (1927), billed cunnilingus as 'the latest importation from Paris.' And fully 37 per cent of the sex films made in that decade incorporated fellatio as a theme (11 per cent of the total offered cunnilingus).[61] Compared with erotic films today, these figures are small (at present virtually 100 per cent of such films present oral sex). Compared with representations of sexuality in the seventeenth century, though, these numbers are huge. There is no doubt that, in society's advance towards total body sexuality in the late nineteenth century, oral sex played a key role.

Anal Sex

'The last sexual frontier isn't some intergalactic tactile data fuck,' said sex observer Lisa Palac at the end of the twentieth century. 'It's your ass.'[62] Historically, the anus has been the last area for straight people to explore, and for most of recorded history anal intercourse was simply not on the agenda for anyone except homosexuals. This starts to change a bit towards the end of the nineteenth century.

The historic condemnation of heterosexual anal intercourse – not just by clerics and moralizers but by people who were themselves sexually active – is almost universal. Poet John Donne cleverly alludes to it in an elegy entitled 'Love's Progress':

> Rich Nature hath in woman wisely made
> Two purses, and their mouths aversely laid;
> They then which to the lower tribute owe
> That way which that exchequer looks must go.
> He which doth not, his error is as great
> As who by clyster gave the stomach meat.'[63]

The two purses mean the vagina and the anus. Donne's idea must have been that those interested in the vagina (anatomically 'the lower') would pursue their own path. Those interested in the anus would be making as big a mistake as drinking from an enema syringe ('clyster').

Sixteenth-century Florentine sculptor Benvenuto Cellini recalled in his autobiography with horror an accusation of anal intercourse against him in 1543 in Paris. A young woman, Caterina, had denounced him to the court for sodomy.

The judge turned to her and said, 'Caterina! Tell us all that occurred in your relations with Benvenuto.'

Caterina told the judge she had had relations with Benvenuto 'after the fashion of Italy.'

Benvenuto pretended not to know what she was talking about: 'If I had intercourse with her after the Italian fashion, I should have done so solely with the desire of having a child, as you [French] all do.'

The judge replied, 'She means that you have had connection with her by another method than the natural one.'

Benvenuto responded that this must be the French fashion, 'since she knew it and I did not.'

Benvenuto made Caterina tell the judge exactly how he, Benvenuto, was supposed to have entered her, and after she had repeated the intimate details three times, Benvenuto began yelling, 'To the stake, to the stake with her,' which effectively ended the case.[64] People could actually be executed for anal intercourse, and it was not a sexual option one would have chosen without reflection.

Among the wayward priests prosecuted by the Inquisition in seventeenth-century Spain, anal sex was apparently quite unusual.[65] Something hellish clung to the entire idea, for in an anticlerical Dutch print of 1735, showing a Jesuit sodomizing a young woman, devils look on in the background.[66]

Even in the world of prostitution, anal sex, strictly against the law, had a hellish aspect to it. Of the 197 men arrested by the London city constables in the 1720s for having hired prostitutes, only one had engaged in 'unheard of lewdness' with a woman, which Trumbach surmises to mean anal intercourse.[67] The Marquis de Sade approached six prostitutes in Marseille on a fateful July day in 1772 (for an orgy that got him sentenced to death); yet only one consented to be anally penetrated by either Sade or his valet – and she refused the first time she was asked.[68]

Even the grand libertines who otherwise stopped at little drew up at the anus. As Brantôme pointed out in the sixteenth century, 'There are some who are denatured and crazy right up to the ass, even some women. One should be scrupulous about touching it, for many dirty reasons that I shan't point out. Because the fact is that two rivers gather down there and almost touch each other, and there's a danger of missing the one and navigating the other, which is just too awful [*par trop vilain*].'[69] Two centuries later Casanova, who accidentally found himself at a drunken orgy in Rome in the early 1760s, politely refused the opportunity to sodomize some of the young women who had been invited for the occasion: 'In this whole incredible party I felt not the slightest arousal.'[70] Of course, one could argue that the other guests were all avid to penetrate the young women anally, yet Casanova said he'd never seen anything like this previously, and never would again – so it could not have been a common impulse.[71]

Yet the slate is not a complete blank. If anal intercourse is part of the total body sex package, it must have been represented historically in some form (for heterosexuals, that is: for homosexuals it was common coin). It appears in two forms, one as a very occasional theme in premodern pornography, and secondly, in the Italian boot.

Anal sex was certainly not the quasi-universal pornographic theme that it would become by the beginning of the twenty-first century. And some of the most popular erotic works shunned it completely. John Cleland allows the courtesan Emily in *Fanny Hill* to be horrified as a client attempts to penetrate her. And Fanny herself reacts to her friend's misadventure with revulsion: 'I could not conceive how it was possible for mankind to run into a taste, not only universally odious but absurd.' The brothel-keeper, Mrs Cole, smiles at Fanny's naivety.[72]

Yet there are allusions. Henry Ashbee's *Bibliography of Prohibited Books* (1877) offers numerous examples of pre-1850 erotic literature incorporating anal themes (for example, in one 1790 tract the woman wore a feather in her anus).[73] In Nicolas Chorier's *Dialogues on the Arcana of Love and Venus* (c. 1660), 'Tullia' declares that, 'We Italian and Spanish women have ... Venus's door too wide.' 'The back Venus [anus] is therefore more satisfactory in this respect. The invading tool finds it difficult of access, and when it has forced its way in, it not only occupies the whole space but even strains it ... What is more, the place suits the guest as the muscles may be tightened or loosened at will.'[74] In the 1770s the Swiss-English artist Johann Heinrich Füssli (Henry Fuseli) created a drawing entitled 'Change of Roles' that showed a woman with a strap-on penis penetrating a man from behind.[75] Anal sex was, in any event, on Füssli's mind.

Which brings us to the second theme: the curious reputation that Italy has maintained historically as the continent's elective site for buggery: not just homosexual, for which there is ample evidence, but heterosexual as well. After William Lithgow visited Italy in 1609 he thundered, 'The people for the most part are both grave and ingenious, but wondrous deceitful in their actions, so unappeasable in anger, that they cowardly murder their enemies rather than seek an honorable revenge, and so inclined to unnatural vices, that for bestiality they surpass the infidels.'[76] This can only be a reference to sodomy, though among whom exactly he leaves vague.

A few years later Chorier the pornographer summed up the reputation of the Italians – the Florentines, in particular – in the sex world: Octavia says to Tullia, 'The Florentines, you know, are in the habit of defrauding Venus. Rumour has it that they enjoy having to do with young lads and that they love those maidens who do not mind playing the part of boys and supplying the boyish part of the business.' Tullia then describes her own experiences with letting her paramours 'drive their tools into me by whatever furrow they wanted ...' Happily, however, at the end of the scenario, 'they then went along the straight path to the honourable Venus.'[77]

Interestingly, the Marquis de Sade chooses to set some of Juliette's most extravagant anal sex scenes in Rome rather than Paris. Juliette says that her two Italian lovers – supervised by the Princesse Olympe – 'devour me, but in Italian style. My ass becomes the sole object of their attentions. Both of them kiss it, tongue it, bite it. They cannot get enough; they can scarcely believe that I'm a woman.'[78]

Was it true that Italian women were partial to anal sex, or was it just a pornographers' smear? In a study of court cases involving homosexuality in fifteenth-century Florence, historian Michael Rocke has found that women generally resisted anal intercourse. One accuser said that the wife of Benedetto Sapiti, a 'very great sodomite,' had abandoned her husband because she refused his demands for anal sex.[79] (In any event, according to a systematic survey of sexual behaviour in the

Veneto region today, few traces remain of the purported Italian fondness for heterosexual sodomy.)[80]

In sum, it is likely that in the world we have lost, regular anal intercourse among heterosexuals – outside of the context of birth control[81] and the perfervid imagination of the pornographers – was extremely rare.

Then towards the end of the nineteenth century, heterosexual sodomy ceases to be highly unusual. It would be hard to think of a more straight-laced setting than Freud's Vienna, and Freud's friends and patients – many of them Jews of Orthodox Polish and Russian origin – were anything but libertines. So Freud must have been speaking on the basis of what people had told him, of his impressions of normal and abnormal, when he accepted anal intercourse as more or less equivalent to vaginal. As he wrote to editor Friedrich Krauss in 1910, 'Psychoanalysis constrains us to observe that the anus – in a normal manner and among non-deviate individuals – is the seat of erotic sensitivity and in a certain sense responds quite like the genitals. Talk about anal eroticism, and an anal personality that arises from it, causes physicians and psychologists to explode in indignation.'[82] Surely anal sex among the Viennese middle classes could not have been uncommon for Freud to declaim so confidently about it.

In 1909 Joyce wrote to Nora – perhaps 'sighed' would be a better verb – that he longed to hear her fart. 'At such moments I feel mad to do it in some filthy way, to feel your hot lecherous lips sucking away at me ... to stick it up between the cheeks of your rump and bugger you.'[83]

By the 1920s even the English middle classes must have had some passing sexual familiarity with the anus, for Lawrence, in his 1928 novel, *Lady Chatterley's Lover*, permits Mellors the gamekeeper a bit of anal play with Connie Chatterley. Mellors praises Connie's behind in general terms: 'All the while he spoke he exquisitely stroked the rounded tail, till it seemed as if a slippery sort of fire came from it into his hand. And his finger-tips touched the two secret openings to her body, time after time, with a soft little brush of fire.'

Mellors comments on the topography: 'Tha' got a proper, woman's arse, proud of itself.'

Mellors then lays his hand firmly over the anus.

'I like it,' he says. 'I like it!'[84]

The world of erotic art in the 1920s and 1930s brims with material on the anus. The French illustrator 'Rojan,' known primarily for his children's art, produced a series of thirty hand-coloured erotic lithographs that surfaced around 1934, many of which featured anal eroticism: for example a gentle-man in a car inserting his finger in the anus of a sweet young thing, her face a mirror of pleasure (his of concentration).[85]

The Parisian physician and author Céline, real name Louis Destouches, was a bit of a wild man with women. He was thirty-eight when in 1932 he wrote to his girlfriend Erika that there would be 'no lovemaking without a condom, or else *par-derrière*' – with your behind. He added that VD and preg-nancy were both undesirable, but the subtext of the remark was that both people were perfectly familiar with anal sex.

Later he writes to her, 'It helps enormously to make men happy without any risk."[86]

Nothing in these letters suggests that for Céline and his girlfriends anal sex was anything other than what Freud had suggested: a perfectly conventional substitute for the vaginal version.

When in the late 1920s the above-mentioned survey of the sex lives of middle-class New Yorkers was conducted, the 100 women in the poll were queried, 'Has your husband ever had intercourse with you by entering your rectum?' Three said yes. Three more said yes in various ways: One, 'Yes, once, and it was horrible to her.' Another had done it with her first husband but not with her second. A third said, 'Yes, when he was drunk.' Five said, 'Yes, incompletely.' That makes a total of eleven women in this sample of 100 who had encountered anal sex: more than 10 per cent. (Kinsey found that 6.7 per cent of college-educated men had at least tried it in marriage, and that it had been tried on 10.7 per cent of the married women.)[87] By the late 1920s significant minorities of middle-class men and women were experimenting with sodomy.[88]

If the pornography of a society offers some indication of its erotic range, the Kinsey Collection of photographs at the Institute for Sex Research in Bloomington, Indiana, should permit an assessment of the importance of anal sex in erotic imagery between the 1880s and the 1950s. In fact, of the 1,699 photographs in that collection depicting sex relations between heterosexuals (and that can be dated), the fraction showing anal intercourse oscillates between 15 per cent (in the 1880s) and 6 per cent (in the 1950s). Averaging the decades out, the overall figure is 8.9 per cent.[89] Because the composition of the collection depends so heavily on happenstance, little may be made of trend figures. Yet in the American erotic imagination over this period, heterosexual anal imagery appeared in one photo out of ten: not a lot, but not negligible either.

Masturbation

Around 1900, Parisian psychiatrist Pierre Janet saw a fifty-two-year-old patient, B., who complained of fear of open spaces but whose real problem, in Janet's view, was chronic masturbation. 'From the age of twelve he started to masturbate with a true frenzy,' said Janet.

B. said, 'I couldn't live if I didn't do it at least once a day and sometimes three or four times. I tell myself: I'm exhausting myself, I'm going to kill myself, but I can't stop from doing it.'

Janet did not seem surprised at the story and wondered only that B's 'poor wife' had stood up so bravely.[90]

Masturbation is an appendage of total body sex, permitting individuals to enlarge the range of fantasies they would like to experience with their newly sexualized bodies. Masturbation's remote history remains shrouded. We know that it once formed part of the sexual baseline experience that has always existed, yet we know little of frequency. Then in the middle of the eighteenth century a tremendous wave of medical castigation of masturbation arises, possibly indicating an increase in the frequency of the practice (as doctors previously had for the most part been silent about it). Yet this is scarcely conclusive proof.

Of great interest is that in the last third of the nineteenth century, subjective testimonies about masturbation become more common, individuals confiding intimate details either to their doctors, as B. did to Janet, or to pollsters, or to their diaries. In the first year of high school in Berne, Switzerland, Paul Klee, then eleven and later to become a noted painter, witnessed his pals masturbating: 'During class I saw in front of me one of my fellow students practising onanism in the shadow of the table.'[91] Painter Salvador Dali recalled from the decade before the First World War his school chums making of masturbation 'a regular habit.'[92] These are mere postholings from a vast field of turn-of-the-century eyewitness testimony about masturbation.

In these years, Vienna psychologist Siegfried Bernfeld encouraged adolescent pupils to keep diaries. Typically, they provided two kinds: proper diaries of all their daily activities and 'sinful' diaries of their masturbatory endeavours. Robert, fifteen, offered the following entry for one day in 1914: 'I met my old grade-school teacher K. We talked about lots of stuff and he asked me whether I am familiar with sexual love. I responded not yet with fulfilment along natural lines, and we continued to talk about sexual matters. He said that self-abuse brings self-ruin, but the fulfilment of sexual desire often brings, which is still more awful, syphilis. I was supposed to choose the right way. I drifted for a long time between masturbation and natural fulfilment ...' Robert almost chose the latter but then at the last minute, he confided to his diary, he went for masturbation. Bernfeld editorialized, 'There remain few psychologists who can doubt of the ubiquity of masturbation in puberty.'[93]

Polls from the United States in the 1920s suggest that adult masturbation was almost as common as juvenile. A survey of 518 male college students in the western United States around 1915 found that 62 per cent had at some point masturbated (of a New York City group, by contrast, only 35 per cent said they did so).[94] When in the early 1920s Katharine Bement

Davis, general secretary of the Bureau of Social Hygiene, quizzed 1,183 unmarried female college graduates, she found almost exactly the same results as for the western males: 31 per cent did so currently; another 30 per cent had once done it but now stopped. (She found some confusion among respondents about what 'masturbation' meant; some were unfamiliar with the term 'orgasm.' Also, the poll may have been tilted towards the liberal side, as more than four-fifths of the women who received the questionnaire failed to respond.)[95] A survey in the late 1920s of middle-class married New Yorkers under forty found that matrimony had dimmed the onanistic fury somewhat: only 16 per cent of married men masturbated once a week or more, 11 per cent of married women. (A mere 6 per cent of the men had never masturbated, 30 per cent of the women.)[96] One of seven married men did it oftener than once a week. This was certainly more frequent than Pepys.

The New Physicality of the Body

Clearly, late in the nineteenth century and early in the twentieth, new zones of the body were becoming sexual playgrounds. Yet there was more. People in general were acquiring a new sense of the very physicality of their bodies, an awareness of the body as a source of play and pleasure, not just as the weary frame – the eighteenth-century 'machine' – that one was destined to drag about until an uncorporeal life in the hereafter began.

As the Russian dancer and choreographer Vaslav Nijinsky was planning his ballet *Jeux*, which would premiere in Paris in 1913, he said, 'The man that I see foremost on the stage is a contemporary man. I imagine the costume, the plastic poses, the movement that would be representative of our time ... When today one sees a man stroll, read a newspaper or dance the tango, one perceives that his gestures have nothing in common with those, for instance, of an idler under Louis XV, of a gentleman dancing the minuet, or of a thirteenth-century monk studiously reading a manuscript.'[97]

Although Nijinsky was not a historical scholar, he had enough of a folk memory to realize that there was something different at the turn of the century in how people carried their bodies, felt about them, and attended to them. The natural sensuality of the brain was energizing the body with a new physicality, a hitherto concealed electricity. This is partly what is meant by the 'sensualization' of sexuality.

This new body sense manifested itself in many ways. As early as 1855 American poet Walt Whitman had picked it up in 'I Sing the Body Electric':

> The expression of a well-made man appears not only in his face,
> It is in his limbs and joints also, it is curiously in the joints of his hips and wrists,
> It is in his walk, the carriage of his neck, the flex of his waist and knees, dress does not hide him,
> The strong sweet quality he has strikes through the cotton and broad-cloth,
> To see him pass conveys as much as the best poem, perhaps more,
> You linger to see his back, and the back of his neck and shoulder-side.

What images then, did Whitman, with his strong homo-erotic verse, find arousing?

> The swimmer naked in the swimming-bath, seen as he swims through the transparent green-shine, or lies with his face up and rolls silently to and fro in the heave of the water,
> The bending forward and backward of rowers in row-boats, the horseman in his saddle.
> ...
> The march of firemen in their own costumes, the play of masculine muscle through clean-setting trowsers and waist-straps.[98]

Although poets over the centuries have celebrated the muscularity of the body, there is something new here. Whitman caresses the body not as an example of God's benevolence or nature's wonder, but because it gives him an erection. That same year he wrote elsewhere: 'I am the poet of the body ... If I worship any particular thing it shall be some of the spread of my body ...'[99]

Whitman strikes here historically new themes. He revels in the body as a sensualist not as a philosopher, pioneering the corporeal awareness of flesh and sinew that would in the coming decades be part of the new physicality.

This thrill of the physical runs through the intimate reflections of many writers of the day. As the Viennese novelist Robert Musil, whose novels are filled with images of muscularity, wrote in his diary around 1900 at age twenty, 'A precondition of art is intoxication. Sexual excitement, big desires, parties, competition, extreme physical movements are the key to it: feelings of the limitlessness of power and of fullness.'

In the view of young Musil, this kind of body-power thinking was very new. A few years later in his diary he added, 'People think that in the mind and soul there's nothing new under the sun, that a thousand years ago greatness had the same measure as now, that age-old passions merely recur in new places and that the same actions merely repeat themselves, only with new tools. But that's wrong. There are new moods, new delectations of beauty, new values of sensuality. Erotic love, a sense of nature and humanity: all have changed.'[100]

Just to get away from the heady intellectuality of the Viennese coffee houses, we find American writer John Dos Passos at age nineteen cavorting with friends on the beaches of Newfoundland around 1915: 'We were absolutely the only living things about except white cawing sea gulls,' he wrote to a friend. 'The water was pale green, and simply stung when you got in – but it was like a bath in champagne! After it we danced about the beach like Greek fauns or nymphs. You can imagine what fun it was.'[101] Before the late nineteenth century, the common people simply did not think in these images – the tide flooding over their naked skin like a bath in champagne, or hopping about naked on the beach, because they were modest about their bodies, and couldn't swim, and feared that cold water would give them colds. People in general did not relish the extreme physicality of this kind of experience.

Women too delighted in this new physicality. There was, for example, the discovery of one's own body in the mirror. Until age sixteen in 1906, Nina Hamnett, later a writer and socialite in England, had never seen herself nude. 'I drew from the nude at the Art School, but I had never dared to look at myself in the mirror, for my Grandmother had always insisted that one dressed and undressed under one's nightdress using it as a kind of tent. One day, feeling very bold, I took off all my clothes and gazed in the looking-glass. I was delighted. I was much superior to anything I had seen in the life class ...'[102]

It was in front of the mirror that Marie Bashkirtseff discovered, as a girl of fifteen in Russia in 1878, the contours of her body: 'I looked all of a sudden so beautiful, after I had taken my bath this evening, that I spent fully twenty minutes admiring myself in the glass. I am sure no one could have seen me without admiration.'[103]

The reader may think that young women (and men) have always wanted to be admired for their bodies. Perhaps they have. Yet previously the most appealing parts of the body were invisible under layers of clothes. Now they emerge to send sensual messages to onlookers and to the owners themselves. (It is piquant that Marie had earlier wailed, 'My form like that of a Greek goddess ... my bust small and perfect in shape – of what use are they, since no one loves me?')[104]

This emergence takes place not just in London and Moscow, but all over Western society. Here is Sibilla Aleramo, later writer and feminist, at fifteen in a north Italian industrial city around 1891. She goes to the beach and loves to show off her body, asking herself as the men look at her, 'Will I fall in love?' 'The game pleased me, and seemed to give a new savour to the life that I was already living with such enthusiasm. Letting myself be cradled in the waves for hours and hours under the blazing sun, I mocked danger by bathing away from the shore ... I unified myself with nature and gave vent to the exuberance of my body. I was a person, a little person who was free and strong; I felt it, and I felt my breast filling with a kind of ill-defined joy.'[105] Few Italian women of a century earlier would have penned such lines.

Later, Italian women do become filled with the rhetoric of the sleek power body. This theme of power, energy, and icon-smashing innovation resounded heavily among the Italian futurists generally in the years before the First World War. And it certainly echoes in the 'Futurist Manifesto of Lust' of 1913 by Valentine de St Point, one of the few female futurists. 'Lust, when viewed without moral preconceptions and as an essential part of life's dynamism,' she wrote, 'is a force.' She proceeded to dilate upon the virtues of lust. 'Lust excites energy and releases strength ... Today it drives the great men of business who direct the banks ...'

What about the body? 'We must stop despising desire, this attraction at once delicate and brutal between two bodies, of whatever sex, two bodies that want each other, striving for unity.' She had no time for 'the histrionics of love,' romanticism, and 'the rhetoric of parting and eternal fidelities.' Thus for Valentine de St Point the new era of physicality brought with it incandescent bodies: 'Lust is a force, in that it refines the spirit by bringing to white heat the excitement of the flesh. The spirit burns bright and clear from a healthy, strong flesh, purified in the embrace.'[106]

This sensation of a new physicality emerges perhaps most powerfully in the New World of pleasure, in the United States. Is it that in the New World the hindrances to the expression of desire were fewer, despite the fabled American puritanism? That traditions of privacy were better established; that the legitimacy of individual self-expression had a currency unknown in the Old World? In any event, in the last quarter of the nineteenth century a powerful body-centred rhetoric emerges among American women. Looking back on her days as a nurse in the 1890s, American novelist Mary Roberts Rinehart realized that something of a cult of the body was in the making. The middle-class women patients whom she saw as a private-duty nurse 'dressed and primped' for the doctors. 'And it was there that for the first time I saw something of the cult of the body; the delicate soaps and powders and perfumes, the soft silk and lace night-dresses and bed jackets.'[107]

There is little doubt that in American society by the 1920s and 1930s women had a kind of erotic energy that was simply absent a century earlier. 'Becky was nineteen,' wrote novelist F. Scott Fitzgerald in a notebook in the 1930s, 'a startling little beauty ... Her body was sturdy, athletic; her head was a bright, happy composition of curves and shadows and vivid color, with that final kinetic jolt, the element that is eventually sexual in effect, which made strangers stare at her.'[108]

Was this the rambling of a dirty old man? What Fitzgerald described corresponded to the way dancer Martha Graham felt in those years. Around the time of the First World War she joined the basketball team of her California high school. 'All the women on the team wore the same brown uniform. I wore my long hair in a single braid that swung across my back as I ran across the gymnasium floor in an attempt to make a hoop. I believe I took quite naturally to this sport because I wanted to move.' She didn't know how to dance at this point; she just wanted to experience the sheer physical pleasure of her body in motion. 'I think this is one of the reasons I took up basketball in the first place.'[109]

In this new emphasis on the body, one theme emerges for both men and women with dramatic clarity: muscles. Both genders want them.

For men, the modern history of bodybuilding begins with a Prussian strongman named Eugen Sandow, who, as a student at Göttingen in the 1880s, underwent physical training, becoming, in the words of his admiring biographer, 'one of the most perfectly built men in existence.' He toured for a bit as a wrestler on the Continent, then from 1889 on began showing in England and the United States, where he became a huge sensation. For one of his Saturday night shows at the Westminster Aquarium, 'the theatre was packed with a very fair specimen of athletic humanity, men who could give a literally striking account of themselves in a scrimmage.' With Sandow's arrival in England, 'the worship of muscle became a cult,' said his biographer, 'and every phase of athleticism ... was minutely and unweariedly discussed.'[110] To be sure, interest in 'hard, bulging muscle,' as historian Patricia Anderson puts it, had been building in Anglo-Saxon society for some years, the 'tall, dark and handsome' hero becoming steadily more muscular towards the fin-de-siècle: 'Most important of all, he had a strong, well-built body.'[111] Yet the huge amount of press that Sandow garnered made him a cynosure for men interested in their bodies: in becoming muscular for its own sake.

It is striking to encounter this desire for muscularity in women as well, not necessarily in bulking up as Sandow did (though there were 'Sandow women') but simply in becoming strong. Muscles are not new on women. Anyone who has visited a swimming pool in a country town on a Sunday afternoon knows that the farm wives have backs like stevedores: lats and delts bulging against the straps of their bathing suits. Indeed, when Fanny Burney visited the English coast in 1773 she saw a rowing match between the women of Shaldon and Teignmouth involving participants 'who have a strength and hardiness which I never saw equal before in our race.' Their husbands were away fishing nine months a year in Newfoundland, and the women were 'strapping owing to their robust work.'[112] But the traditional middle-class woman was always a 'pencil-neck,' as they say in the bodybuilding world, and women in general have always been less strong than men. Towards 1900, this started to change.

In 1902, the Parisian novelist Sidonie Gabrielle Colette,

creator of the 'Claudine' series, allows Claudine to muse about 'the slow and agreeable corruption' that she owes to her lover Renaud. 'Renaud revealed to me the secret of giving and feeling sexually [*la volupté*], and I've kept it, and I enjoy it passionately, like a kid playing with a revolver. He revealed to me the power, certain and frequent, of my long, supple, muscled body ...'[113] A few years later Colette had taken up boxing. As she teased her friend Christiane Mendelys (who also was taking boxing lessons) in 1911, 'You're going to come back with bulging muscles everywhere, athletic and bronzed, in the hope of getting me all jealous.'[114]

There is no doubt that the fin-de-siècle male found these strong female bodies exciting. In his 1884 novel *À rebours* (*Against the Grain*), French novelist Joris-Karl Huysmans allows his fictional hero des Esseintes – whose basic interests were more on the homoerotic side – to muse about the muscled body of his former mistress 'Miss Urania': 'an American, her well-built body, her quick legs, her muscles of steel, her arms like cast iron.' She had at first been a circus acrobat and, driven by he knew not what impulse, des Esseintes returned to the circus again and again to see her.[115] Thus, Huysmans's wide readership started to become accustomed to the idea of muscular women.

Céline also responded to physically fit women, and his girlfriend Cillie, a gymnast from Vienna, is described as 'very muscular' (*tout en muscles*).[116] In many settings, therefore, in the 1880s and after, we start to encounter lithe muscular women and not just plumpish fainting Victorian heroines in their hoop skirts.

In sum, as we tap towards total body sex at the turn of the century, we do so with bodies of both sexes that are turning out to be hard and firm from head to toe.

Towards Total Body Sex

The concept of total body sex, with every part of the body sending sensuous signals to the brain, emerges only in the

1960s. Yet in this initial fin-de-siècle efflorescence of sensuality it's adumbrated: sketched in meagre yet recognizable detail. As the hindrances to these underlying neural drives come away, the drives themselves begin, timidly at first, then with ever-gathering force, to power to the surface.

They surfaced for young English writer Arthur Symons in the late nineteenth century after he moved from the provinces to London. Previously, 'I was ignorant of my own body; I looked at the relationship of man and woman as something essentially wicked ... I had a feeling of the deepest reverence for women, from which I endeavoured to banish the slightest consciousness of sex.'

City life changed him, and he became something of a sensualist. 'I fell casually in love with woman after woman, who, as a matter of fact, had little attraction to my senses.'

Then he becomes attracted to evil. 'One begins by taking a purely spectacular interest in vice and disorder; with things evil, with things forbidden, with things unforbidden. One hears of them, longs for them, reads of them, succumbs to them.'

To what, exactly, did he succumb? 'Sex ... has been my chief obsession.' Symons described how slowly and sensuously he undressed his girlfriends: 'One gets a glimpse of those tempting and clinging white drawers which invariably excite one's senses, knowing exactly what they conceal, but not yet aware of the shapeliness of the legs.' When one of his lovers is almost undressed, Symons looks at her naked back, and at her breasts that stand out temptingly even as she unlaces her shoes. 'Then the girl I refer to rose to her feet, without the least shame, but excitedly, let me devour passionately all that there is in such pure and perfect nakedness.'

This is a prototypical description of total body sex: every aspect of her body excites him, and he touches and embraces virtually every part. 'My aesthetic instincts became perverted,' he tells us. 'I relished nothing that was not vicious, morbid, fantastic, abnormal. When I was in the company of men and women, of thieves and prostitutes, I made no excuses – no excuses were ever needed.'[117] Symons flagellates himself as a kind of sexual outcast, yet the point is that, a hundred years later, all this behaviour had become normal.

Or almost normal. The turn-of-the-century sexologists, for the most part prudish physicians who found every deviation from the missionary position to be evidence of degeneration, were not pleased by these trends. Said Albert Eulenburg in 1895, a Berlin psychiatrist with an extensive middle-class private practice, 'There are women who are abnormally excitable in sensual terms, or who are spoiled with excessive and perverse sexual pleasures. For them, everything becomes an "erogenous" zone ("tout est con dans une femme" [women get off on everything], as a nymphomaniac actress once observed about herself).'[118] Yet these trends must have been evident or the sexologists would not have scorned them so emphatically.

This march towards total body sex is similarly seen in the progression of erotic art. A large private collection in Frankfurt, the Döpp Collection, accumulated by an experienced private collector and donated to the Art Society of that city, provides a kind of narrative. According to this material, before the eighteenth century erotic art rarely showed anything more than genital sex, though often in non-missionary postures (the pornographers' preference – as Peter Weiermair points out – because such poses make it easier to visualize the genitals). After the 1780s occasional exceptions to this rule occur, such as a French drawing in 1830 showing a maiden performing oral sex on a satyr while being penetrated by another satyr. A series of lithographs around 1840 show Napoleon being fellated. Yet the other nineteenth-century images are highly conventional and rely upon intercourse in the missionary position.

Now we skip forward sixty years in the Döpp Collection to the Munich illustrator Peter Geiger during the belle époque. The tone is totally different, featuring aggressive, hard-bodied women with armoured nipples. In 1907 another German illustrator, Franz von Bayros, shows one lesbian woman playing with another's nipples. Around 1920 German artist Max Liebermann depicts a woman tonguing a man from behind: the scene is a celebration of female voluptuousness. On and on goes the erotic artwork of the pre- and interwar years: it is a triumph of alternative sexualities, female pleasure, 'lesbian' playfulness, and heterosexual threesomes. There can be no doubt at all that the pornographer's vision has shifted dramatically and that now the entire body in all its erotic potential is being valorized.[119]

It was a vision that Connie Chatterley, in Lawrence's 1928 novel, shared after the gamekeeper Mellors had caressed her mouth with deep kisses, her legs, her nipples, her vagina, and her anus: 'The human body is only just coming to real life,' she said. 'With the Greeks it gave a lovely flicker, then Plato and Aristotle killed it, and Jesus finished it off. But now the body is coming really to life, is really rising from the tomb. And it will be a lovely, lovely life in the lovely universe, the life of the human body.'[120]

CHAPTER SEVEN

The Great Breakout for Gays and Lesbians

By 1900, gays and lesbians had begun the same sexual breakout from a single restricted focus that straights experienced as they left the missionary position behind. The same sense of sensual excitement that D.H. Lawrence felt on the balcony in Bavaria looking at Frieda's naked body churning in the water infused homosexuals as well, creating a note that is as unlike the brutish sodomy of previous times as the lyre is from clogs on a wooden floor.

'Live!' Lord Henry Wotton apostrophizes Dorian Gray in Oscar Wilde's famous 1890 novel. 'Live the wonderful life that is in you! Let nothing be lost upon you. Be always searching for new sensations ... A new Hedonism – that is what our century wants.'[1] And just as heterosexuals everywhere began responding to the call for the new hedonism with deep kissing, nipple play, and oral and anal sex, gays and lesbians responded too, widening the gamut of gay sex from buggery to oral eroticism, tongue kissing, and an adoration of the physique that would soon imbricate the entire body.

Like heteros, homosexuals were casting loose the ties to small-town life and piety in search of physical pleasure. In London's Jermyn Street they could if they wished flounce about like Wilde in short pants and dress up for drag balls. In Wilde's novel, Dorian Gray, on the verge of marrying, expresses doubt about Lord Henry's theories of hedonism. Lord

Henry responds, 'Pleasure is the only thing worth having a theory about. But I am afraid I cannot claim my theory as my own. It belongs to Nature, not to me. Pleasure is Nature's test, her sign of approval. When we are happy we are always good, but when we are good we are not always happy.'[2] Henceforth, the sexuality of gays and lesbians would be directed increasingly by the pleasure principle, experimenting with the entire body as they quite rightly felt nature had ordained it. Historian Alain Corbin asserts that late-nineteenth-century gays 'pioneered the model of purely hedonistic sexuality, cut away from procreation.'[3] Whether they were really in advance of everyone else is uncertain. Yet they shared fully in the pleasures of the transformation of sexuality.

Gays: From Anal to Oral

Just as straights broke out from the narrowness of whatever had been deemed appropriate in the second floor above the village shop, male homosexuals as well were liberated by the freedom and anonymity of urban life. It's true that nobody had forced them to do only buggery, ignoring other parts of the body. Yet the new positive emphasis on the body of the late nineteenth century – the new interest in athleticism, in bicycling, in weightlifting, and in the joy of dance movement – encouraged a fresh consciousness of the whole body throughout society. The shifting in tone at Oxford and Cambridge late in the nineteenth century, for example, from heterosexuality to homosexuality, seems to have occurred in the context of rising interest in fitness and sport.[4] The physical verve and energy that the Russian Ballet displayed in its Paris debut in 1909 made director Sergei Diaghilev 'overnight a leader of the Paris homosexual set,' in the words of Diaghilev's biographer.[5] Towards 1900 in Berlin, Magnus Hirschfeld noted how enthusiastic gays were about the amateur athletics and physical culture scene.[6]

It is likely that gays experienced this new physicality as an inducement to reach beyond their restrictive focus on the

anus. The sources leave unclear exactly when the shift towards oral sex and body physique began, but there is no
doubt that after the 1880s it was in full swing throughout
Europe and the United States.

Like so many upper-middle-class English gays, Joe
Randolph Ackerley related best to working-class men and to
men in uniform – sailors, soldiers, firemen, and policemen,
basically straight individuals who were not unwilling to have
oral sex performed upon them but who shunned the anus. In
his posthumous memoir, Ackerley, who lived with a young
sailor for four years, is often explicit about what they did
together. 'He liked dancing with me to the gramophone,
readily accepting the female role,' Ackerley wrote. 'And often
when I had ascertained that he too was in a state of erection
we would strip and dance naked, so unbearably exciting that
I could not for long endure the pressure of his body against
mine.' Their pleasures were, as Ackerley said, 'fairly simple,
kisses, caresses, manipulations, intercrural massage.' Yet
Ackerley did not want his partner to think him 'queer.' The
memoir contains no references to anal sex (though Ackerley
did occasionally permit others to bugger him),[7] and indeed
the relationship broke up after Ackerley, against his better
judgment, fellated the disgusted sailor. 'I suppose I acted
towards my sailor thus because his body was so beautiful
and desirable that I simply wanted to eat it.'[8]

Ackerley was probably typical of the English gay sex scene
by 1900. Havelock Ellis, who interviewed twenty-four homosexuals in a systematic study, said in 1897 that buggery was
not characteristic of this group: thirteen of them did practise
anal intercourse, but only six of those declared it the 'preferred method.' Nine had some erotic contact up to the level
of mutual masturbation, and three were partial to fellatio.[9]
Oscar Wilde and Lord Alfred Douglas did not apparently get
beyond frenzied kissing and mutual masturbation, which we
know because in the late 1930s a young American gay man
named Samuel Steward went over to England, made an appointment to see the now famous Lord Alfred, took him out

to a pub, then seduced him. Steward fellated Douglas: 'Head down, my lips where Oscar's had been, I knew that I had won.' But maybe Oscar's lips hadn't been there at all, for Lord Douglas immediately clamped his hand upon Steward's penis: 'You really needn't have gone to all that trouble, since this is almost all Oscar and I ever did with each other.'

The astonished Steward stammered, 'B-b-but ... the poems, and all ...'

'We used to get boys for each other,' Lord Alfred said. 'We kissed a lot, but not much more.'[10]

Anal sex clearly had not been abolished in the British Isles. It seems to have been the main interest of such figures as the Irishman Roger Casement (later tried and executed in 1916 for leading the Easter Rebellion), whose diary notations from 1910 abounded in such references as '*very* deep thrusts' and 'deep screw and to hilt' – he apparently giving them.[11] Yet by these years the emphasis in England was manifestly away from the anus and towards other parts of the body.

For Paris we have, in fact, a statistical study conducted by a visiting German scholar (evidently gay psychiatrist Paul Näcke) in 1910. The author analysed the graffiti in fifty-two pissoirs (open public urinals), virtually all of which carried messages from gay men seeking partners. Of the 114 graffiti specific enough to analyse for sexual tastes, 35 offered to perform oral sex; receiving passive anal sex (29) was the second commonest desire.[12] Parisian observers confirmed these findings: André Raffalovich, a gay sexologist, considered anal sex 'a heterosexual deviation' rarely practised by homosexuals (who mainly exchanged caresses, according to him).[13]

Näcke watched the Berlin gay scene quite closely and characterized its sexual practices around 1904–5 as follows: deep kissing was probably the primary sexual activity. According to an unnamed gay correspondent writing to Näcke, 'Most of the men I associate with as well as myself, who scarcely deserve the term sensualists, believe that the tongue kiss is part of the sex act.' Why insist on it? 'In gay sex the possibility of an intense connection is not present, as with man and woman, but the desire is certainly there. And this desire finds its expression in the kiss, which consists of more than a superficial contact with the body.'[14]

On the basis of several surveys, only around 8 per cent of all German gays practised anal sex.[15] Magnus Hirschfeld thought that German gays did mainly embracing and masturbation, with little anal traffic.[16] Even though he was writing for a mainstream audience and trying to pretty up the picture, other insiders agreed with him. According to scene-insider Max Katte, anal intercourse was not common among German gays, who mainly preferred mutual masturbation ('immissio penis in anum' occurring 'only seldom').[17]

In the United States, gays around the time of the First World War thought of oral sex as 'the twentieth-century way,' to use a term then popular on the West Coast. According to a police investigation in Long Beach, California, the fifty gay men arrested in 1914 for 'vagrancy' practised overwhelmingly oral sex rather than anal.[18]

Claude Hartland, from a small town in the South and author of one of the earliest American gay memoirs, came of age sexually in the 1890s. His rather extensive homosexual experience seems to have included mainly kissing, hugging, and mutual masturbation; throughout his recollections there are no references to oral or anal sex.[19]

When Gilbert Hamilton collected a non-random set of sexual histories from 100 married New York males in the late 1920s, he found that an astonishingly high 57 per cent of them had had some kind of adolescent same-sex encounter: 41 per cent of those entailed mutual masturbation or some unspecified activity, 13 per cent rubbing their penises against another male's leg, 12 per cent fellatio, and 12 per cent sodomy. The overall level sounds suspiciously high, yet the distribution of homoerotic activity rings true for the time.[20]

What clinches the triumph of oral over anal in the United States are the Kinsey data, which centre on the generation of men who came of age between the two world wars. Kinsey found that, whereas only 18.6 per cent of gay men had anal sex in half or more of their sexual encounters, 62.7 per cent had oral sex in more than half of their encounters. (Receiving oral and anal sex is meant.)[21] It is clear that in the United States, in the years of the great breakout of sexuality, the anus was no longer the preferred mode of caressing the gay man's body.

In assessing this swing away from buggery, let's not forget about one small circumstance that made total body sexuality more appealing for both gays and straights: better hygiene. These were the years of paeans to the scent of young working-class male bodies. 'This odor,' said one informant to sexologist Bloch, 'is the peculiar possession of young men who live in the open and have natural occupations, and is never found in women. The perspiration of such youths is fresh, quite unlike that of young girls in a dance hall: it is more refined, more ethereal, more penetrating.' There was something about the clothing of these stout chaps, the informant insisted, that 'emits an indefinable scent combining cleanliness and sexuality.'[22] Though some of this may have been wishful thinking – or scented with the nose of faith, as it were – such encomiums to the bodies of working-class youth would have been inconceivable if the young men had not bathed periodically or had their mothers wash their clothes, which otherwise would have stunk with fetor. One doesn't want to overplay the importance of such a mechanical factor as periodic washing in a mental change of vast dimensions, yet such things can make a difference.[23]

Gays: The Physique Focus

Gay men have never been indifferent to physique. Michaelangelo's magnificent fifteenth-century statue *David* is considered a gay icon par excellence. But it is towards the end of the nineteenth century that muscularity starts to acquire a total-body focus for gays. Indeed, muscles do bring the body together, from bulging forearms, to 'ripped' abs, to pecs that could lift a locomotive. Muscles on men and women send powerful physical messages.

In the belle époque Frederick Rolfe, a gentleman adventurer from London, loved to go sporting among the north Italian adolescent males who hired themselves out as prostitutes, letting gay men such as Rolfe fellate them. In 1909 Rolfe found his way to a ring of young male prostitutes in Padua, where he met Amadeo, age sixteen. 'First, sir, see my person,' said Amadeo, quickly disrobing, 'so that his breast and belly and thighs formed one slightly slanting line unbroken by the arch of the ribs,' as Rolfe exulted to a friend back home. 'His beautiful throat and his rosy laughing face strained backward while his widely open arms were an invitation. He was just one brilliant rosy series of muscles, smooth as satin, breasts and belly and groin and closely folded thighs ... with a yard [penis] like a rose-tipped lance.'[24] For sheer exuberance about the physicality of the body, I am unaware of many such accounts before the 1860s or so. Thereafter they are legion.

What is particularly interesting in this context is the rise of 'beefcake' – homoerotic photography featuring the male body in seductive poses. Beefcake is almost as old as photography itself, and as early as the 1880s gay men such as John Addington Symonds – himself a worshipper of handsome, trim, working-class males – were exchanging bundles of sex photos with one another. (During Robert Browning's funeral service in Westminster Abbey in 1889, one gay literary critic kept glancing furtively at a photo Symonds had sent him.)[25]

In the 1890s, male beefcake acquired wider distribution, as Florenz Ziegfeld in New York featured the German strongman Eugen Sandow on stage. Theatre strongmen passed from mere weightlifting on stage to the striking of muscular poses, and it was out of this vaudeville stream that the male beauty pageants of the 1920s were born: 'Mr Olympia, Mr America, and Mr Universe.' Bodybuilders such as Charles Atlas and Joe Weider retired from these in the 1930s to build their business empires. Muscle building appealed, of course, to all sexual orientations, but muscle magazines as such had a specifically homoerotic clientele.[26]

The 'physical culture' magazines, though not intended solely for gay readers, were nonetheless snapped up by them in an era when sending erotic photos of naked men through the U.S. mails was illegal. In 1899 Bernarr MacFadden began publishing *Physical Culture*, the most famous of the gay photo mags, which by 1919 had a circulation of 151,000.[27] The expressly gay Swiss beefcake magazine *Der Eigene* ('The Distinctive One') began publication in 1899 as well, often offering photos of nude boys.[28] *Physique Pictorial*, founded in 1950, acquired a huge gay following even though it published pictures not of 'ridiculously overmuscular men' (as one gay man said appreciatively just as it hit the stands) but of 'sensibly built, good-looking fellows.'[29]

Simultaneously, an elite corps of gay art photographers arose, among the first of whom was the German Baron Wilhelm von Gloeden, who in the 1870s situated his studio in the Sicilian spa Taormina. It was said that Kaiser Wilhelm himself would sail down to Sicily, where he would anchor his yacht in the harbour and seduce von Gloeden's young male models. By the 1890s von Gloeden had established himself, in Norton's words, 'as *the* master of male nude photography.' His photos circulated widely throughout the European gay subcultures; they also came to represent 'the British concept of what constitutes "the romantic Mediterranean."'[30] In the 1920s and after, such photographers as George Hoyningen-Huene in Paris and George Platt Lynes and Paul Cadmus in New York pioneered 'the streamlined look of smooth-bodies and sleek hair' for such bodybuilders as the Ritter brothers and dancers such as Lincoln Kirstein and George Balanchine. All posed naked. (Lynes removed the Ritters' posing straps, saying, 'We use shadows.')[31]

Of course one could argue that there weren't photos of male nudes before the 1860s because there were no cameras. Yet there are deeper erotic themes here – a revelling in muscular sensuality (as opposed to the formal magnificence of Renaissance statuary) that one has not seen since ancient times.

Effeminacy?

We are in a gay bar in Paris in the late 1920s frequented by a now enormous portion of the gay spectrum: the effeminate 'queers.' John Glassco, a Canadian exile in Paris, recalled the 'pale weedy youths in shabby tight-fitting suits, sporting so many rings and bracelets, these heavy men with the muscles of coalheavers, rouged, powdered and lipsticked ... all conveyed the message of an indomitable vitality, a quenchless psychic urge. Never had I felt the force of human desire projected with such vigour ...'[32]

By 1900, effeminate gays had grown from a small minority theme on the margins of the traditional homosexual universe to a massive presence – as much as half of all homosexuals, according to Bloch,[33] having their own dances, bars, and lingo. A French ex-cop visiting Berlin around 1904 was astonished to see monthly drag balls, authorized by the police, with 400 to 500 men in attendance, half of them dressed as women. The dances weren't 'modern,' meaning no quadrilles or cake-walks, but waltzes, scottishes, mazurkas, and polkas. There was nothing like it at the time in Paris, he said.[34]

Yet by the 1920s Paris, too, was offering an annual drag dance at the Magic City music hall, a huge queer event for 'the aunts.' Said one gay sophisticate rather scornfully, 'The pharmacist from Périgueux finally gets a chance to dress up as a woman and make his début in Paris. There's something painful and pathetic about the whole thing.'[35] Perhaps. Yet not to the participants themselves at the City of Light's numerous drag dances.

By 1900, Venice had become a Mecca for 'delicate types,' a code word for effeminate gay. 'You find everything there in the Western world that is at all reminiscent of aesthetes, dandies, and decadents,' said gay scholar André Koeniguer – himself hostile to effeminacy – who attributed this to a 'retro' vogue in the gay world that had 'transformed the city into a hospice and rest home for decadent neurasthenics.'[36]

Across the ocean, effeminate American gays didn't necessarily go to drag balls. The whole idea was rather downscale. But middle-class 'queers' would present themselves as 'a persona of highly mannered – and ambiguous – sophistication,' incorporating, if all went well, 'the elegance and wit attributed to the English gentry.' The analysis is George Chauncey's, historian of gay New York.[37] The city was so big it embraced every possible style.

But elsewhere in the United States the pressure on a gay man to act 'queer,' without necessarily being a cross-dressing 'fairy,' was quite intense within the gay community. One self-identified 'sissy' in Chicago said of his coming out in the 1930s, 'I did every possible thing to imitate the effeminacy of the queers that I had come in contact with. I began to wear flashy and obvious clothes, and use cosmetics to a greater extent.'[38] In San Francisco in the early 1940s, 'If you called yourself gay, you were supposed to be a swish.' 'The bars in those days were dominated by queens,' the source recalled. 'People would say, "Well, Jimmy, if you're gay, act gay."' Jimmy tried. 'I put on a little cosmetics and nearly rubbed my skin off trying to see that it didn't show. And I would try to swish but my hips just didn't swivel right ...'[39]

In sum, by the first third of the twentieth century, public gayness had become heavily identified with effeminacy. The queers and fairies, as they called themselves, had their own institutions and speech, their quintessential gestures – parodied as the limp wrist or the lisp – and their private vocabularies, which leaned heavily on calling one another 'Mary,' and the like. Private gayness is a different matter. Most gay males told Kinsey they preferred 'masculine' partners and denied exhibiting obvious characteristics 'that would make someone suspect you were a homosexual.'[40] Yet we're talking about the bar scene here, the public persona. It is not that the effeminate men who haunted this scene felt like women, or were an intermediate step between men and women, as several of the nineteenth-century sexologists believed. Rather, they had chosen to take a minor theme in the history of homosexuality and puff it into mainstream.

Meanwhile, a large number of virile gay males furiously resisted this onslaught of effeminacy, identifying with what André Gide called in 1911 'normal pederasty.' Gide did not think of himself as a 'uranist,' a term for effeminate gays coined in 1864 by the German homophile activist Karl Heinrich Ulrichs, himself said to be quite effeminate. Gide had no interest in the whole Venice-decadence aspect of gay Europe and thought of himself – in his 'Corydon' persona – as 'solid and well-built: my appearance scarce told the tale of my misery. None of my friends suspected, and I would have sooner been drawn and quartered than reveal it to anyone.'[41] When, considerably later, a young American gay man named Donald Vining visited Paris, he was 'delight[ed]' that the gays he saw weren't effeminate. 'I don't think I've had to shy away from a single one on the score of excessive daintiness.'[42]

But back home in the United States, 'Trade did the fucking; trade never sucked,' was the rule for virile gay men. 'Trade' in this context meant masculine gay men who bore none of the stigmata of effeminacy (as opposed to 'fairies'). 'Trade wasn't queer,' said historian John Loughery of the 1920s.[43] Masculine gays, in theory, did not let themselves be penetrated, nor did they give blow jobs. One Californian who had moved to New York in the early 1930s absolutely could not stand the 'pansies-on-parade' aspect of the gay balls and street scenes. 'I hated it, just hated it. They had the same kind of thing going on in the clubs in [Los Angeles]. Queens prancing around in the street was bad enough, I always thought. No discretion. No dignity. Before a crowd of straight men in a cabaret, being laughed at – I mean, what good did that do us?'[44]

'I like gentleness, love it in a youth or man,' confided a young gay in Washington, D.C., to his diary in 1927, 'but effeminacy repels me. Thank God I have been spared that. Homosexuality may be curse enough ... but it is a double curse when one has effeminate ways of walking, talking, or acting.' Jeb, the author of those lines, hated being scorned as a 'fairy.'[45]

So did many American gays. Why therefore in the last decades of the nineteenth and the first of the twentieth were there so many 'fairies'? The effeminate homosexual had been rare historically, and in the 1970s and after would become rare again. How do we account for the rise and fall of the fairy? I think that only towards the end of the nineteenth century do gay men acquire enough public permissiveness – acceptance is not really the term – to start experimenting with lifestyles. (Berlin, for example, had 123 gay bars by 1930, where this kind of experimentation took place: such a large concentration would have been unthinkable without a large measure of public toleration.)[46]

The vanishing of the fear of being burned at the stake liberated the mind powerfully; it represented the lifting of a great historic hindrance. There had always been a small number of effeminate gay men: Jeb thought the quality inborn.[47] But given some latitude for public experimentation with one's image, this small number offered a role for a much larger number of gay men to experiment with. Why the effeminacy role was chosen over other possible roles (policeman, lumberjack, etc.) is not clear. But for a brief historical period, effeminacy became a kind of gay template, which those men who were biologically inclined to effeminacy enforced on those generically inclined to homosexuality. Then in the 1970s other roles entirely offer themselves; effeminacy is abandoned by most (save, perhaps, among those effeminate by nature).

Lesbians at the Breakout

One night in 1917, a thirty-year-old unmarried woman, Mary MacLane, sat before a candle in Butte, Montana, aching with desire. 'Sex-desire comes wandering in dusk-time and gulfs me as in a swift violent sweet-smelling whirlwind.' She wanted another woman, a repetition of her first and only lesbian encounter five years earlier, apparently in New York: 'I have lightly kissed and been kissed by Lesbian lips in a way which filled my throat with a sudden subtle pagan blood-flavored wistfulness ...' So what was the problem? Was it the undoubted lack of a lesbian bar in Butte and the shortage of any potential candidates except Josephina the cleaning woman? ('Josephina's sex [pudendum] looks porcinely obvious and uninteresting like her large dubious breasts.' There was also a hygiene issue: 'Josephina would seem never to have had a bath.')[48]

Or was MacLane's own resistance to pleasure, her unwillingness to let go, holding her back? She considered herself 'wanton,' in proof of which she sat there in Butte at eleven at night wishing for 'a thousand careless kisses.'[49] Yet she remained a closet lesbian.

As lesbian women stood in 1900 at the threshold of their own breakout towards total body sex, they were hindered by a thousand years of internalized resistance to pleasure. This is a theme that appears in virtually no gay male memoir: a timidity about approaching pleasure because one has been socialized against it. For men, the force of desire was invariably overpowering. Yet an almost antihedonistic resistance to pleasure constitutes a definite theme in gay women's stories and may account for the considerable lesbian lags in the surge towards new forms of sexuality.

French author Colette is often held up as a lesbian icon. Yet however sensuously she may have behaved around men – she had three husbands and three male lovers – she evidently had problems letting herself go around her numerous female lovers. In *The Pure and the Impure*, written in 1941 – thirty years after the end of Colette's lesbian period – she allows her alter ego 'Charlotte' to express dubiety about orgasms.

Charlotte is asked by a lesbian woman, 'And what you're missing, is it really so difficult to find?'

Charlotte replies haughtily, 'Possibly not. But I would be embarrassed to show the truth after so many lies [faking orgasm]. I don't know, Madame, ummh, you can imagine, just abandoning myself to pleasure, like some imbecile, no longer knowing what you're letting show in either gestures or words. Anything but that. Oh, I could never accept that idea.'[50]

What Colette liked about lesbianism was the subtleness of intimate relationships that she found impossible to achieve with men, not the sensuousness.[51] She is the exact opposite of a standard-bearer for the new lesbian desire.

But there were many Colettes, women who felt uneasy about the details of same-sex desire. 'Diana Frederics' was the pseudonym of a woman who described her agonized and largely unsuccessful attempts early in the 1930s to come to terms with her lesbianism. It was already a big victory when she could shout at the boyfriend, 'Do I have to say it again? I'm a *lesbian*!' Yet she was turned off by the pants-wearing butches she encountered as a graduate student at Smith College. Her sexual encounters with women were timid and inhibited. She said, 'I hadn't realized how hard it had been to endure sensuality until it was over.'[52] The point is not that whoever wrote under the pen name Diana Frederics was a prude; rather, she, like Colette, put up great resistance to letting same-sex physical desire sweep over her, and a world filled with Diana Fredericses would never have known what was later to be called 'sex-positive feminism.'

Yet the world was not filled with them. Quite the opposite. On the whole, lesbians participated just as enthusiastically in the great breakout as did gay men and straights. For one thing, many more women came out as lesbian in the last third of the nineteenth century. This was visible in Paris as early as the 1880s. In Zola's novel *Nana*, Nana herself begins a lesbian relationship, and as the hapless Muffat protests, 'she shrugged her shoulders. What cloud was he coming from? This was going on everywhere, and she listed her girlfriends; she swore that anyone a little bit sophisticated was lesbian.'[53] Ten years later, in 1891, journalist 'Leo Taxil,' a pseudonym for conservative Catholic journalist Gabriel Jogand-Pagès, complained that 'one sees lesbians [*tribades*] everywhere. They are in all the brasseries, these young women who affectedly dress like twins in exactly identical dresses and whom the students tease by calling them "little nuns."'[54] Jogand-Pagès was admittedly a hostile witness, yet he had a sharp eye for social detail, and his testimony suggests that by the turn of the century lesbianism had become a common phenomenon in the French capital.

As for the United States, the terrific American success of Radclyffe Hall's novel *The Well of Loneliness*, about very mannish lesbians, published in London and New York in 1928, would suggest that an ever-growing audience lay out there waiting. By January 1929 more than 20,000 copies had been sold, and the book was near the top of the U.S. best-seller list.[55] Other evidence: on the basis of almost 6,000 interviews with American women, Kinsey estimated that women born before 1929 had a 20 per cent lifetime chance of some experience of lesbian sexual contacts, 13 per cent progressing to orgasm.[56] Very close to these numbers was the survey of Katharine Bement Davis, general secretary of the Bureau of Social Hygiene, who in the early 1920s asked a systematic sample of 2,200 women – chosen arbitrarily from members of clubs and organizations and from lists of college graduates – about their sex lives. Of the 1,200 who had remained single, 19.5 per cent said they had experienced fully erotic lesbian relationships involving mutual masturbation or more. Of the 1,000 who had married, 14.9 per cent had had explicit lesbian relationships. Davis concluded 'that the phenomena described in this study are much more widespread than is generally suspected, or than most administrators are willing to admit.'[57]

Just as the erotic scope of heterosexuals was broadening in these years to all zones of the body, and that of gay men to oral sex, the sexual activities of lesbian women as well were expanding from mutual rubbing and hugging to include cunnilingus. By the 1920s, the density of references to oral sex among lesbians had become very substantial, in contrast to references a hundred years previously, which were virtually non-existent.

The first references to lesbian oral sex of which this author is aware stem from the Parisian milieu of the can-can and its sexy cousin the chahut in the 1880s. The women who executed these rapid, athletic dances in the clubs were often lesbian, and it was widely known that the two nicknamed La Goulue and La Môme Fromage lived together and enjoyed oral sex.[58]

Lesbianism was widespread among the prostitutes of Paris, and Jogand-Pagès asserted that some of the streetwalkers, called the 'Little Miss Down-on-Your-Knees,' often satisfied their female clients orally.[59]

However abstemious Colette may have been, there is suggestive evidence that other prominent Parisian lesbians were enthusiastic about oral sex. Colette hints as much for Renée Vivien (real name Pauline Tarn), and the famous sapphic vedette Natalie Barney waxes so lyrical about the 'infinite variations' of lesbian sex that it's unlikely she omitted the oral variety.[60]

What was it that English lesbians did together around the turn of the century? 'The passion finds expression in sleeping together, kissing and close embraces, with more or less sexual excitement,' said Ellis. 'The extreme gratification is cunnilingus ...'[61]

At least two of the twelve aquarelles of Danish painter Gerda Wegener, published in Paris in 1925 to 'illustrate the work of the divine Aretin,' depict oral sex between women, one showing the merrymakers in a 'sixty-nine' position (mutual oral sex).[62]

From the United States, finally, we have a solid piece of statistical evidence on lesbian sexuality. Of the 145 'experienced' lesbian women from whom Albert Kinsey was able to extract information about techniques, 77 per cent did deep kissing, 85 per cent oral stimulation of breasts, and 78 per cent oral stimulation of genitalia. 'Genital apposition,' or frottage, the traditional lesbian sex technique, was avowed by only 56 per cent.[63]

These anecdotes and statistics paint a picture of lesbian

women pioneering a path towards total body sex as certainly and resolutely as gay males and heteros. When French sex novelist Louis-Charles Royer was undertaking a fact-finding tour of Magnus Hirschfeld's Institute of Sexual Science in Berlin in the late 1920s, he started discussing his own concepts of lesbian sexuality with one of the co-workers:

Royer: 'In general, women get sexual pleasure only by being kissed on certain limited parts of their bodies, such as the mouth, the breasts, and so forth. But here it seems to me that the lesbians are responsive all over their bodies. Is there some special practice that lesbians here favour?'

Answer: 'Among all lesbians there are multiple erogenous zones ... Quite apart from the zones that you mention, centred on the mucous membranes, we believe that most of the regions of the epidermis, when involved frequently in sex play – for example, through tickling or sucking – are capable of yielding sexual pleasure.'[64]

There it is: The voice of German science saw it coming.

Butches and Femmes?

With butchy lesbians we run into exactly the same question as with effeminate gay men: nature or nurture? The polarity between butch and femme has had an astonishing vigour within the history of lesbianism.[65] Just as effeminacy was the order of the day for several generations of early-twentieth-century gays, the lesbian world was filled with tough, or let us say mannish-looking, 'dykes,' a favourite self-description, who tended to pair with highly feminine women. Some biological evidence speaks in favour of butches, at least, being a natural category: they are more tomboyish in childhood than heterosexual women and demonstrate high testosterone levels.[66] Yet there are many fewer 'bulldykes' today than formerly, and we have here, exactly as with effeminate gays, a classic rise-and-fall problem.

That the butch-femme scene had become huge by the 1920s and 1930s there's no doubt. Paris photographer Brassaï's friend Fat Claude took him to the lesbian bar Le Monocle: 'From the owner ... to the barmaid, from the waitresses to the hat-check girl, all the women were dressed as men, and so totally masculine in appearance that at first glance one thought they were men.'[67] Unlike the usual pairings, the butches at Le Monocle danced with each other and not with feminine-looking partners.

In Berlin, with its great array of homosexual services, night clubs for butches were part of the gamut. Around 1928, women did not go out in public looking like men, but in 'closed circles' the middle-class mannish lesbians might wear a tight black wool skirt and a male-style jacket, and underneath it a silk blouse with a collar, cuffs, and a tie, possibly a monocle as well.[68]

Femmes appeared in the Berlin scene, as Ruth Roellig, the author of the above, pointed out: 'The inborn chivalrousness of the virile woman is noteworthy, which is all the more convincing because it almost always speaks from the desire of the heart to serve the courted feminine partner; the femme's pronounced desire for protection expresses itself as tenderness towards the loved one and is capable of creating absolute erotic miracles.'[69] At the women's club Monbijou, 'boys' sat on one side of the room, 'girls' on another, the butches having little gongs with which to summon their partners across the floor for the 'gong dance.' Or there might be a dance for the 'sweet mammas,' in contrast to the butch 'daddies,' standing there in tuxedos.[70]

The phenomenon of the tough fighting butch did exist – working-class lesbians able to handle themselves in street fights, even against men, and to protect their femmes from predators. Yet most mannish lesbians were not tough; they did not see themselves as ersatz men, and the middle-class butches had a horror of the kind of bar scene in which the brawling butches flourished. Vita Sackville-West, a lover of Virginia Woolf (and many others), practised masculine-style domination. In April 1918, anticipating a visit from the femme Violet Trefusis, Vita tugged on a pair of trousers. 'In the unaccustomed freedom of breeches and gaiters,' she said, 'I went into wild spirits ... in the midst of my exuberance I knew that all the old undercurrent had come back stronger than ever and that my old domination over her [Violet] had never been diminished.'

'You alone have bent me to your will,' wrote Violet to Vita after the encounter.

On one occasion Vita did blacken the eye of another lover – Dorothy Wellesley.[71]

Butches and femmes abounded in American lesbian society, and not just its upper reaches. A lesbian club in Salt Lake City, Utah, in the 1920s and 1930s consisted of ten butches, eight femmes, and five members who fluctuated.[72] But at the upper reaches, as well, there were plenty of mannish figures, such as the New Yorker Marion 'Joe' Carstairs, who excelled at motorboat racing and became an object of hostile comment in the press for her tattoos and her muscles (all of which qualities would be unremarkable in a woman today; yet we are talking about the 1920s).[73]

In brief, butch and femme were as American as apple pie. These roles dominated the international lesbian scene as well for perhaps a century, only to fade, like the 'fairy,' into unfashionableness in the 1970s and after: unfashionable roles perhaps, but nonetheless real to those who feel called to them.

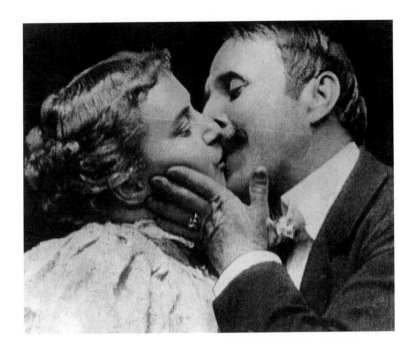

New erotic zones: Parts of the body formerly ignored or tabooed began to emerge in the late 19th century. Deep tongue kissing was still barely on the radar in 1896 when Edison's brief kinetoscope 'The Kiss' shocked viewers by showing actors kissing on screen for the first time. (The Picture Desk, The Kobal Collection)

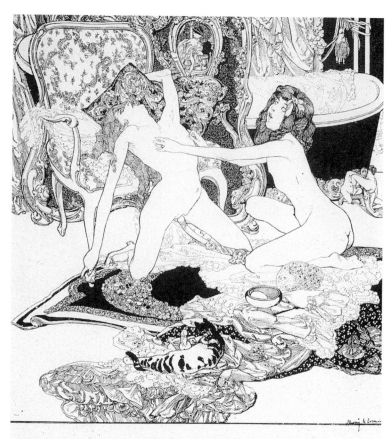

"Tu n'as qu'à y penser,
et tes tetons deviennent aussi durs que le cautchouc de notre bon-ami!"
"L'extase."

New erotic zones: Women's enjoyment of nipple-play started being acknowledged in erotic art. Depicted here is a 1907 fantasy portrayal of lesbian lovemaking by the Marquis Franz von Bayros. (Men's interest in their own nipples emerged more slowly.) *Die Grenouillère* (1907), Franz von Bayros.

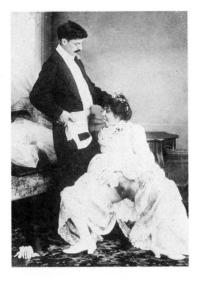

New erotic zones: Growing interest in oral sex in the late 19th century is reflected in the Kinsey Collection of photographs at the Institute for Sex Research in Bloomington, Indiana. 'Wedding night' scenes showing newlyweds experimenting with a wide range of sexual activity were a popular theme in the 1880s and 1890s. (The Kinsey Institute for Research in Sex, Gender, and Reproduction, Inc.)

New erotic zones: Anal sex between straights also began to emerge as an erotic theme at the end of the 19th century. The Kinsey Collection includes numerous images of heterosexual sodomy from the period, such as this 'wedding night' scene from the late 1890s. (The Kinsey Institute for Research in Sex, Gender, and Reproduction, Inc.)

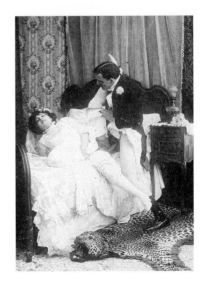

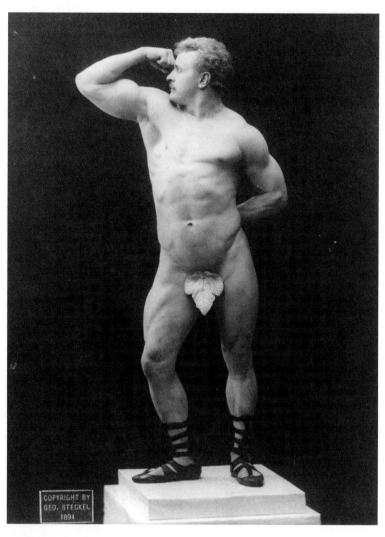

COPYRIGHT BY
GEO. STECKEL
1894

The physique focus: 'Beefcake' photography emerged in the gay underground as early as the 1880s, and entered the mainstream a decade later as German strongman Eugen Sandow popularized physique posing. Eugen Sandow (1867–1925), the most celebrated bodybuilder of the late 19th century appears in a photoprint dated 1894 by George Steckel. (Courtesy of the Library of Congress, USA)

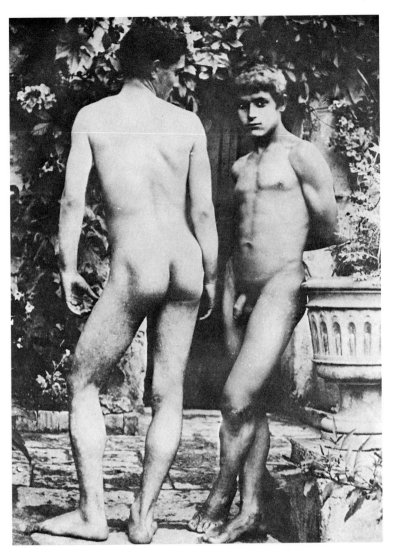

Homoerotic art photography also emerged during the latter part
of the 19th century with the work of Baron Wilhelm von Gloeden
(1856–1931), who set up a studio in the Sicilian spa town of
Taormina. Von Gloeden's studies of young male models circulated widely throughout the European gay subculture. (Leslie
Lohman Gay Art Foundation)

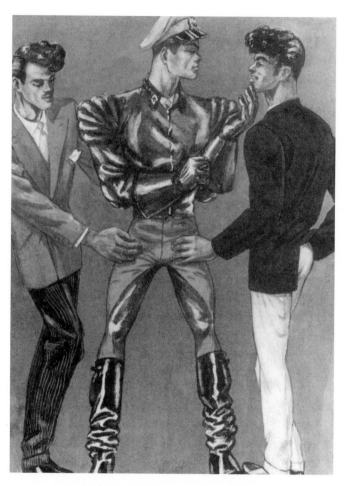

Trade and fairies. Many virile gay men ('trade') rejected the effeminate 'fairy' persona popular in the first half of the 20th century. The early version of the the leatherman portrayed in this 1947 illustration by Tom of Finland wears the canvas officer's cap and brown leather jacket and gloves of the day, but by around 1950 Tom had replaced the entire ensemble with black leather. (Protected under international copyright law. Permission for inclusion granted by the Tom of Finland Foundation, Los Angeles, CA; www.tomoffinlandfoundation.org; email: administration@tomoffinlandfoundation.org)

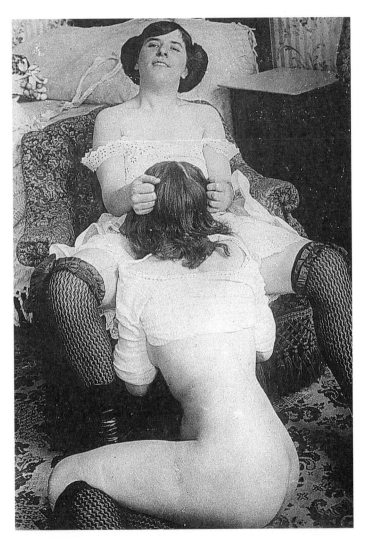

Lesbians at the breakout: By the late 19th century the sexual horizons of lesbians were expanding to include oral sex. Like most depictions of lesbian activity before the 1960s, however, this image from the Kinsey Collection was produced for male consumption rather than representing genuine lesbian self-eroticism. Photograph ca. 1889–92. (The Kinsey Institute for Research in Sex, Gender, and Reproduction, Inc.))

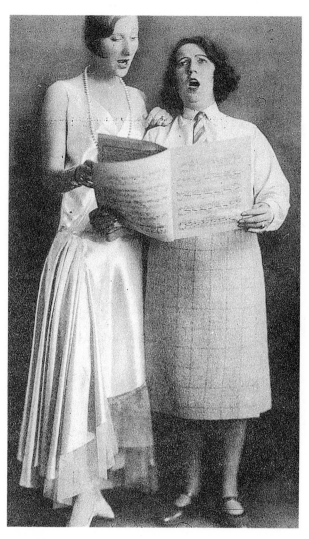

Butch and femme. By the 1920s and 1930s the large lesbian subcultures in Paris and Berlin consisted of mannish 'dykes' who frequently paired up with very feminine women. During these
years, butches did not go out in public in full male drag, but
favoured severe suits and such masculine touches as the shirt and
tie. Claire Waldoff and Margo Lion singing, Berlin, 1920s. (ullstein
bild Berlin)

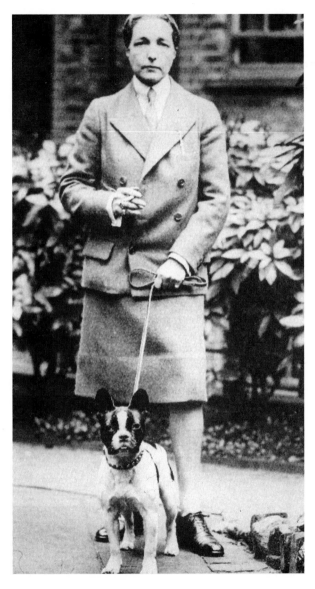

Radclyffe Hall, whose 1928 novel *The Well of Loneliness* featured very mannish lesbians not unlike herself. In this 1927 portrait she is standing in her garden with her dog, Colette. (CORBIS [© Bettmann])

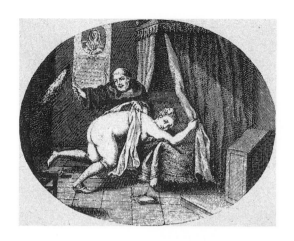

Traditional SM: Until the late 19th century, the erotic scope of SM was as narrow as in other aspects of sexuality, rarely moving beyond simple flogging. Dutch caricature of a monk flagellating a servant, ca. 18th century. (Eduard Fuchs, *Geschichte der erotischen Kunst* [Munich: A. Langen, 1908])

Domineering women were also a popular theme in traditional SM flagellation scenes, such as 'Lutz Arden's' illustration, *Die gestrenge Gouvernante* (The Strict Governess). (Paul Englisch, *Irrgarten der Erotik* [Lykeion, 1931])

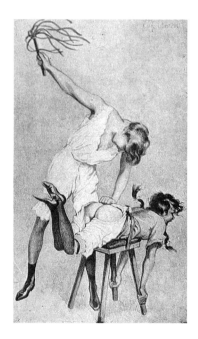

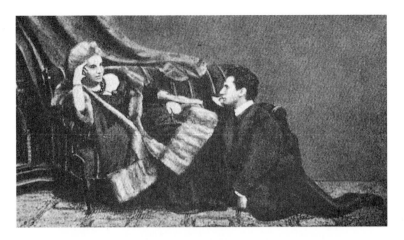

SM and fetish begin to break out: Leopold von Sacher-Masoch
kneels at the feet of Fanny Pistor-Bogdanoff, the fur-clad dominatrix portrayed as Wanda in his 1870 novel *Venus in Fur*. (Carl Felix
von Schilitegroll, *Sacher-Masoch und der Mascochimus* [Dresden:
Dohn, 1901]).

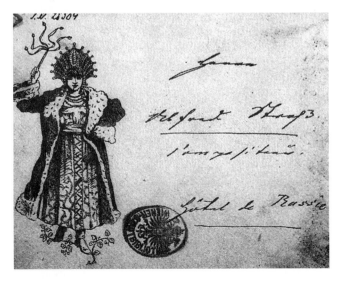

Sacher-Masoch embraces a fetish/SM lifestyle: His letterhead,
featuring Wanda dressed in fur and wielding her whip.
(Stadt- und Landesbibliothek Wien)

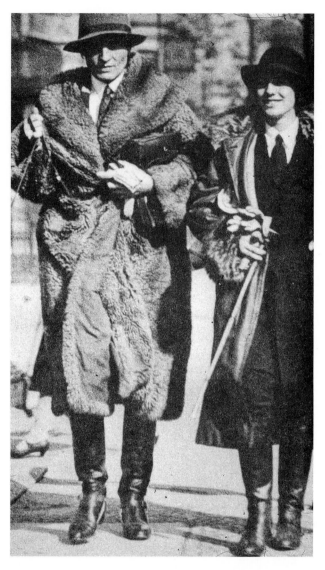

Fur and boots as fetish objects: In a late example of the domineering woman in fur, this German lesbian couple, photographed
in 1931, sport furs along with their fedoras and ties. Here the use
of leather is still confined to their boots. Renee Sintensis with
friend, 1931. (ullstein bild Berlin)

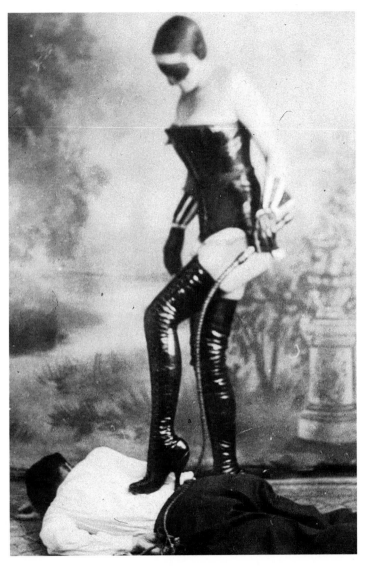

Emergence of leather in the SM/fetish scene: The first depictions of the leather-clad dominatrix appeared in the mid and late 1920s, including this image from the Kinsey photograph collection of a booted domme topping a man. (The Kinsey Institute for Research in Sex, Gender, and Reproduction, Inc.)

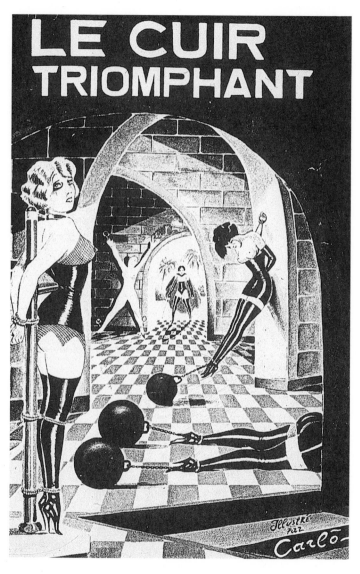

By the 1930s the leather domme was firmly established in the erotic imagination: 'Carlo's' cover illustration for Alan MacClyde's *Le cuir triomphant* (Triumphant Leather) (Paris: Librarie Generale, ca. 1934) is one of the first representations of the dominatrix (and victims) in leather bondage gear.

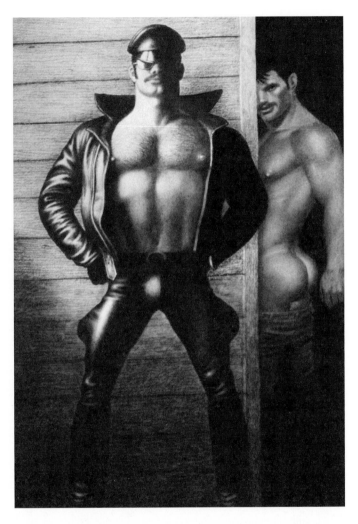

Triumphant leather: Leather gear and the hypermasculine gay
scene came together in the 1970s and after as the fairy gives way
to the hardbodied macho man celebrated by Tom of Finland. The
leatherman's gear emphasizes the erotic unity of the entire body,
from his biker's cap to his booted feet. (Protected under international copyright law. Permission for inclusion granted by the Tom
of Finland Foundation, Los Angeles, CA; www.tomoffinlandfoun-
dation.org; email: administration@tomoffinlandfoundation.org)

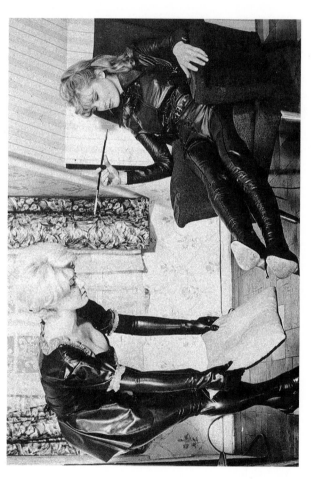

SM/Fetish joins the mainstream: By the late 1950s, commercial leather and latex clothing produced by aficionados was beginning to make the dominatrix look a practical reality for the average person. In this 1960s photo advertising rubber fashions, fetish/SM images begin moving from the underworld to the mainstream, a process that has continued right up to the present. (The Kinsey Institute for Research in Sex, Gender, and Reproduction, Inc.)

CHAPTER EIGHT

Towards Total Body Sex

At some point in the year 2000, Professor Elaine Hatfield asked the students in her human sexuality class at the University of Hawaii about their sex behaviour during the last month. Of the 191 who were currently dating, 89 per cent did French kissing. That is up from the 63 per cent of the college grads in the Kinsey survey fifty years earlier who had French kissed *in their entire lives.*[1]

Eighty-six per cent sucked their partners' nipples – presumably the men doing the women. It remains rare today for sex surveys to ask about men's nipples.

Seventy per cent of the women had given their boyfriends fellatio in the last month. A similar percentage of men had performed cunnilingus on their girlfriends.

Anal sex? Here the participation falls off dramatically, though one student in ten had experimented with it in the last month.

How about spanking? Equal percentages – one student in five – had spanked or been spanked.[2]

These statistics are evidence that the sexual scene has changed very dramatically. These young people are experimenting with total body sex.

The most striking demonstration that our own sexual energies are fuelled by biology is the steady, unidirectional, and irreversible drive towards total body sex that has taken place throughout the twentieth century and rockets into the twenty-first. Starting from modest levels at the time of the initial breakout from the missionary position in 1900, the number of people experimenting with sexual zones involving the entire body has risen steadily until our own time. It is the relentless, remorseless nature of the climb – every year seemingly more than the previous one – that suggests some deeper human drive is being unleashed rather than the cyclical ebbing and flooding of fashion. Fashion implies a pendular movement: the skirt hems go up and down. But sexuality has gone in one irreversible direction across the tides of fashion and the cataclysms of a century involving two world wars, the destruction and migration of entire peoples, and roller-coaster rides from prosperity to poverty and back. Human sexuality is in the control of biology, and Master Desire is flogging the beast forward.

Beginning in the 1960s, this surge towards total body sex began to accelerate considerably. This is apparent from many sources, not the least of them advice manuals for women with a very different tone from the nice-girl guides of yore. In 1969 Terry Garrity, under the pseudonym 'J,' wrote the first explicit sex manual for women, *The Sensuous Woman*. The sensuous woman learns to explore her lover's entire body with her hands: 'Memorize all the variations of skin texture, from the roughness of his legs to the miraculously velvety feel of the head of the penis. Get to know that funny little bump on his left shoulder blade, run your fingers through the hairs on his chest, feel the muscles in his arms expand and contract ... There is so much of him to discover.'[3] The hardback version was on the *New York Times* bestseller list for forty-eight weeks, number one for ten weeks (the paperback for much longer).[4]

Garrity, a staff member at the publishing house Lyle Stuart, was just reporting from the microworld of her female lunch pals what a group of sex researchers based at the University of Chicago would later discover in 1994 after a random massive nationwide survey of the American population: 'Beginning in the 1920s, the sexual script for opposite-gender sex has become increasingly elaborated to include more kissing, more caressing of the body, more manual genital contact, and, more recently, more oral sex.'[5] By the beginning of the twenty-first century, total body sex has spread from the small beachheads it had established a hundred years ago to become a massive reality in the nation's bedrooms.

'The Most Sexually Turned-On Country in the World'

The story has two aspects, quantitative, or how much? And qualitative, or what body parts? We skip lightly over the quantitative story – at what age people begin having sex, and how often they do it in marriage and outside of marriage, because that is basically a chronicle of releasing restraints: social restraints on the ability of young people to express themselves sexually, the restraints that stress and weariness put on marital sexuality, and the sanctions that society places on adultery. In the history of desire, the qualitative story is more interesting because it shows the brain nudging human behaviour ever closer to some approximation of what the brain most desires: the sexual utilization of – that is, pleasure signals from – the entire body.

Still, the quantitative changes have been remarkable. For one thing, the United States, rather than France, is now the most sexually turned-on country in the world. According to the Durex Global Survey, the average American makes love 135 times per year, the average French person only 128. The average American is 16.2 years old at first intercourse – the earliest among fifteen major countries surveyed – as opposed to a global average of 17.6.[6]

In terms of the average numbers of sex partners ever, Americans also do very nicely. A random national survey of 2,765 persons in 1988, the *Janus Report*, found that 53 per cent of all men and 48 per cent of all women have had between eleven and sixty sex partners.[7] The tables in the source compel this rather cumbersome form of reporting, yet the gist is that the typical American man and woman are now having lifetime numbers of sex partners similar to those of Casanova.

As for the initiation of one's sexual career, the average age for women has been getting steadily younger. The 1995 National Survey of Family Growth of the U.S. government found that for women aged 40 to 44 years at the time of the survey, the average age at first intercourse was 18.6; for the 35- to 39-year-olds, 18.0; for women 30 to 34, 17.8; for women 25 to 29, 17.5; for women 20 to 24, 16.6.[8] In other words, the daughters are starting sex two full years earlier than their mothers. Sixteen was often the average age at the onset of puberty in the world we have lost: the first sexual experience would have occurred much later.

Sex before marriage has now become virtually universal. In the United States as a whole, almost 70 per cent of grade 12 girls have had sex, somewhat more, in fact, than grade 12 boys. By grade 12, as many girls as boys have had 'multiple sex partners.'[9] Said cultural commentator David Frum of the 1970s, 'The sudden and total disappearance of the ideal of bridal virginity has to be reckoned one of the more astonishing psychological developments in recent American history.'[10] Yet there it was: young women had acquired the same right to pleasure as young men.

Once paired off, people have sex often in the week. The above-mentioned study of American sexuality, done at the University of Chicago in the early 1990s, showed that 27 per cent of the married respondents had sex three times a week or more, 54 per cent of those cohabiting.[11] The behaviour of unmarried people living together is probably the model for the future. Three times a week, plus, means that going to bed or waking up is basically focused on sex. That more than half of couples are this active suggests that the typical post-1990s American couple is becoming highly eroticized.

Extramarital sex, another quantitative dimension, occurs quite frequently today. According to the University of Chicago study, men born in the 1930s had a 23 per cent chance of an extramarital relationship, women an 8 per cent chance. Yet the 'adultery rate' has dropped since then, mainly because marriages in which either partner is tempted by infidelity tend now to break up before anyone actually has an outside relationship. The median duration of marriages involving adultery plunged from 27 years for men born 1933 to 1942, to 15.1 years for those born 1943 to 1952, to 9.7 years for those born 1953 to 1962, to 2.8 years for those born 1963 to 1974.[12] So 'fooling around' can be misleading as a quantitative index of the eroticizing of marriage. What is really of interest is that, as the charms of Eros fade, the union breaks apart.

In sum, people are beginning sex earlier in life; sex is tending to become the focus of their late evening or early morning; and they seem to break up as soon as they decide they're no longer interested. Yet the qualitative side also has news to report.

Zones

In total body sex, many hitherto silent zones of the body become eroticized. The body as a whole becomes an engine of sexual pleasure.

The nipples of both men and women had historically been scorned, women's seen as a source of baby nutrition, men's as uninteresting warts on the chest. Around the turn of the twentieth century, interest in nipples begins to quicken a bit, but the great acceleration of nipple sexuality does not commence until after the Second World War.

In the Kinsey Collection of erotic photographs in Bloomington, male nipples do not come sexually into play until the mid-1930s. The first such photograph, in which a woman pinches the man's nipples while fellating him, dates from the period 1935 to 1937. The frequency of such images thereafter increases.[13]

When Kinsey and associates rather plumply asked their interview subjects about premarital petting – 'Was there mouth on bare female breast?' – 45 per cent of the college men remembered the answer as yes (40 per cent of the women).[14]

So women's interest in their own nipples was accelerating. (It is inconceivable that men would have offered this service if the women had been uninterested.)

The evidence that men were discovering the erotic potential of their own nipples is largely anecdotal, since the sex researchers uniformly shy away from this theme. Yet the anecdotes are interesting. In the 1950s, rock-and-roll singer Little Richard was not exactly a model of sexual propriety. He was tight with Buddy Holly, and Buddy was attracted to Little Richard's girlfriend Angel. Recalled Little Richard of one meeting, 'Buddy came into my dressing room while I was jacking off with Angel sucking my titty. Angel had the fastest tongue in the West. Well, she was doing that to me and Buddy took out his thing ...'[15] Nipples had clearly become part of men's own arousal in this admittedly rather fast set.

The whole concept of male nipple eroticism seems to have spread its wings by the time 'J' wrote *The Sensuous Woman* in 1969. On the subject of 'man's erogenous zones,' she quizzed her readers: 'Did you know that fifty to sixty percent of men have either partial or full nipple erections?' Counselled 'J,' 'Run your tongue around the nipple a few times, then across his chest to the other nipple, excite it and then back up to his mouth. No man could stay indifferent with a mouth like yours tantalizing him.'[16]

It's not news that oral sex became part of the basic package for both men and women. The nationwide study done by the University of Chicago found on a lifetime basis that about 60 per cent of men in their fifties had performed or received oral sex (44 per cent of women that age had performed it; 62 per cent had received it). Younger people, by contrast, have had a much more ample experience of orality: 85 per cent of men 25 to 29 had performed cunnilingus; 76 per cent of the women had performed fellatio. As those individuals grow older, these percentages might even rise. Said the authors of the study: 'If there has been any basic change in the script for sex between women and men, it is the increase in ... fellatio and cunnilingus.'[17] One bears in mind that among the Kinsey generation, meaning mainly the men and women who came of age in the years between the world wars, people were not entirely unfamiliar with oral sex; yet of the college-educated – sexually the most liberated of those whom Kinsey interviewed – only 24 per cent of the men practised cunnilingus, and only 27 per cent of the women fellated their husbands.[18] These recent figures are much higher.

The pornography of the twentieth century gives some indication of society's expanding erotic range. Whereas only 37 per cent of stag films in the 1920s featured fellatio, 77 per cent of those in the 1960s did so, the percentage having increased steadily every decade in between. Cunnilingus rose from 11 per cent of the stag films of the 1920s to 64 per cent of those in the 1960s.[19] In the Kinsey Collection, let's look at the statistics for just one position for oral sex: men performing oral sex on kneeling women: there is one representation of this posture from the 1880s, three from the 1890s, eight from the 1920s, and twenty-five from the 1950s (similar statistics could be produced for each of the numerous positions possible in oral sex). 'It's advisable to include a lot of oral lovemaking in your picture,' pornography film maker Steven Ziplow counselled novice porn directors in 1977. 'Blow jobs are always a big hit with the porno crowd.'[20]

But we're dealing with something here that goes far beyond pornography. At the start of the new century today, qualified trainers are holding workshops for women on performing oral sex. In one news account, 'Audrey,' who had been educated at some of the top-notch schools, including the Sorbonne, said that her boyfriend had insisted, and that she simply 'had to overcome her distaste ... So Audrey set her black-wire spectacles firmly in place and went out to take perhaps her toughest class.'[21]

The mouth has thus become every bit as much an erotic zone as the vagina was in the eighteenth century: it gives and accepts pleasure and affirms the notion that sexuality now embraces the entire body.

Total body sexuality now encompasses the anus, though to

a lesser degree. (The author of a 1981 book on anal sex couldn't even find a bindery for it, so taboo was the theme.)[22] The University of Chicago survey found that 25.6 per cent of all heterosexual men had encountered anal sex on a lifetime basis, 20.4 per cent of the women. These are surprisingly high figures for both genders. Nor was anal sex necessarily limited to a single hideous night of experimentation: 9.6 per cent of men have experienced anal sex within the last year, 8.6 per cent of women.[23] This is in contrast to the Kinsey generation, of whose college graduates only 2.6 per cent of the men performed it at least some of the time in their marriages (4.5 per cent of the female college grads reported anal penetration).[24] It seems that for mature adults, anal sex may have more than doubled in frequency between the 1930s and the 1990s.

In the 1980s these couples began coming into the San Francisco sex shop Good Vibrations asking about dildoes and harnesses. 'This is what I call one of the biggest secrets of the last two decades,' said feminist sex writer Susie Bright, who worked in the store at the time. 'The popularity of anal sex has become outrageous.' 'Men want their female lover to fuck them in the ass.'[25] These were young couples, and polls among students today suggest that the frequency of anal sex may increase in the future. In 2000, two investigators mailed questionnaires to 1,779 undergraduates at the University of California in Santa Barbara, half of whom responded. After those over thirty (and those without sexual experience) had been omitted, it turned out that 22.9 per cent of the remaining sample of 647 reported anal sex at some point in their lives.[26] These are not lubricious anecdotes, or statistics on bizarre populations of hippies; this is information on young people from the heartland who will go on to have middle-class careers. The practices they adopt are likely to endure.

The women's magazines offer a sure-fire guide to the arrival of new sex ideas, and by the end of the twentieth century they were just starting to discuss the anus. What might a guy say to you in bed if he really wants you to turn him on?

asked *Redbook* in June 1999. In addition to 'Suck my toes and chest [nipples],' and 'Hold my penis while we're just lying around doing nothing,' *Redbook* suggested that Mr America might request, 'Play with my anus.' (Twenty-eight percent of the males responding to a poll on the magazine's website indicated an interest in anal sex.)[27] Emboldened, perhaps, by the success of this issue, three months later *Redbook* gave readers advice about finding his 'G-spot,' meaning his prostate gland, though the magazine did not use that term: 'Insert a lubricated finger in his anus and move up the front rectal wall ...'[28] These findings suggest that for Mr and Ms America some form of anal involvement is becoming part of the standard sexual repertoire and that interest in this theme has been growing now for decades.

Anal sex has also become part of what average people enjoy watching as well. The representation of anal sex in blue movies began to rise in the 1950s and 1960s.[29] In 1977, porn-film maker Ziplow could still counsel aspirants, 'Not every male is turned on by anal sex, but enough are to make its inclusion a pleasant experience for a large portion of viewers.'[30] Yet twenty-five years later, women's appreciation of these themes seems to have climbed as well. The porn-video market is now definitely aimed at both sexes – women accounting for as much as 40 per cent of the rentals[31] – and current videos feature such female-positive, and previously unheard of, positions as 'RC,' or 'reverse cowgirl,' the woman straddling the man on top but facing away from him, and 'RAC,' or 'reverse anal cowboy,' this time featuring anal penetration.[32] Tristan Taormino, in her *Ultimate Guide to Anal Sex for Women*, published in 1998, advised readers, in preparing for anal masturbation, to 'Bring out that favorite vibrator or dildo, turn on a hot porn video or a steamy movie ...'[33] The fantasies that accompany anal sex have clearly become equal-opportunity experiences.

Does facial beauty matter for nothing? With all this talk of nipples and anuses must we abandon the notion that sheer loveliness is a turn-on? As one reader of the manuscript of this book sniped at me, 'You apparently believe that people who regard the face as the most interesting portion of the anatomy are pretty benighted. Well, to each his own, but personally, I don't find nipples and anuses to be very expressive – or even particularly appealing, if the person bearing them has a disagreeable face.'

The evidence says that prettiness remains an important element of sexual attraction – in acquaintanceship, let's say, getting to know somebody else. A couple won't find themselves in bed unless mutual attraction – on the basis of handsomeness – brings them there. After that, other factors take over today in maximizing the pleasure of the sexual experience they enjoy together.

There's one more point. The delectation of the entire body comes together, finally, in the form of masturbation, in which celebrants may address many other body parts in addition to the genitals. 'J' urged readers of *The Sensuous Woman* to sensitize their entire bodies for the act of masturbation: 'To awaken your body and make it perform well *you must train like an athlete for the act of love.*'[34] According to the University of Chicago study, more than a third of men in leading-edge relationships – cohabitation without marriage – masturbate once a week or more (and one in seven women in such relationships).[35] This stands in contrast to married men, only 16 per cent of whom masturbate this often (and one married woman in twenty).

So that is point one: masturbation is associated with the kinds of relationships that tend to be sexually quite active. Thirty-one per cent of the married women who told a *Redbook* poll in 1974 that they masturbated said they did so as an 'enjoyable addition to intercourse' (by contrast, only 18 per cent of the female masturbators declared coitus 'unsatisfying').[36]

Point two is that, married or cohabiting, people in relationships today masturbate much more often than in Kinsey's time. In those days, fewer than 1 per cent of married, college-educated men masturbated once a week or more (there were comparable figures for college women; the non-college re-spondents masturbated even less).[37]

It's a shame that we are so poorly informed about the techniques people use in masturbation. They likely involve simultaneously touching the nipples, or simulating male pelvic thrusting, and people do all this much more often than in Kinsey's day to say nothing of the long, narrow centuries previously. Betty Dodson, who began offering masturbation workshops to women in 1973, drew the anus into play: 'We did anal self-massage by oiling and then gently pressing around the outside of the anal opening before we inserted a finger. Breathing into the sensation, we further relaxed the sphincter muscles while concentrating on letting go of all tension and negative feelings we had about our "sweet little rosebuds." Once relaxation occurred, pleasurable sensations followed. The poor anus was the last part of our bodies to ever get any love and attention.' Or else, Dodson and the workshop members might oil their bodies thoroughly; or, in the 'women's masturbation circle,' have the participants stroke each other's entire bodies. 'We were moving past two thousand years of sexual repression in one afternoon,' said Dodson.[38] The bottom line is that masturbation seems to offer the finishing touch to the whole sensuous packet of total body sex.

The Women's Narrative

There is no reason to think that women plunged into post-1960s sexuality any less enthusiastically than men. Yet what changed in the 1960s was not the desire but the secure assurance of not conceiving. One thinks of the poet Sylvia Plath, panting with desire in adolescence at the beginning of the 1950s. After a date, the recent high-school graduate complains about the burden of her conscience: 'I hate, hate, hate the boys who can dispel sexual hunger freely, without misgiving, and be whole, while I drag out from date to date in soggy desire, always unfulfilled.'[39]

Why were so many women in the early 1950s unfulfilled?

The story for women does run a bit differently than for men – and women's adoption of new sexual styles in the 1960s is all the more dramatic – because of their particular risk of conception. The knowledge that virtually any sex act could result in a conception acted historically as a powerful brake on women's sexuality. This brake was definitively loosened in 1960 when the U.S. Food and Drug Administration approved the first birth-control pill, Enovid. The number of Enovid prescriptions increased tenfold from 1960 to 1962, from 191,000 to 1,981,000. By 1969, the National Prescription Audit estimated that 8.5 million American women used the pill each month. By the time of the National Fertility Study in 1970, of the women using some form of contraception, a third were relying on the pill.[40]

The pill opened a new era in women's access to pleasure.[41] Since about 1957, Mary Quant, 'the mother of the miniskirt,' had been selling young women short tight skirts and black stockings in her shop on King's Road in London. Women who associated short hemlines with sexual liberation frequented her boutique. Quant later said of the pill, 'Women had been building to this for a long time, but before the pill there couldn't really be a true emancipation. It's very clear in the look, in the exuberance of the time – a rather child-like exhilaration: "Wow – look at me! – isn't it lovely? At last, at last!"'[42]

The pill introduced a major discontinuity into the history of women's sexuality. They were suddenly able to act on the basis of desire, something men have always been able to do. In the 1960s, this was referred to as a sexual revolution for women, a term later scorned by some who felt the so-called revolution merely increased women's vulnerability to men. Yet as feminist theorist Gayle Rubin looked back on the 1960s she felt the decade entailed 'enormous social and sexual gains for women. There was a fresh, post-Victorian discovery of the female orgasm. Many women were actually able to change the way that men made love with them ...'[43]

The 1900s had started the revolution in women's sexuality, but the 1960s vastly accelerated this unhesitant willingness to grab sex for the sheer sake of physical pleasure. It started to become normal that women would act as men had always acted. Naomi Wolf: 'We need sluts for the revolution.'[44] This is a delicious echo, in real life, of the feminist pleasure manifesto in Sade's 1796 'Story of Juliette,' where Mme Clairwil declares, 'Whoring is the virtue of women; we've only been created for fucking.'[45]

The sexual revolution worked its way into women's lives in various forms. Led by such widely read magazines as *Cosmopolitan*, which Helen Gurley Brown took over in 1965 to celebrate sex as 'the determining force in a woman's life,' a new sexual directness began to dawn for women.[46] As Barbara Ehrenreich and co-writers said later, 'Brown explained that the number one reason for a single woman to start an affair was because "her body wants to."'[47]

Women started to express themselves more frankly. In the early 1980s, Susie Bright, exasperated that 'lesbianism had become a political stand, not a sexual preference,' decided to 'bend the stick the other way.' As noted earlier, in 1984 she and Debi Sundahl founded the self-styled 'blatantly pornographic' magazine *On Our Backs* – the title itself a take-off on the sexual primness of the official feminism of the day with its antiporn Washington, D.C., newspaper *off our backs*. At the time, said Bright, 'Women were scared shitless of writing about their sexual lives in ways that didn't portray them as victims or props.'[48] In the 1980s, sex-positive feminism found its voice and began to nudge the official antipornography movement out of the spotlight. As Linda Williams, author of a work on women and sex, said in 1989, a central feature of any pornography is that 'the body is recalcitrant; it has desires and appetites that do not necessarily conform to social expectations.'[49] It didn't matter any more that women were sex objects. What they wanted to be was sex subjects.

Women themselves often conceived this new openness to desire in the language of total body sex. In Rossana Campo's

1997 novel, *The American Actor*, the protagonist describes her feelings while undressing a fabulously handsome actor: 'When I discovered all that beautiful meat, every cell in my body was bursting with happiness. My ears were ringing, and, guys, when we started really to get into it I'm sure that I was reaching some superior state of consciousness ...'

'I know I'm always exaggerating,' she added, 'but what do you want? I'm a woman and I've got a tendency to mix sex with mystical ecstasy. Who ever said there was anything wrong with that?'[50]

Yet amid this celebration of physicality, which is very new in the context of women's sexual history, there was one source of continuity in women's post-1960s drive towards pleasure: muscles. At the beginning of the breakout of desire around 1900, developing muscles played something of a role for many women (see chapter 6). As the drive towards total body sex intensified after the 1960s, muscles mattered for men, of course, and workouts at the gym were supposed to translate into success in the meat market. But powerful and wealthy men have never experienced much trouble finding partners, even without muscles, and the interesting continuity here is women's interest in their own muscular bodies as a source of pleasure to *themselves*.

On 7 February 1997, a young woman named Cook in Portland, Oregon, wrote in her Internet diary about getting an eighty-pound punching bag in order to work out her anger. 'I just came back upstairs after beating the living daylights out of it! My shoulders feel more relaxed than they have for months ... I need to learn how to hit it the right way. But I don't care. I feel fucking GREAT! I have a damn punching bag of my very own!'[51]

Muscles for women have become part of the sexual ether of the early twenty-first century. This has been building for a while. In 1982 *Time* cheered, 'Spurred by feminism's promise of physical, domestic and economic freedom, you have done what few generations of women have dared or chosen to do. You have made muscles – a body of them – and it shows. And you look great.' At that point Danskin, a manufacturer of tights, leotards, and other workout dress, was doing about $100 million in sales annually.[52] 'In the middle of the last Olympics,' said writer Sallie Tisdale in 1994, 'I noticed a sudden change in the population of my fantasies. Everyone in them, male and female both, sprouted muscles. So did I, in my dreams: big, shiny muscles bulging out of tank tops and nylon running shorts.' She had been lifting weights a bit, 'learning to grunt from the lower belly with each lift, then coming home to watch the skiers with their potent thighs ... It all blended together, health and sex, hygiene and sweat.'[53]

Yet women have come only recently to serious muscle. While men had engaged in bodybuilding as early as Sandow in the 1890s, it was only in 1977 that Ohio YMCA director Henry McGhee founded the United States Women's Physique Association and organized the first bodybuilding contest for women. The sport came to national attention with the first Women's World Bodybuilding Championships in 1979 in Los Angeles and has since taken off.[54] As the *New York Times* pointed out in 1996, 'women have acquired muscles that their mothers never had.'[55]

The connection between muscles and sexuality doesn't just exist for the benefit of the men watching reruns of *Xena: Warrior Princess*. Women bodybuilders report that they feel more turned on. Eighteen of twenty elite female bodybuilders interviewed in one study reported feeling sexier and more feminine. One of them commented, 'I never felt womanly before I began to bodybuild. Too skinny, no shape ... I really enjoy the sexual attention I now get from men. Bodybuilding has really enhanced my sexual power.'[56]

Nor are women in the real world who work out on weights totally insensible to these pleasures. The number of women lifting free weights frequently (100 days or more) soared from 1.4 million in 1987 to 6.6 million in 1997 (an almost fivefold increase, in contrast to a threefold increase for men).[57]

For these women, muscles make the body come together into a whole, an instrument for pleasure far more honed than that of poor Mlle de Lespinasse in the eighteenth century, who spoke so piteously of 'my machine.'

Gay Men Move towards Total Body Sex

The inexorable migration of gay men away from buggery and towards total body sex was mapped on the body of young Donald Vining, born in 1917 in a small town in Pennsylvania and living from 1942 on in New York City. Vining, who spent an entirely unremarkable life as a clerk, left behind a riveting diary that would represent the founding document of the history of gay men, just as Anne Lister's diary would have done for gay women had it not come so late in time. After a few tentative attempts at cruising back in Pennsylvania, Vining really started to get into gay sex in the showers of a New York City YMCA. On New Year's Eve 1942 he noted of the move to New York, 'My sex life was radically altered. After years of resisting the repulsive idea [of gay sex] and letting my puritanical impulses strangle my unconscious desires, I finally found out what I want sexually ...'

Yet at first Vining found the notion of actually kissing other men repellent. Not until 1945, when he picks up an apparently straight man ('trade'), does he discover the pleasure of kissing: 'Tho he was trade, he kissed as I have never seen trade kiss. I have never cared for kissing but I made an exception for John. His lips were lush without being overly so.'

Vining's next surprise was the pleasure of kissing men all over their bodies. First, he discovers the thighs. Later in 1945, with Quentin, 'Ears attract him and legs attract me, so that he madly kisses my ears and I just as avidly kiss his thighs.' Shortly after this encounter, Vining starts to discover French kissing, though at first he doesn't care for it much.[58]

In 1946 Vining met the man, Ken, who was to become the great love of his life. Vining was a masculine gay, and previously his sexual experience seems to have been confined to receiving oral sex. Yet a few months later Ken has apparently taught Vining a thing or two because Vining is now giving Ken blow jobs.[59]

By the late 1960s Vining is well into middle age and is now quite rounded sexually. On 3 December 1969, apropos the Freudian theory that homosexuals like to draw male organs into them because they feel uncertain of their masculinity, he writes, 'I, for instance, like to suck AND fuck, but do not care much for being fucked and am so indifferent to being sucked that I frequently cannot reach orgasm that way.' He felt that his own mixed tastes refuted the theory. Yet most of this could have happened in 1900 and fit perfectly into the sexual scene of Oscar Wilde's day.

In 1972, however, Vining's sexual horizons begin to expand as he goes to Beacon Baths in Manhattan, although at first with much trepidation about being caught in a police raid. 'In the end I made myself go ... and it turned out even better [than in one previous bath trip in Paris], much better.' He went back and forth between the shower room and the steam room. 'Every one was manly but my God, the things that went on in that steam room, let alone in the private cubicles, which I never investigated.' Vining accepted only the overtures of bearded men: 'I can't understand how I could sit in that steam room with at least two people watching and blithely let the first bearded one go down on me and then turn and unconcernedly go down on him. A veil of sorts was drawn by ... the steam but I knew perfectly well that I was being watched and I didn't give a damn.'

Here we encounter an important new theme in the development of gay sexuality: the sexual abandon that the all-enveloping climate of steam, water, and white tile make possible. These men let their entire bodies be permeated by the hot steam and drenching water, and then, naked among a group of others similarly in the thrall of hydro-oceanic experience, they start to sense that anything is possible. On one day Vining felt he had met with an almost revolutionary experience: 'Another time I went in [to the steam room] and found a huge bearded boy being done from all sides. He was beautifully shaped and every erotic zone including his nipples was being worked on by someone and he was in a seeming transport but not so transported that he couldn't reach out a hand to grasp me.' This is very different from fifteenth-century Florence. 'This whole gay revolution is a matter of the last five years,' said Vining.[60]

As the 1970s progressed, the bath scene became wilder and wilder, sprouting 'orgy rooms' and the practice of fist fucking (hand and indeed entire forearm in someone else's rectum). The fearful toll that AIDS would take in the 1980s and beyond was being prepared. Yet the point for us, in this book about pleasure and desire, is that in the 1960s and 1970s gay men progressed far indeed at the baths on their historic journey towards total body sex. Vining was merely experiencing in Manhattan what was going on in many other places.

Vining was pleasantly surprised to find that, as an older gay man, he was still getting lots of action. For gays in general, the frequency of sex seems to have increased greatly in the course of the last hundred years, largely as a result of more opportunities. Three things changed in particular, an increase in the number of public toilets beginning in the 1930s, a rise in the kind of gay bars called 'pig parlours' where men could actually have sex, and a growing number of baths catering to gays in the 1950s.

Since the eighteenth century at least, 'tea-room' sex, or sex in public urinals, has appealed to the spectrum of the gay community who value totally anonymous sexual activity. Lacking bars or other sheltered places, gay men have always sought out the protection of the public washroom, the older and less appealing fellating the young and handsome, men then shifting from one category to another as they grow older. The federal works programs of the 1930s led to the construction of many new public urinals, and as the automobile made it possible to reach them easily, tea-room sex underwent a boom. One scholar, who conducted a survey of tea-room sex in the late 1960s in St Louis, noted how often middle-class men would stop off at the urinals for a blow job on their way home. As older patrons remembered the 1930s, 'It just seemed like half the men in town met in the tea-rooms.'[61]

In 1946 Kinsey took his new co-worker Paul Gebhard for a visit to the public urinal in Grand Central Station in New York. Gebhard had been dubious that the level of homosexuality could be as high as Kinsey thought. Kinsey and Gebhard stopped about halfway down the stairs, 'just far enough to be able to see everyone in the room,' as historian James Jones reconstructed the story. Kinsey turned and asked Gebhard how long it took for someone to relieve himself.

'Oh, I don't know. A couple of minutes, I guess,' said Gebhard.

What Gebhard saw instead was 'eight or nine men migrating from one urinal to another, washing their hands, drying them, milling around, and then coming back to the urinals.'

Kinsey told Gebhard, 'Those are homosexuals. They are looking for partners. So, now what do you think about the incidence of homosexuality?'[62]

The proliferation of gay bars in the 1960s moved many men, of course, out of the tea rooms. Bars for gay men to congregate in had always existed, some in four-star hotels, others in theatre districts or in slums. With the rise of 'pig parlours' in the late 1960s, bars where men could have sex, the nature of these meeting places changed. The first pig parlour in New York, the 'Zoo,' started up in 1969 or 1970, an after-hours bar in the Village that opened about midnight. Wrote one early patron to a researcher, 'They have liquor, dancing, fuck movies, and a dark room behind the juke box JUST FOR SEX. I "came" five times between 1:30 a.m. and 6 a.m.'[63] The first group of pig parlours in New York was closed down by the police in 1971, but then a new group opened in 1975, scandalizing an entire generation of lifestyle journalists with tales about fist fucking in leather swings and the like.

But not only journalists were scandalized. 'For me New York gay life in the Seventies came as a completely new beginning,' said author Edmund White, who in January 1970 had moved to Rome for ten months. As he returned, an old friend met him at the airport, gave him an 'up' (amphetamine) to pop, and took him on a tour of the 'brand-new back room bars.' One was Christopher's End, where a go-go boy, stripped down to his shorts, peeled them off and tossed them at the crowd. 'A burly man in the audience clambered up onto the dais and tried to fuck the performer but was, apparently, too drunk to get an erection.' White and his friend drifted into the back room, where they stared 'through the slowly revolving blades of a fan into a cubbyhole where one naked man was fucking another ...'

Even outside the bars, said White, historic street cruising gave way to 'half-clothed quickies.' White overheard someone saying, 'It's been months since I've had sex in bed.' White comments: 'All this was new.'[64]

Gay men had been frequenting baths ever since they were introduced as adjuncts of public hygiene in the mid-nineteenth century. Towards 1900, New York had plenty of gay baths, and London was said to offer nothing compared to the Everard baths in Manhattan or the Palace Baths in San Francisco.[65] In turn-of-the-century Paris a steambath in the rue de Penthièvre was said to be exclusively for gays; another in the rue Notre-Dame-des-Victoires drew a mainly middle-class crowd; a third appealed more to youths and workers.[66]

Yet the scene that developed in the big American cities after the 1960s really was a new world, offering hitherto undreamed-of levels of hedonism in private cubicles, where men could lie with cans of Crisco beside them (for fist fucking). The baths also appealed because they offered a zone of safety, the police raids of the past gradually coming to an end in the new climate of tolerance. In 1965 Cleveland's Jack Campbell founded the Club chain, which by 1971 had fourteen bathhouses in cities such as Atlanta, New Orleans, and Newark. His baths were situated in out-of-the-way settings easily accessible by car. 'For men who were married or didn't have a place to take somebody, we were a godsend,' said Campbell.

'And there wasn't any nonsense about straight managers or attendants looking down on the men who went there.'[67]

'Bathhouses were the most obvious gauge of the new atmosphere,' wrote historian John Loughery. 'Men who would never have imagined setting foot in a gay bathhouse in the 1960s, or who would have had to travel a great distance to do so, became "Buddy Night" regulars a few years later.'[68] When Karla Jay and Allen Young did a survey of gay and lesbian sex in the late 1970s, based on almost 5,000 questionnaires returned by participants at conferences and other settings plus readers of *Blueboy* magazine, 35 per cent of the respondents said they went to gay baths for sex 'somewhat frequently' or even more often (as opposed to 17 per cent who used public rest rooms).[69]

Parisian philosopher Michel Foucault, who visited Toronto in 1982, had never imagined anything like the bathhouses he found in Ontario's capital. The story is a bit more complicated because Foucault discovered the leather SM scene in Toronto as well, which also enchanted him. Yet Foucault later pontificated about the baths as such: 'I think that it is politically important that sexuality is able to function as it functions in the bathhouses. You meet men there who are to you as you are to them: nothing but a body with which combinations and productions of pleasure are possible. You cease to be imprisoned in your own face, in your own past, in your own identity.'[70] Foucault experienced physical abandon in Toronto just as Donald Vining had met it in New York.

The availability of these new venues contributed to gay men becoming sexually far more active than either straight men and women, or lesbians. In statistical terms, they are virtually off the scale in terms of the number of times per week and number of partners. Whether these very high frequencies of sex partners held true for gays in the dim past is impossible to say, but already in 1951 Cory was commenting on it. Gay men, he thought, were unsatisfied by a single loving relationship. 'The result is that, instead of desiring the same man again, there is frequently a desire for a second one, followed by the third, the fourth, and the hundredth.'[71]

In the early 1980s Philip Blumstein and Pepper Schwartz discovered in a nationwide random survey that, whereas only 26 per cent of married men (and 33 per cent of male cohabitors) had experienced non-monogamous sex since the beginning of their current relationship, 82 per cent of gay males had done so.

Further: The number of different partners during your current relationship? Let's say twenty-plus? Only 7 per cent of husbands had had so many partners, 4 per cent of male cohabitors, 43 per cent of gay men.

Number of times you have sex a week? As high as three times a week or more? Forty-five percent of the newly-weds (together two years or less) had sex that often, 61 per cent of the newly cohabiting, and 67 per cent of the newly partnered gay men.[72]

These frequencies drop off greatly for longer relationships. Edmund White cuttingly described the typical gay couple of the 1970s in Manhattan as 'two men who love each other, share the same friends and interests and fuck each other almost inadvertently once every six months during a particularly stoned, impromptu three-way.'[73]

On the qualitative side, what changes have there been in the sexual behaviour of gay men? Here the answer seems to be that they do everything, only a lot more often than fifty years ago. Nipples, for example, have come to the forefront. In the Kinsey Collection in Bloomington, we encounter the first gay nipple action in an image from 1936, in which a man fingers his partner's nipple, all the while touching the partner's penis with his foot, while the partner masturbates him.[74]

After the 1960s, nipple play becomes a standard theme in gay sex, at a time when it is still a decidedly minor chord for heterosexual males. Of the non-random but surely not unrepresentative sample studied by Karla Jay and Allen Young in the mid-1970s, 59 per cent said that stimulation of the nipples was 'very important' or 'somewhat important' to them. (Only

11 per cent said 'very unimportant.')[75] By the 1970s at the baths, some gay men were demanding 'heavy nipple work,' entailing pinching, biting, sucking, and clamping; they were identifiable as nipple fans because their own tended to be large and distended.[76] In August 1990 the gay magazine *Drummer* advertised 'Tattooed Tit Enhancement,' suggesting that before getting the aureole about the nipple tattooed, candidates engage with their lovers in 'colorization foreplay,' decorating the chest with felt-tip pens and experimenting with the 'design, color and size of the aureole.'[77]

John Preston's classic 1983 novel of gay cruising, *Mr. Benson*, opens with Mr Benson, a masterful figure, coming on to the protagonist in a bar. Says the first-person protagonist: 'My nipples were almost flat in those days. They were nickel-sized circles of brown flesh until Mr. Benson started to take a personal interest in their education. But still, when he reached up and his hand started to rub a thumb back and forth across their surface, it sent flashes of sensation through my whole upper torso. I forced a deep breath and unconsciously spoke, "Oh, please, Sir!"'[78]

Thus for gay men, in the surge towards total body sex, the nipples are definitely part of the picture.

In the post-1960s world, oral sex still led anal in the gay community in terms of popularity. In the Jay-Young survey in the 1970s, 74 per cent always or very frequently practised 'sucking your partner's cock' (the same order of magnitude for 'getting your cock sucked'); 23 per cent practised anal sex.[79] Twenty years later the big University of Chicago poll found that 94 per cent of gay men had had oral sex in the last twelve months, 77 per cent anal.[80] In other words, the trend is towards huge majorities of men doing both. All kinds of pleasure have increased!

In the hypermasculine gay world of the 1970s, being penetrated became acceptable for manly figures. John Loughery commented, 'Prejudices about specific activities in bed collapsed as hard-muscled young men made it clear they wanted to be the passive as well as the active partners in anal sex and stigmas about penetration by a man as a feminine desire became untenable.'[81]

Simultaneously, effeminacy began ebbing from the gay scene as the macho man roared in. Here we're doing social history rather than biology, because the dominant style of gayness is clearly linked somehow to larger social trends. The rise and fall of the 'queen' would be inexplicable in biological terms alone. Similarly, the muscled, bearded 'clones,' meaning gay men dressing as lumberjacks or urban tough guys, must have somehow spun off from the larger society, for there is no lumberjack gene.

The masculinizing of gay culture had started as early as the Second World War, exposing large numbers of gay young men to military models. Historian George Chauncey writes of New York, 'Jeans, T-shirts, leather jackets, and boots became more common in the 1940s, part of the "new virile look" of young homosexuals.' Chauncey believes the term 'gay' specifically branded these young butch types, in contrast to the lisping 'fairies.'[82] In the 1950s such magazines as Bob Mizer's *Physique Pictorial,* with its muscled hunks, fed the beefcake market, replacing camp and swish. The new line was, 'I'm a gay man, but I'm as butch as any of you.'[83]

In the 1950s, pockets of drag queens still remained. Rock singer Little Richard recalled the black queens of Macon, Georgia, in the early 1950s who all called each other 'Miss Thing.'[84] Yet Miss Thing was doomed. Said Tom Burke in *Esquire* in December 1969, 'Love in homosexual terms used to be essentially feminine. Now, they don't have a gender. Movies were camp, and queens could only identify with women. Today, gay kids identify with males – with Peter Fonda, or Dustin Hoffman.'[85] So, no more 'third sex.'

On Christopher Street in Manhattan, reported one journalist in 1978, 'The universal stance is a studied masculinity. There are no limp wrists, no giggles, no indiscreet hip swiveling ... This is macho country.'[86]

As Edmund White travelled about the gay scenes in the United States in the 1970s, he realized that a whole new look was evolving, identified with Castro Street in San Francisco. 'The Castro Street Clone,' he said, was characterized by 'the open V of the half-unbuttoned shirt above the sweaty chest; rounded buttocks squeezed in jeans, swelling out from the cinched-in waist, further emphasized by the charged erotic insignia of colored handkerchiefs and keys; a crotch instantly accessible through the buttons ... legs molded in perfect, powerful detail; the feet simplified, brutalized and magnified by the boots.' Interestingly, White found this costume directly associated with 'the three erotic zones – mouth, penis and anus.' 'More recently still, the nipples have also been sensitized, indicated by the gold ring sunk through them.' Why had this image triumphed over all competitors? According to White, it is the costume 'that "natural selection" has favored for cruising. It is an image of homosexual desire potent enough to have crowded out all others.'[87]

The queens? The Jay-Young poll in the mid-1970s found that only 24 per cent of respondents 'camped it up' somewhat frequently or more often. More enjoyed watching others do it, almost as though at a circus.[88] By contrast, when asked whether the respondents chose sex partners who wore 'very masculine' clothing, uniforms, and the like, 44 per cent did so 'somewhat frequently' or more often.[89]

Martin Levine was doing field research in Manhattan in the early 1980s as the clone look swept over the previous fairies. One source told him, 'Over the last few years, I have watched many of these girls [men] as the times changed. A couple of years ago, they had puny bodies, lisping voices, and elegant clothes. At parties or Tea Dances, they came in dresses, swooning over Garbo and Davis. Now, they've "butched up," giving up limp wrists and mincing gaits for bulging muscles and manly handshakes, giving up fancy clothes and posh pubs for faded jeans and raunchy discos.' One afternoon Levine went to Ty's, a popular bar on the clone circuit. 'A group of suburban homosexuals walked in. These men wore designer jeans, LaCoste shirts with the collars flipped up, and reeked of cologne. They were obviously *not* clones. As they passed by, the man I was chatting to nudged me and said, "Look at those trolls! They must be Tunnel and Bridge ... Who let them in?"'[90]

These charming anecdotes tend to stop in the 1980s, when AIDS ripped through this community. Indeed, many of the gay men cited in this chapter are now dead. Yet the underlying exuberance of gay sexuality, released now completely from its historic hindrances, continues unabated into the twenty-first century. Homosexual men have duplicated exactly the evolution of heterosexual ones.

Lesbians and Total Body Sex

What is striking about the evolution of lesbian women towards total body sex is their relative slowness, in the context of gay and straight sexuality. These leads and lags were already visible around the turn of the century, as the anus and even oral sex seem then to have been non-themes for many lesbians. A lesbian lag emerged clearly in the last third of the twentieth century, exasperating such sex-positive feminists as Pat Califia. Speaking to potential writers for lesbian-owned sex magazines in 1988, Califia urged contributors not to be so timid: 'Lesbian writers have got to loosen up, drop our drawers, spread our cheeks, stick out our tongues, get nasty.'[91] She wanted to bring erotic writing for lesbians up to the same speed as that for gays and straights. Although at the beginning of the twenty-first century there's evidence that this lesbian lag is rapidly being overcome, it emerges as a significant factor in the history of the sexuality of gay women.

The social construction of sexuality does go on, and here lesbian politics played a role. In the 1970s, when lesbianism burst forth as a public presence, the doctrine prevailed that the movement was not about sexuality but about 'female bonding.' Such official lesbian spokespersons as Lillian Faderman, an academic at California State University in Fresno, tended to see lesbianism as a feminist 'political choice,' indeed almost a choice of personal convenience. '[Nineteen-seventies lesbians] preferred to make their life with another woman because it was a more viable arrangement if one were going to pursue a career,' said Faderman.[92]

In 1970, Jeanne Cordova, a young butch in her junior year at UCLA, went to a meeting of a group that advertised itself as 'Lesbian-Feminists.' What a disappointment! There was no one there wearing heels or make-up. 'I knew no bona fide femme would go out in public without makeup or heels.' Worse, 'There were no butches.' 'Concluding that they were some kind of crackpot sect,' Cordova rose to leave. 'As I stomped across the wood floor, enjoying how the chains on my boots clanged through their meanderings, the one called "Radical Rita Right On" shouted at me, "What kind of lesbian are you?"'[93]

There could not have been a more total disconnect between sexuality and politics. One researcher noted the strange absence of sexual language in much lesbian fiction in those years, asking, 'Do lesbian writers "bypass" the way our bodies act?'[94] Karla Jay later looked back in dismay at the efforts of official lesbians in the 1970s 'to downplay erotic energy and to define ourselves as political creatures.' 'In retrospect, our error ... was in glossing over the fact that most of us had tons of sexual energy as well as rage.'[95]

The sexual nadir of official lesbianism was the efforts of straight women to experiment in bed with real lesbians. As historian Martin Duberman said, reporting widespread opinion in the lesbian community in New York, 'These political lesbians, as they were known, tended to be lousy sex partners. Despite themselves, they brought their homophobic leftist baggage with them to bed, and were likely to find their sexual experiences with women disappointing.' 'They were really boring in bed,' one lesbian told Duberman. 'It was like eating matzoh.'[96]

Starting in the 1980s, the sex-positive lesbians began to send out the message that the force of Eros bypassed politics. When in 1984 Susie Bright and Debi Sundahl started *On Our Backs*, it was with the goal of mocking officially sanctioned lesbian 'erotica' and producing porno that readers would find arousing. The editors later branched into videos for the adult lesbian market. Partner Debi Sundahl saw *On Our Backs* as a kind of 'boot camp, so many women came through and learned all these skills: editing, erotic fiction writing, designing, distribution, publicity ... a huge labor pool to grease the wheels of the women's erotica industry was groomed there.'[97] There are very few occasions when what is publicly written or spoken influences behaviour in the private sexual realm, but this may have been one of them. The grip of official feminism's deadening hand slackened, and sexual experimentation was not just legitimated but came to count as forward-looking. Said Cherry Smyth, a lesbian writer in London, of the late 1980s, 'As the focus shifted from a fear of objectification to a revelling in ourselves as sexual subjects, suddenly fisting [fist fucking], role-play, rimming, sex toys, female ejaculation and cruising were being workshopped ... It had all the momentous mood of a second sexual revolution.'[98]

In retrospect, many observers considered it a huge mistake to have confused lesbianism with feminism. Lesbian theorist Gayle Rubin pointed out that, 'By conflating lesbianism (a sexual and erotic experience) with feminism – a political philosophy – the ability to justify lesbianism on grounds other than feminism dropped out of the discourse.'[99]

These political issues help to explain the otherwise puzzling lesbian sexual lag. In quantitative terms – how much sex and when – lesbians after the 1960s emerged as considerably less active than gay men. In the Blumstein survey in the early 1980s, only 3 per cent of lesbians in stable relationships (together two to ten years) had sex more than three times a week, compared with 32 per cent of stable gay men, 38 per cent of cohabitors, and 27 per cent of married couples. Lesbians in relationships had much less non-monogamous sex than did gay men: 28 per cent versus 82 per cent. And of those lesbians who did stray from monogamy, fully 53 per cent had only a single outside relationship, versus 7 per cent of gay men. The facts add up to a kind of staggering lesbian sexual timidity, at least compared with gay men.[100] Even somebody like Judy Grahn, an important lesbian poet and certainly no shrinking violet, said that lesbians don't trick (the gay male expression for making pickups) but rather have serial monogamy. In her fantasies, she said, she'd adore to be 'sucked for the seventh time in one night by a seventh handsome dyke – if only to know what that experience could possibly feel like.' But the reality in 1984, when Grahn, age forty-four, wrote those lines, was that 'whores can trick and faggots can trick, but not dykes.'[101]

Why not? Here we see the influence of a thousand years of modesty on women. What would she wear, Grahn pondered, as she backed up against a tree in Washington Square Park in Manhattan? A kilt? 'How could I display myself erotically to strangers with clothes that place emphasis on my genitals and hips and breasts without attracting men instead of women? No, it cannot be done in this society.'[102] In the 1980s, lesbians weren't yet going to bathhouses.

Since the 1980s there is some evidence that lesbian women have started to cast off the shackles of modesty. Of course the height of immodesty, in a manner of speaking, is the bathhouse, where everybody is naked and feeling sensual. It is therefore of interest that a lesbian bathnight scene has been developing. In 1991 novelist Jane DeLynn commented, 'There are [lesbian] baths now in San Francisco, and backrooms. I don't like to have sex standing up and in the space of five minutes so it's not for me, but I think that's where lesbians are going right now.'[103] In Toronto, one club began offering bathhouse all-nights for lesbians in 1998, the events proving 'wildly popular.' The pre-event tickets for a bathnight that was raided by the police in September 2000 had been sold out in ten minutes.[104] In Seattle, the South End Steam Baths had routinely offered 'Lesbian Night' until 1999, when the baths were torn down.[105]

DeLynn is not untypical of a whole new generation of lesbian women whose sexuality is just as unconstrained as anyone else's. 'I have slept with a lot of women,' she said, 'virtually all of them on the first date or the first night I met them. There are plenty of people who will sleep with you right away and the pretense that they don't is nuts.'[106]

Indeed, after the 1980s the lesbian scene radiated sexual vigour, in contrast to the rather prim, business-suited lesbian images of the early days. Said Lynn Flipper in 1996, a member of the San Francisco 'all-dyke band' Tribe 8 ('Tribade'), 'Right now there's a lot of sexual energy in the dyke community. Everyone's having sex all the time. Maybe their relationships suffer, but this is a whole new world for dykes.'

So lesbians have only recently, but rapidly, been bringing their sexual behaviour into line with the American mainstream, behaviour that older generations might have qualified as promiscuity but that now is merely thought of as 'going for it.'

What lesbians do in bed has been melding with the mainstream as well, in the form of large, recent increases in the various forms of total body sex. Oral sex was once shunned by most lesbians. Said Grahn of the West Texas college town where she came of age in the late 1950s, 'We knew about cunnilingus, though only the boldest among us practiced it.' Even after Grahn broke through this barrier with her girlfriend Von, it would take the 'freewheeling, loudmouthed sixties' to free both of them up enough to use such expressions as 'eat each other out.'[107] Within the world of working-class lesbians in Buffalo, New York, oral sex had just started to become accepted in the 1950s, and the ideal of the unmoved, untouchable 'stone butch' still held sway in which lesbian sex meant tribadism (mutual rubbing of pelvises) or the butch masturbating the femme.[108]

In the 1960s, oral and anal sex started to become quite popular among lesbians as the old butch-femme roles were put on the shelf and both partners turned into hippies. By the time of the Jay-Young poll in the mid-1970s, 57 per cent of all lesbian respondents were practising oral sex 'always' or 'very frequently.'[109] By 1995, in a poll in the magazine *The Advocate*, this figure was up to 75 per cent.[110]

What about lesbians and the anus? In the Jay-Young poll, 12 per cent said that their partner stimulated their anus 'always' or 'very frequently,' and a further 14 per cent said 'somewhat frequently.'[111] This means that by the 1970s over a quarter of all lesbians in the United States (if the poll was representative) had broken through the strong anal taboo that had hung over lesbianism for centuries. Yet the language of the taboo still clung to *The Advocate*'s survey in 1995. The editors tell us that 'More than half will neither perform nor receive anilingus, and almost as many express dislike of anal penetration.'[112] (But is the glass half-empty or half-full?)

Much higher rates of anal sex were reported among Norwegian lesbians: in a random sample of 10,000 people in 1987, 48 per cent of the bisexual lesbians were having anal sex on a lifespan basis, and 14 per cent of the heterosexual women.[113]

A sort of epiphany in the lesbian anal sex story was achieved in 1998 when Tristan Taormino – herself a lesbian and editor of *On Our Backs* – published *The Ultimate Guide to Anal Sex for Women* and followed it with a how-to video featuring 'Buttman,' who, camera in hand, did street interviews convincing pedestrians (porn actresses) to show him their tits and ass and then to rendezvous on the video set for the main bill. So unconventional did the theme seem to many porno producers that Taormino initially had difficulty commissioning her video. Yet it turned out a great hit among female viewers.[114]

Just as for effeminate gays, the post-1960s world represented a major defeat for the butch-femme system. These particular roles became scorned by lesbian feminists, who insisted that all should be equal and that the bulldyke with her 'D.A.' hairdo and sturdy oxfords belonged to the dustbin of history's sexist stereotypes. Middle-class lesbians shrank away from the bulldyke image just as they cringed at the fighting butches in the working-class bars and at dildoes. Throughout the 1970s and 1980s the butches sank down, as Joan Nestle put it, to 'the Uncle Toms of the movement.'[115]

Yet many women retained a feeling that their butch and femme instincts were biologically based, else this theme could not have been so enduring in lesbian history – nor so strongly felt by those involved. According to Nestle, 'The saddest irony of all behind this misjudgment of femmes [as carica-tures of femininity] is that for many of us it has been a lifelong journey to take pleasure in our bodies.' When Nestle spoke at a meeting of feminist health workers at the Stony Brook campus of the State University of New York in 1982, she wore 'a long lavender dress that made my body feel good and high, black boots that made me feel powerful.' Standing there in the face of the hostile stares of the new-style femi-nists, Nestle noted that it took a certain courage for her to express, and embody, a form of lesbianism that everybody else wished abolished but that she herself felt very deeply. She said later, 'The butch-femme tradition is one of the oldest in lesbian culture.'[116]

In fact, like effeminacy in gays, the butch-femme style did not die out but merely went on the back burner for a couple of decades. In the Jay-Young poll of the late 1970s, fully a quarter of the respondents said that they felt 'very positive' or 'somewhat positive' about their partners' dressing in 'drag butch clothing.'[117] In the 1990s, observers considered that the butch-femme duo were bouncing back on stage again. A 1989–90 survey of 589 lesbians across the United States identified 15 per cent as butch, 18 per cent as femme, and the rest as androgynous or 'none of the above.'[118] Yet what really happened in the world of lesbian lifestyle dress was not the return of the D.A. and oxfords, but the triumph of the leather-woman, the symbol of strong lesbian women for the early twenty-first century.[119]

To wrap up: two millennia of the history of desire, begin-ning in Christian Europe and ending provisionally in our own time, have pushed straights, gays, and lesbians all re-morselessly in the same direction. All began the story with their sexuality crumpled and curtailed by the church, by community regulation, and by centuries-old edicts against

bodily pleasure that inhibited homosexuals from experimenting just as effectively as heterosexuals. Then the anonymity
of urban life, the decline of the power of small-town convention, and the societal acceptance of hedonic behaviour late in
the nineteenth century permitted an initial breakout from
this thousand-year prison. But the spectacular drive towards
total body sex involving all zones of the body would accelerate only in the 1960s and rush past the year 2000 with all the
players – gays, lesbians, and heterosexual men and women –
finding new forms of pleasure in exactly the same ways. In
terms of the erotic potential of the body, the differences among
the sexual orientations have become trivial. All respond now
to the same deep neural drives.

CHAPTER NINE

SM and Fetish

This penultimate chapter is really a bit of an aside, but an interesting one in the history of desire. What is now called role playing, formerly sadomasochism, has never been more than a sidebar in the history of sexuality, but it is a theme whose parallelism to the main narrative is arresting. The SM story begins with a kind of monochrome flogging comparable to the missionary position or buggery as the single main sexual outlet. Then towards 1900 new sources of sexual expression arrive in the SM world, namely fetish – though fetish also has a life of its own unrelated to SM – together with a new interest in the zones of the body. Finally, in our own time SM revels in total body themes just as straights, gays, and lesbians in general have done. This tangent into SM-fetish is therefore not entirely without interest.

In the fall of 1992, Milan designer Gianni Versace stood musing before a reporter. He had just launched his collection of 'S&M dresses,' as the fashion press called them. Versace sniffed at the notion that there was anything especially sexual about them: 'I'd be very rich if I was sexy. If I give this to you,' he said, stroking his black leather vest, 'and you are a beautiful woman, you're still a beautiful woman. If you're ugly, you're still ugly. If I could give sex with this vest, I'd be the emperor of magic clothing.'[1]

But for many it *was* magic clothing.

On the sexual scene today, there has been a huge proliferation of leather fetishism and consensual sadomasochism, Versace's own personal interests. This comes almost out of the blue. The sexual orientations themselves go back for thousands of years and doubtless emerged in the human condition in the course of evolution. But fetish is quite new, and one is hard-pressed to document a history of SM going back more than a few centuries. What is today the main fetish, leather, was simply not on the sexual radar before 1900; nor does its appeal rest upon some imputed quality of the hide itself such as its scent or its 'animal' feel. Latex rubber shares today a similar popularity and has neither of these qualities. As for SM, once considered a hideous perversion, it is now accepted as a more or less legitimate band of the sexual spectrum and is called in polite circles role playing because people do not really hurt one another in the sense of causing tissue damage. The comparison with homosexuality – once also deemed a ghastly perversion and now counted as a normal aspect of human sexuality – is quite interesting.

The SM-Fetish Package

What is arresting about the SM-fetish package is its parallelism to the larger story of total body sex. Originally, the vernacular of SM was limited largely to flogging, just as heterosexuality focused on vaginal intercourse and gay-male sexuality on buggery. Then early in the twentieth century, in the great breakout from the thousand-year carapace of limited sexual expression, SM began to imply a consensual relationship in which the partners switch roles of dominant ('top') and submissive ('bottom') back and forth and use the whole format as a means of experimenting with the issue of control rather than pain. In the 1920s and 1930s, leather appears within the SM relationship and in non-SM relationships as well, perhaps as a way of bringing all the parts of the body together into a single visual and sensual whole. This is a correlate of total body sex: leather gear emphasizes the erotic unity of the entire body, from the hood of the dominatrix or the leather officer's cap of the lesbian top, to the gloved hands of the whip-wielding mistress and the booted feet of the gay Castro Street clone. It is precisely during the accelera-tion towards total body sex that SM themes and leather cos-tumes come to occupy significant portions of bandwidth for straights, gays, and lesbians alike. This chapter discusses only straights, but parallel developments might be noted for gays and lesbians.

Historically, the terms 'masochism' and 'sadism' have been used in three entirely different ways. At one level, sadism means gratuitous cruelty and masochism means a witless inability to look after one's own self-interest, as in the 'sadis-tic prison guards' or the 'masochist' partner in a relationship who is trod upon. Neither of these uses has anything to do with sexual desire. As the late-nineteenth-century English sexologist Havelock Ellis said, 'Any impulse of true cruelty is almost outside the field [of love and pain] altogether.'[2]

At a second level, sadism and masochism mean certain kinds of deep intrapsychic processes first described by Sigmund Freud and considered by psychoanalysts to be vir-tually universal in the human condition. According to Freud, masochism represented the 'punishment for the sense of guilt associated with forbidden Oedipal wishes' (boys' desire to possess their mothers). And sadism suggested the directing outward of the death instinct under the orchestration of the sex drive.[3] As personality components that virtually every-one would have, SM in Freudian terms stood for something far broader than sexual practices. In Ellis's view, all men tended to delight in domination, all women in submission, again a generalization (certainly false, moreover) about the human condition that made little reference to what happened in bed.[4]

At a third level, sadism and masochism – today's role playing – mean the consensual exchange of power in a sexual relationship, in which pleasure derives not from inflicting pain but from the absolute control over another human be-ing, though it is a dominion temporally limited and agreed to in advance. Or pleasure may come equally from the feeling of being controlled. According to Thomas S. Weinberg and G.W. Levi Kamel, among the few academic experts on this subject, 'At the very core of sadomasochism is not pain but the idea of control – dominance and submission.'[5] This is the level of SM that is described in this chapter, though the consensual element may have been somewhat attenuated in the more distant past (before the passage of legislation on assault).

'If we're talking about an SM relationship,' said novelist Kathy Acker in an interview early in the 1990s, 'the ones I know about are just *play*, really, which means if there's some pain it's "scratch" pain ... a little play with dangerous weapons – toys! ... You're curious about your body – how will your body react to this? And it's not only just pain, it's also how you react in terms of being *controlled*.'[6] So control, not pain, is the subject of this chapter.

We might think of the SM-leather package as a kind of 'overlay' on the three main sexual orientations, an additional dimension that rests on top of the basic sexuality of some people within the orientation, though by no means all. Basic biological sexuality acquires such overlays from time to time. One might think of romantic love as an overlay, present at some times during history but quite absent during others. In family life before the eighteenth century, sexuality generally functioned in the absence of romantic love; likewise in the gay scene at the baths today.[7] Another kind of overlay is the doctrine that the partners in a union should be of similar ages. That certainly came to prevail in the nineteenth and twentieth centuries, unlike in the world we have lost. Yet it was quite untrue for the man-adolescent homosexuality of fifteenth-century Florence or ancient Greece. A third sort of overlay is leather fetish and consensual SM – today a massive presence in the sexual scene; yet fetish was virtually unknown before the late nineteenth century, and SM was not visible before the Renaissance. How did the SM-fetish package become so huge?

SM and fetish are actually quite separate concepts, though

they may intertwine. Getting a sexual rush from the sight of oneself geared out before the mirror is not the same thing as restraining one's partner. Yet as overlays they fit together as a pair. What is germane for the larger story of total body sex is that SM exquisitely *enacts* sex over the entire body while fetish *represents* the entire body in a thematic way.

Here an English rubber fetishist, whose tastes were formed in the 1960s, describes what it is exactly that appeals: 'Features for which the fetishist demand is considerable are: high and tight collars, back-fastening straps, buckles and laces; very tight fittings in general ... complete head and face coverings, corsets and waist "cinchers." The fetishist likes to be encased, covered up, and protected ...' An SM theme is apparent as well, the author stipulating that the genitals may be 'difficult of access or, on the contrary, fully exposed.'[8] Evident is the fact that SM-fetish represents an overlay on the wearer's basic sexuality: whether straight, lesbian, or gay remains unchanged. In each sexual orientation, the overlay speaks to the total body.

Where does SM-fetish come from? Does it represent some biological drive? Or are SM and fetish part of the new empowerment that women, for example, have received under feminism, a kind of warrant for the political success in bed of the new woman?[9] This is the same kind of biology versus social-construction dilemma that has bothered us at other points. One thing is clear: any behaviour that appears historically only in the last several hundred years cannot possibly be biological in the sense that one's sexual orientation is, or it would have been known in all times and places, like homosexuality. Yet the players perceive SM-fetish as biological indeed. They believe it to be inborn, so powerfully do they experience these desires in adult life.

In the very first case of SM on record, a friend of the Italian scholar Giovanni Pico della Mirandola in the fifteenth century told Pico that he liked his wife to flog him (see below); the friend also demonstrated this belief in biology, telling Pico that it was 'a taste I acquired as a child,' meaning that at no point was he not aware of it.[10] In John Cleland's eighteenth-century novel *Fanny Hill*, Mrs Cole, the madam, considered flagellation to be an inborn taste; she referred to 'those unhappy persons who are under a subjection they cannot shake off, those arbitrary tastes that rule their appetites of pleasure with an unaccountable control.'[11] The late-nineteenth-century sexologists mainly believed fetish and SM to be inborn tastes. German psychiatrist Paul Näcke posited a biological predisposition for both; French psychiatrist Paul Garnier believed that SM constituted evidence of inborn 'degeneration,' and the more moderate Havelock Ellis thought that a taste for these things resulted from 'a congenital predisposition.'[12] The belief is common today in the SM subculture that, as one group of investigators put it, 'sadomasochistic interests are "natural ones" from childhood, that is, that they are the earliest sexual thoughts that can be remembered.'[13] That so many people think something is so, of course, does not necessarily make it so. Yet the prospect is intriguing that in this area as well nature may have her grip.

Men and Women in Traditional SM

When does this overlay on the various sexual orientations first appear? Whether sexual sadism and masochism are part of the human condition – an added dimension as old as the hills – or whether they are recent add-ons, is an important question. One theme in the SM world does go back hundreds if not thousands of years: flogging. A whole host of refinements then starts to be added on around the turn of the twentieth century. The comparison to the development of the three sexual orientations themselves is striking, for the missionary position similarly limited sexual expression among regular heterosexuals for centuries, and buggery that of gays. An identical constriction of hedonic possibilities in the SM overlay would suggest that the whole picture of basics-plus-overlay does indeed possess a kind of underlying organic unity.

The ancient world, in any event, is out of consideration. Scholars have uncovered virtually no examples of SM in either the Greek or the Roman worlds, discounting the gratuitous cruelty with which the sources abound. John Boswell believes that the Roman emperor Nero was 'possibly the sole classical example of a person indulging in what is now called sadomasochism,' although the example Boswell adduces – Nero dressing up in wild-animal skins and 'attacking' the private parts of men and women bound to stakes – sounds more like assault than sex play.[14]

Flagellation for religious reasons occurred extensively during the Middle Ages, the monks and nuns thrashing each other to achieve penitence before prayers. Possibly this occurred against some dark sexual background that has not survived in the sources. Yet as far as anyone can tell, this religious flagellation had no immediate sexual associations; it was certainly not seen as a source of sex play or interpreted by others as erotic. As Ellis observes, if there had been an association with sexuality, 'this form of penance would not have been approved or at all events tolerated by the Church.'[15]

The first references to sexual flagellation of which the present author is aware begin in the fifteenth century. Elector Albrecht of Brandenburg was said to have 'a tolerant wife, who not only accepted his orgies but enthusiastically participated.' She also participated in his efforts to 'pepper' the participants, his code word for whipping. The day after Christmas 1474, he wrote to her, 'We'll save up the pepper until I get home. If your butt's got big, you're really going to get it ... You whip the virgins good for me, and strike them firmly so that they think of me. If God vouchsafes me a safe return, I'm going to whip you soundly with young Albert [his code word for penis]. Young Albert really wants to get big.'[16] A few years later, in 1495, Pico della Mirandola described the above-mentioned friend of his who, in order to have sex, had to plead with his wife to flagellate him with a whip prepared in advance with vinegar; the more strongly she hit, the more he became excited. 'Moreover,' said Pico, the friend 'was in other aspects not a wicked man and recognized and detested this ailment of his.'[17] These are the earliest cases of erotic flogging on record.

Beginning late in the seventeenth century, references to prostitutes flogging their male clients – or being whipped by them – start to abound. By 1698, a group of London men had formed a club, the Flogging Cullies ('cull' meaning testicles), in which they paid women to come in and cane them.[18] There was a huge subculture of flagellation among the prostitutes of London in the eighteenth century, the clients playing both passive and active roles.[19]

Although SM was not well represented among the prostitutes of eighteenth-century Paris, some did have it on offer, such as a woman named Bourgeois, who advertised herself in 1791 as 'a vigorous person, her lashes are the lashes of a master.' La Chassaigne, by contrast, presented herself as a bottom, 'a tender victim, always open to the lashes of the master and never gets enough.'[20] Louise in the rue Mézières ran a proper whipping salon, 'excellent for those of delicate sensibilities. Mature individuals, who from a desire for penitence or for other reasons want to macerate their flesh, are sure to find here a complete assortment of whips.' Mme Richard supervised a similar house: with a full array of the SM high tech of the day, it was reserved for members of the clergy.[21] It is clear, then, that by the beginning of the nineteenth century, whipping had established itself as the main and perhaps sole practice in the SM repertoire.

At the level of fantasy, the predominance of whipping emerges with even greater clarity in pornography and erotic fiction. In Nicolas Chorier's *Dialogues on the Arcana of Love and Venus*, published around 1660, a leering cleric gets set to 'speedily discharge the pious duty' of whipping Sempronia at the altar, with a whip that she just happened to have in her petticoats. Tullia says reflectively upon hearing of the cleric's plans, 'As pain borders on pleasure, so pleasure borders on pain.' And indeed, moments later Chorier has Tullia herself eager to try the thrills of flagellation.[22]

Johann A.G. Kirsten's 1778 German pornographic novel, 'Lottchen's Trip to Jail,' featuring flogging in a women's prison, inspired W. Reinhard's 1840 work, 'Lenchen in Jail,' written in the sanctimonious tones of social protest but featuring male and female warders flagellating their female charges. Reinhard's story in turn became translated into English as the flagellation classic *Nell in Bridewell*.[23]

So predominant was flogging in SM that even when the pornographers had a chance to involve other body zones they didn't take advantage of it. In the *Letters from Lady Termagant Flaybum, of Birch-Grove, to Lady Harriet Tickletail, of Bumfiddle-Hall*, published late in the eighteenth century and set partly in France, a gentleman comes on to a young lady and explains how fond he is of 'being whipt by a lovely woman. This was an amusement the lady had no objection to, as it was quite common in her country.' When they are alone, she strips him to his shirt, lays him across her lap, pulls up his shirt to his shoulders, and gives him fifty of the best. He turns around and exhibits his 'tarriwags [balls],' which she takes in hand and plays with; then the scene ends.[24] There's no deep kissing, no nipple play. Later generations of pornographers would not have let the opportunity go unused to feature the rest of the body in an SM skit.

John Cleland's *Fanny Hill*, written in 1748, offers one of the best-known flagellation scenes in eighteenth-century literature, yet the erotic scope is as narrow as any other aspect of eighteenth-century sexuality. Fanny first whips a client's back until he reaches orgasm. He then flogs her back lightly, whips her perineum, performs cunnilingus, then administers a graver whipping to her backside. He ignores completely her naked breasts and all other body parts.[25] SM here has been completely reduced to the simple act of whipping.

The apotheosis of SM in erotic literature comes, ironically enough, not at the end of this chain of developments but in the middle. It is the Marquis de Sade, who appears like a great shooting star around 1800; but rather than setting the pace for a newly sensual SM, his themes then slumber in invisibility for the next hundred years, to emerge again towards 1900. Donatien Alphonse François, Count de Sade, had already been in prisons and asylums for many years when in 1791, at age fifty-one, he wrote *Justine*, and seven years later 'The Story of Juliette.' Sade is important in the history of SM for two reasons: one, he discovers the concept of total body sex; two, he understands that the erotic thrill is not the infliction of pain but the exchange of power. Mainly on the basis of what happens to Justine in his novel *Justine or the Misfortunes of Virtue*, Sade has received his lumps from subsequent generations as an unspeakably violent sadist. And it is true that poor Justine does get whacked about a bit (although let's not forget that these are allegories, not true accounts of events, or even masturbatory fantasies; unfortunately Richard von Krafft-Ebing, who popularized the term 'sadism,' wouldn't have recognized an allegory had it hit him on the nose). But Justine had a mirror image: Juliette. And just as Justine was weak, piteous, and victimized, Juliette was strong, self-confident, and utterly determined to inflict her will upon men. She was, in other words, history's first dominatrix.

It's in seeing Juliette and the novel's other female leads, such as Clairwil and Durand, as autonomous pleasure lovers that we understand the exchange-of-power element in SM that so fascinated Sade. The thrill lay in absolute control over the other players, not in being able to torture them as such. At one point Clairwil tells Juliette, 'Ah! My angel. It's just delicious to be the master over the lives of others.'

Juliette replies, 'It's totally true that this is a better thrill than [orgies], because, at the very moment that you started talking to me about this plan [poisoning potential sex partners], I felt my nerves quiver ... and I'm sure that if you were to touch me you'd see me all moist.'[26]

In another scene, one of Juliette and Durand's victims has an orgasm. Durand berates the girl, saying, 'The duty of a victim is to make herself available. She must never expect to share any pleasure.'[27] For Sade, the basic rule of SM was quite clear: the pleasure for the top lay in the certain knowledge that he or she had absolute control over the bottom.

(It would be decades before anyone picked up the point again that SM was about the symbolic, later the consensual, exercise of power, not about pain. In fact, the next writer to bring this to the public's attention was the Viennese psychiatrist Richard von Krafft-Ebing in his best-selling treatise on sex 'pathology,' as he conceived it, *Psychopathia sexualis*, originally published in 1886. By the 1902 edition he had come to the conclusion that, 'It is precisely the concept of submissiveness, which represents the active as well as the passive core of this perverse taste.')[28]

Second, Sade anticipated the notion of total body sex in the SM domain. For Juliette, it begins as she is admitted to a nunnery, where Mother Superior Delbène sets the tone. Juliette asks, 'O dear Sister, isn't it true that the more clear-headed one is, the more one delights in the pleasures of sex?'

'Assuredly,' Delbène replies. 'And the reason for that is quite simple. Sex doesn't accept any limits. You never get off better than when you've broken all the barriers. Now, the more clear-headed you are, the more you break with all restraints. Thus the man with a fresh mind will always be more accepting than anybody else of the pleasures of libertinage.'[29]

Mother Superior Delbène, Juliette, and another woman then embark on a threesome that involves cunnilingus, masturbation, and anilingus. Delbène praises the women's backsides and spanks them, 'causing us to just die with pleasure,' says Juliette. Later scenes involve multiple partners engaged in anal sex as well as oral sex, masturbation, and whipping.[30] All the players participate in the orgies with their entire bodies. The revolutionary nature of Sade's take on SM as an experience involving the whole body, not just the brutish flogging of someone's backside, is amply evident from this material. It's an interesting commentary that his work was found so subversive it was banned for decades in virtually every jurisdiction in which it was translated. It became, quite wrongly, emblematic of horror and despair, a virtual charnel-house of the human spirit. Of course many scenes end with everyone dead except Juliette and her accomplices – as in numerous other works of Sade's. Yet Sade conceived those parts as social allegories, not as stroke manuals, and the celebration of the physicality of SM itself in Sade has survived across the decades to make him, in our own time, a fashionable figure. This may not be everybody's cup of tea, of course, but neither is homosexuality.

The women in Sade's novels, it goes without saying, belong to the male pornographic imagination. Yet in the real world as well, women have had a long though very subterranean involvement with SM. With women, however, we encounter a more diverse picture than whipping. Among the very few historical references are Brantôme's sixteenth-century recollections of his mondaine female friends. He was discussing with them the question of who's on top in bed. The law of nature, said Brantôme, dictates that women should accept their subordination in bed. But there are women who respond, 'Yes, OK. I confess that you're supposed to feel glorious when you have me underneath you and have subdued me. But also, when it pleases me and if the man does not insist on always being on top, I take the top role for fun or a gentle whimsy that I might have, and not because I must. Moreover, when your supremacy doesn't appeal to me, I shall have you serve me like a galley slave, or even better, make you strain against your harness like a true cart horse, and have you – labouring, struggling, sweating, panting – trying to perform the corvées and tasks that I impose on you.'

Brantôme recalled another 'beautiful and worthy woman' whose husband awoke her from a deep sleep in order to have sex with him. After he'd come, she said to him, 'You got off but I haven't.' Continued Brantôme, 'Then, because she was above him, she tied up well his arms, hands, feet and legs.'

She said, 'I'll teach you not to wake me up again.' Then she gave the husband, who was still beneath her, a sound shaking and beating until he cried mercy. Then she made him get erect again 'despite himself, and rendered him so tired, so attenuated and flaccid that he was out of breath ...'[31]

The sexual power of women over men was not an unfamiliar rhetorical theme. The sixteenth-century Lyon poet Pernette du Guillet once fantasized about symbolically assailing her lover while she romped naked in a fountain:

> Entirely naked, I'd leap into the water
> But if he came straight toward me,
> I'd let him approach me boldly.
> And if he wanted to touch me, however slightly,
> I'd throw a handful, at the least,
> Of the clear fountain's pure water
> Straight into his eyes, or at his face.[32]

This is not exactly SM, but it's the allegorical equivalent thereof.

We come closer to women on top with the art of the Swiss-English painter Henry Fuseli late in the eighteenth century. In the 1770s he pencilled a sketch of 'Mistress and Slave' in which a severe-looking woman stands behind a muscular, bound man kneeling before her with an erect penis. In the same decade Fuseli produced another drawing of a man lying on a slab, feet bound to posts and hands bound atop his chest. One woman tongue kisses him; another at his side manipulates his penis. Both women are naked and highly muscular, as is the man.[33]

Turn-of-the-Century SM

Just as the range of sensuality in general had become greatly expanded by the turn of the century, that of SM had as well. It becomes a more nuanced kind of interaction than simple flogging, and subtle psychological exchanges of power come to take the place of the bottom lashed to the bench.

Commoner, too. By the last decades of the nineteenth century, SM had evidently become familiar enough in real life that it started spilling into art and medical practice. Zola in his 1880 novel makes Nana a kind of proto-dominatrix as she puts poor Muffat through his paces. They had started out playing 'bear' on the rug of her room and gnawing at each other's ankles. Then a kind of furor of sensuality overcame them. 'One day, when [Muffat] was playing bear, she pushed him so abruptly that he fell against a piece of furniture and ended up with a bruise on his forehead. From that time on ... she treated him like an animal, whipping him, persecuting him with kicks.

'"Gee up! Gee up! You're a horse. Whoaaa! Fucking horse, can't you move!"'

On other days, he might be a dog. She would throw her perfumed handkerchief across the room, and on his hands and knees he had to run and pick it up with his teeth. Then one evening she had the idea of making him dress up in an official outfit that he had and took him out in public, laughing at him and kicking him in the Tuileries gardens. Back in her room, she ordered him to undress, and as the suit lay about the room, 'she cried at him to jump, and he jumped; she cried at him to spit, and he spat; she cried at him to walk all over the gold braid, the epaulettes, and the medals, and he did.'[34] Zola saw Nana and her behaviour as the embodiment of evil, yet others might interpret it as role playing, she the top, he the bottom, acting out a scene that, in the end, gave them both pleasure.

By the 1890s, SM had apparently become so frequent that Krafft-Ebing was seeing patients in his practice who had psychiatric disorders and who were also given over to role playing, or sex-play masochism, or whatever (which is how these practices became medicalized, or, if one will, psychiatrized. People who do them show up for other reasons in doctors' offices and the doctors, appalled at stories they never learned about in medical school, make the behaviour itself the diagnosis. This is precisely how homosexuality became a 'medical' condition for about a hundred years). In 1891 Krafft-

Ebing interpreted 'masochism' in women to mean 'voluntary submissiveness of the fair sex as a physiological phenomenon.' The evidence? 'Beneath the varnish of our salon manners, women's instinct for servitude is visible everywhere.' One of Krafft-Ebing's patients, a woman of twenty-one, fantasized continually about 'being the slave of her lover; as he punishes her, she desires to kiss his feet.' Or she fantasized about being admitted to a private nervous clinic where, as she had heard elsewhere, the director might pull her from bed by the hair and flagellate her, or 'the coarse, untrained female orderlies will punish me mercilessly.'[35]

Krafft-Ebing also allowed it was possible – though totally perverse – for a man to submit to the will of what Krafft-Ebing was calling a 'Domina,' a woman who towered over him sexually: 'There is no doubt that the masochist feels himself in a passive, feminine role in the face of the Domina, and that his sexual satisfaction is dependent on the success of the illusion of submission to the will of the Domina.'[36] The tremendous commercial success of *Psychopathia sexualis*, first published in 1886[37] then followed by many successive editions, made the terms 'masochism' and 'sadism' household words.

As for England, in 1903 Havelock Ellis said that 'the love of active flagellation, and sadistic impulses generally, are not uncommon among [English women].' He found that in 'normal' sadism – meaning sex play – 'it is nearly always the male who is the victim of the female.'[38] Ellis had interviewed a large number of people about their sex lives, and such a judgment is interesting.

SM positively pullulates at the fin-de-siècle. In 1909, as James Joyce gathered material for *Ulysses* (serial publication of which began in March 1918), he toyed with SM fantasies. On 13 December he wrote to his wife, Nora, 'I am your child as I told you and you must be severe with me, my little mother. Punish me as much as you like. I would be delighted to feel my flesh tingling under your hand. Do you know what I mean, Nora dear? I wish you would smack me or flog me even.' Joyce then developed the fantasy of wishing that Nora were a big strong woman, and that he perhaps had committed some offence, and she would call him into her room, where he would find her sitting 'with your fat thighs far apart and your face deep red with anger and a cane in your hand.' Then she would tear off his clothes, tug him into her lap 'until your big full bubbies almost touched me and [I would] feel you flog, flog, flog me viciously on my naked quivering flesh.' So obscene did this fantasy seem to Richard Ellmann, the editor of the Joyce papers, that Ellmann omitted it from the first two-volume edition and inserted it only in a later selection of Joyce's letters.[39]

In *Ulysses*, the protagonist Bloom shows a taste for SM at various points, as women threaten to flog and humiliate him, and Bella Cohen, the brothel madam, rides about on him horseback. (By this point Bloom has been magically changed into a woman and 'Bello' Cohen into a man.) Bello tells Bloom of his enslavement: 'By day you will souse and bat our smelling underclothes, also when we ladies are unwell, and swab out our latrines with dress pinned up and a dishclout tied to your tail. Won't that be nice? (*[Bello] places a ruby ring on [Bloom's] finger.*) And there now! With this ring I thee own. Say, thank you, mistress.'

Bloom: 'Thank you, mistress.'[40]

In Germany, SM had become sufficiently common by 1900 that the Berlin newspapers were full of ads on behalf of male bottoms seeking female tops: 'Strict disciplinarian sought for an older lad. Women who are familiar with English discipline will receive preference.' Or, 'A gentleman, 37, with weak character, seeks marriage with a lady of strict, dominant nature.'[41]

In an astonishing autobiography, a Viennese schoolteacher named Edith Cadivec related her experiences with SM around the time of the First World War. Like Donald Vining or Anne Lister, she was an absolutely unexceptional person, but she happened to get caught abusing her pupils in the private boarding school in Vienna of which she was headmistress, and in 1924 became the object of a sensational trial. Full of indignation after serving a six-year sentence, in the early 1930s she published a two-volume autobiography. Although she was basically lesbian, she did have one encounter with a man, Franzl, because she wanted a child. She met him through a newspaper ad in 1909, and she was the top: 'My dominating will had power over this man. I took his body and his soul as an object belonging to me and made them erotically serviceable and subject to me. Franzl became wholly an object of my sexual desires ... wait[ing] only to be taken by the authoritarian woman to whom he will-lessly subjected himself ... He became a component part of my self and obeyed blindly.' She proceeds to describe how she forced him to cross-dress, whipped him, and directed him to delay orgasms until she had one.[42]

In the United States in these years, novelist Theodore Dreiser was only a bit surprised when his girlfriend Helen Richardson pulled 'spanking and beating' out of her bag of tricks. It was on Monday, 25 October 1920, in Los Angeles, that Dreiser started to discover that the twenty-year-old had 'a streak of perversion in her.' On the following day, Helen 'outlines her scheme for extracting more bliss out of sex. Is to get me girls & watch me manhandle them.'[43] Months later, 'We play about in a most delicious fashion before getting up. Helen beats me with one of her pink wool slippers and I finally spank her.' We are a long way from flogging here: SM is being kneaded onto a turn-of-the-century sensuousness that is vastly expanded from a hundred years previously.

Given that SM and fetish are attached to their hosts' main sexual orientations, you would expect to see them undergo the same transmutations that the hosts experience. In fact that seems to be true, although the evidence is so thin that nothing like a time series is possible. Over the years, SM seems to become much more complex behaviour than simple flogging, embracing the entire body in the way that the host orientations migrate towards total body sex. Particularly when the women top the men, they indulge, like Nana, in elaborate scenes or, like Edith Cadivec, in scenarios that extend for hours or indeed permeate the entire lifestyle. Classical SM, however, received a kind of swan song from a woman whose sexuality was minted in the 1920s and 1930s, Dominique Aury, the author of *The Story of O*. Aury, born in 1907, had been involved in an affair with Paris publisher Jean Paulhan. Fearing that she was losing Paulhan – and knowing that Paulhan was 'an admirer of the Marquis de Sade' – in the early 1950s she endeavoured to rekindle his ardour by writing an SM novel. It was published in 1954, under the pen name Pauline Réage, as *The Story of O*. An interviewer coaxed from her the admission that she drew also upon her own erotic fantasies, begun during a lonely childhood. She didn't see the bondage and discipline scenes in *O* as male fantasies: 'All I know is that they were honest fantasies,' she said. Intriguingly, in another, literary work of her own she had defined 'love' very much in exchange-of-power terms as 'the spectacle of the total possession of one person by another, without any sense, reason or justice.'[44] And this exchange of power, the total surrender of one person to another, remained the classical red thread of SM.

Although *O* was hailed as a spectacular breakthrough into Eros by a woman writer, it represented, in fact, a continuation of themes at least four hundred years old: the psychological subjugation of one person by another, physical confinement, special gear, flogging – themes current in SM since Brantôme and Sade. 'It was the sex [penis] that O saw first, then the whip ... the whip was stuck in his belt, then she noticed that the man was masked in a black hood completed by a section of black gauze hiding his eyes ...'[45] Insiders would perhaps have noticed the continuity. But for the reading public the revelation of a woman possessing this kind of fantasy life was sensational. In four decades *The Story of O* has never been out of print; at a point in the 1960s it was the most widely read French contemporary novel outside of France. Translated into two-dozen languages, it sold millions of copies.[46]

But there was one curious note in *O* not representative of

the previous SM tradition. At some point another bottom named Jacqueline is brought into the scene. Jacqueline was dressed wearing a golden choker and two golden wrist bracelets. 'O caught herself in the midst of imagining that she'd be lovelier with a collar and with bracelets of leather.'[47]

Fetish

Fetishes are mechanical contrivances that add to the enjoyment of sex. 'Mechanical' may be understood as a piece of clothing or a technique of restraint, something that nature itself does not originally bring to the sex scene. The origins of a taste for fetish are obscure: once-popular psychoanalytic theories about fetish as a way of compensating for castration anxiety are now widely discredited (many women turn out to be just as interested in fetish as men). As in SM, fetish fanciers themselves often incline towards biological explanations, for the fetish grips them so strongly it seems as though inborn. Although fetish often overlaps with SM, the two are certainly not coterminous, and today many friends of fetish have little interest in the exchange of power. It is harder, today, to find SM enthusiasts who are not partial to leather in some way, if only as techniques of restraint. Yet historically, SM existed for centuries with no hint of fetish involvement: there is, to the author's knowledge, not a single reference to leather in the works of the Marquis de Sade.

Fetish seems to arise in the last quarter of the nineteenth century and the first of the twentieth, exactly at the time of the initial breakout from the sexual narrowness of Christian Europe, a theme often visited in these pages. Clearly, the growing interest in fetish was related to the increasing sensualization of sex of those years, part and parcel of the beginning of total body sex. If we search for the origin of fetish, it fits somehow into the experience of total body sex, and with leather it fits ideally. Yet fetish does not begin with leather.

Before 1870, there were of course other reported instances of fetishes. Nicolas Restif de la Bretonne, in his 1798 pornographic novel *Anti-Justine*, displays a sort of curious shoe and foot fetishism that apparently has little to do with leather as such. But the novel was written to demonstrate that peaceful pornography is possible in contrast to Sade's violent sort. As a political document, *Anti-Justine* lacks sexual authenticity, and the fetish element works like a theme that has been dragged in to make a point rather than being desire driven.[48]

After Restif, the fetish platter is bare for almost a century, with a few exceptions: a Victorian Englishman named Arthur Munby had a most extraordinary fetish for soot-blackened cleaning women.[49] There were corset fetishes, as well. One scholar has argued that the commonplace corset represented a fetish object for late-nineteenth-century Englishmen and that women responded sexually to tight-lacing as well.[50] A whole range of phenomena that might now be called obsessive-compulsive disorders were viewed in the nineteenth century as fetish equivalents – as, for example, a patient of the French neurologist Jean-Martin Charcot who felt a compulsive need to look at women's derrieres.[51] These are slim pickings.

What thrust the phenomenon of fetish onto centre stage was Leopold von Sacher-Masoch's 1870 novel about fur fetishism and SM, *Venus in Fur*. Born in 1836 of an Austrian noble family, Sacher-Masoch was a professor of history at the University of Graz before he decided to try his hand as a novelist. In 1861 he met Anna von Kottowitz, and SM was evidently a theme in their relationship; he then encountered in the late 1860s Fanny Pistor-Bogdanoff, who was the explicit model for Wanda, the dominatrix portrayed in *Venus in Fur*. After the novel's success, he apparently decided to take on a fetish-SM lifestyle, courting Angelica Rümelin, who changed her name to Wanda after she married him. He encouraged her to wear fur about the house and to give him the occasional thrashing, until she left him in 1884.[52] Sacher-Masoch had sent a copy of the novel to Krafft-Ebing, who gave Sacher-Masoch immortality when in 1891 he used this ancient Austrian noble name as an eponym for what today is called 'bottoming.'

The fictional Wanda's creed in the 1870 novel was, 'I am young, rich, and beautiful, and being like this I live for plea-sure, for sensation!' In the novel it is Wanda who sports the gorgeous furs that attract young 'Severin' to her. She de-clares, 'I make a good despot – I also possess the necessary furs.' But it wasn't just fur that turned Severin's crank but suffering as well, and he tells Wanda that 'Nothing is so calculated to inflame my passion as the tyranny, the cruelty, and above all the faithlessness of a beautiful woman. But I can't imagine this woman ... without fur.' Wanda and Severin sign a contract in which he will be her slave, and only at this point do we understand that for Severin the real thrill is not necessarily Wanda in fur (the fetish part), but Wanda with absolute control over him (the SM part). As she flogs him she cries out, 'Only now do I understand you! It is truly exquisite to have someone so completely in one's power, and in the bargain a man who loves me – you love me don't you? [Whack] No? Oh, I'll tear you to ribbons. With every stroke I feel my pleasure mounting.'[53]

With the success of Sacher-Masoch's novel, the subject of fetish was now in the air. In 1887 Paris psychologist Alfred Binet, the inventor of the first intelligence test, published an article on 'sexual fetishism' that shifted the long familiar term 'fetish' from the area of religion to that of sex. Binet listed a wide variety of what he considered fetishes, ranging from a fascination with odour, to jewellery, underwear, men's voices, and an intense attentiveness to certain parts of the body such as the female hand.[54] In 1891 Krafft-Ebing, picking up on Binet's work, announced that fetishism represented yet an-other form of perversion.[55]

Virtually everything imaginable became identified as a fetish in the following years, with the exception of leather. A book on 'All Kinds of Fetishes,' published in Paris (in Ger-man) around 1900, listed as fetishes beautiful feet of women, combs, wigs, underwear, and red hair.[56] Because Sacher-Masoch had fixed the attention of the public on fur fetishism, in the following years there were a number of reports of fur as the fetish object. Pornographic pamphlets flourished with such titles as 'Fur and Whip' (by 'Frau Mistress').[57] From the Paris jails three women who'd been masturbating with silk came to the attention of Gaétan Gatian de Clérambault, a staff doctor in the psychiatric emergency department of the Paris hospitals. 'The classic idea that fetishism has not yet affected women is wrong,' noted Clérambault in 1908. Yet for men, he continued, fetishism meant fur: 'It is remarkable that in almost all cases men have fur as their object of predilection.'[58] In October 1909, James Joyce volunteered to buy Nora 'a splendid set of sable furs, cap, stole, and muff. Would you like that?' he asked hopefully.[59] Finally, in a passage from one epoch of fetish to another, it was as a symbolic dominatrix in fur that Marlene Dietrich vamped on screen in a string of films from *The Blue Angel* in 1930 to *The Devil Is a Woman* in 1935.[60]

The concept of fetish was taking time to crystallize in the sexual imagination. But the underlying fetish impulse had been roused by the new fin-de-siècle sexuality, and the individual psyches of many people were groping in an unfocused way towards the master fetish: leather. But about thirty years would pass between *Venus in Fur* and the initial appearance of leather as a sexual fetish. Thereafter, leather swept the field clean. Today, a Yahoo search on the Internet for 'fur fetish' produces one site match ('adult toys, such as dildos, vibrators ... fur') and 1,840 web pages; a search for 'leather fetish' produces 120 site matches and 17,500 web pages. There is no doubt that by the twenty-first century leather had conquered fur as the lead fetish. How did this happen?

Before the late nineteenth century, leather was simply off the scope, non-existent as a sexual theme.[61] The great bibliographies of pornography such as Henry Ashbee's and Hayn and Gotendorf make no reference to leather bondage gear, leather dominatrix clothing, or leather corsets. Nor does the theme of leather fetish appear in any of the autobiographical accounts. The hundreds of photos and illustrations in one exhaustive survey of French houses of prostitution from the

French Revolution to the 1950s feature leather and SM virtually not at all.[62]

If anyone were apt to import leather into the sexual scene, it would have been the American actress Adah Isaacs Menken, who in the early 1860s rode about on stage lashed to a horse with leather straps – and wearing a wide leather belt – in a dramatic re-enactment of Byron's poem 'Mazeppa.' Already the scene sounds as though it had a hard kink edge. But was it perceived as sexual? Menken was called to the bedside, in a manner of speaking, of the English poet Charles Swinburne, who was basically gay and a devotee of flagellation. The idea was that Menken, with her courtesan's skills, was to rescue Swinburne for heterosexuality. Adah, 'in her Mazeppa persona, knew more about leather bonds and pretty little whips than any of the professional highly rouged ladies of St John's Wood [flagellation houses in London frequented by Swinburne],' as one historian puts it. So, was leather a theme in Adah's brief relationship with Swinburne? Apparently, not at all. The ardent poem that he dedicated to her, 'Dolores (Notre-Dame des Sept Douleurs)' – termed 'almost a national anthem for flagellants' – makes no reference to it.[63] The two of them must have staged straight flogging scenes.

Yet it is via such dominatrixes as these that leather begins to penetrate the SM scene, first in the form of fetishy shoes and boots. Interestingly, the first image of a booted dominatrix the present author has encountered is when Sacher-Masoch dresses Wanda up like a bondage doll (though the reference is very fleeting and unlikely to have been a big theme for him, in whose works leather is otherwise invisible). It is in the mid-1870s, just after Wanda has given birth and is interested in anything but SM sex play, that Sacher-Masoch reserves a hideaway hotel room for them in a small town and dresses a rather resentful Wanda for the trip in a giant black fur and a pair of high riding boots.[64] This is the first unambiguous reference to the sexualization of leather.[65]

In the last third of the nineteenth century, mentions of boot fetishism begin to increase. In 1868, Zola drops a passing reference to boot worship in his novel *Thérèse Raquin* (Laurent kisses her boot briefly in an afternoon's outing) but makes little of it.[66] In 1891 Krafft-Ebing, looking over the medical literature, found shoe and boot fetishism to be among 'the commonest forms' of the phenomenon.[67]

Then, however, the dominating women in the high-heeled boots began to spill into pornography. In 1909 an English printer offered *Figure-Training and Deportment by Means of the Discipline of Tight Corsets, Narrow High-Heeled Boots, and Clinging Kid Gloves*, the first such reference for England in a pornography world otherwise awash with titles about flagellation, sexually aggressive women, and the like.[68] An English magazine called *London Life* that appeared between 1923 and 1940 featured fetish high-heel shoe and boot wearers, the women usually with their backs to the camera, the so-called 'letters to the editor' doubtless composed by the editors themselves to arouse interest.[69]

After the First World War, Berlin was fetish heaven. In 1920 the twenty-year-old German painter Rudolf Schlichter had just moved there, creating in that year a folio entitled *Love Variations*. The sketches showed, among other variations, a booted, severe-looking woman in a tight bodice with a riding crop flagellating the buttocks of another woman, who in turn is holding the penis of a man clothed in a business suit.[70] By the late 1920s, the prostitutes in Berlin were regularly wearing boots as a sexual come-on. Louis Royer, a visiting French sex novelist, discovered in the red-light district legions of young women with red and purple boots that laced up to the knee. As for the johns, 'Their fetish is the boot. Their happiness, their passion is when the woman is pacing up and down her square of asphalt, to caress the boots with their loving fingers, to breathe them in, to lick them. Alas! I'm not making any of this up.' Royer took one prostitute back to her place. She lay down on the divan with her boots in his face. When he remained motionless she surmised that he wanted something else, and she opened the appliance cabinet with the whips and restraints.[71]

It is from this stew of dominating women with whips and boots that the archetypcal figure of the SM-fetish scene emerges: the leather-clad dominatrix. Dominatrixes, as we have seen, had been known since Sade; Krafft-Ebing diffused the term.[72] But only in the great cities of Europe in the years after the First World War does the image of the domme, dressed from head to toe in bondage gear, begin to sharpen. It is this image that, for the first time, unifies all the zones of the body in the symbolic representation of total body sex.

In the Kinsey Collection in Bloomington, Indiana, the first leather-clad dominatrixes appear in the mid-1920s. The first image shows two side by side; one is in fur, one in leather, both are booted. An image from 1928 shows a booted domme topping a man.[73]

By the 1930s the domme has become a crisply delineated figure in the erotic imagination. 'Alan Mac Clyde's' *Le cuir triomphant* ('triumphant leather'), published in Paris some time in the early 1930s, must be among the earliest pornographic visualizations of the domme. On the cover, she stands at the doorway of the dungeon, feet in thigh-high boots and wide apart, a leather corset encasing her midriff, opera-length black leather gloves on her arms, a black leather cape about her shoulders, and a whip in her right hand. Her 'victims,' three nubile young women themselves clad in boots, corsets, and gloves, are chained to posts or heavy objects, awaiting their punishment.[74] It is, of course, totally for the male pornographic imagination, yet by the 1930s this was an imagination that now thirsted for leather, and for dominating women dressed in it. Every part of the dommes' glistening bodies comes together in a whole, the embodiment of total body sex.

SM-Fetish Joins the Mainstream

If fetish and SM became indissolubly linked in the 1930s in the form of the dominatrix, it was after the 1950s that the joint concept, later known in the acronym of the Internet category 'BDSM' (bondage and domination, sadism and masochism), began its ascent to the mainstream in American society. There was an overarching logic that held together all the sub-communities in the BDSM universe: the rubber and leather fetishists, the SM-enthusiasts, the 'superbitches' or female dominants, and even the transvestites and transsexuals. It was the logic of total body sex. Wrote one scholar in 1982, 'Since around 1960 there has thrived a fetish for total envel-opment of the naked body in a "second skin" of rubber and leather ...'[75] A study of the Institute of Psychiatry at the University of London found that, statistically, the members of these various interest groups overlapped. Of 568 players in-terviewed, the most popular fantasy among SMs – rubberites, leatherites, and transvestites alike – involved being excited by clothing or material, in contrast to the 75 controls, whose commonest fantasy was 'intercourse with known partner.' Spanking and pain were either way down on the fantasy lists of rubberites, leatherites, and transvestites or not present at all.[76] The common denominator was not leather or rubber as such – to say nothing of flogging, pain, or any of the rest of the historical inheritance of SM-fetish – , but what one ob-server called 'pressure fetishism ... where the sensation of tight-fitting clothing arouses sexual pleasure.'[77] But of course the nineteenth-century corset fit tightly. What distinguishes fetishism in total body sex is the bringing together of the various tight-fitting pieces – gloves, mask, boots, corset, wrist and arm bands, the lot – into a single unified visual and sensory image of the entire eroticized body. It is interesting that even such staunch feminist theorists as Barbara Ehrenreich came to recognize approvingly the intrinsic logic of this rela-tionship. Said Ehrenreich and associates in 1986, 'S/M owes its entrance into the sexual mainstream to its paraphernalia.' 'The gear is not just an optional enhancement, it is essential to the act.'[78]

This rise of SM-fetish into the sexual mainstream had a number of way stations. Beginning in 1951, New York pho-tographers Irving and Paula Klaw started shooting a young model from Tennessee named Bettie Page in bondage gear.

Typically featured in opera-length black leather gloves, a matching corset, and high heels, Page soon became a cheesecake darling of the day, her pin-ups appearing in more than a thousand magazines. She was depicted in one of two formats: either Bettie was the charming All-American pin-up in a sexy pose, or she was the bondage lady (she never managed to look truly severe) tying up some other model in ropes. Said to have been courted at one point by aficionado Howard Hughes, she vanished from the scope in 1957. There are today Bettie Page fan clubs all over the world, and it would be fair to say that she brought the SM-fetish scene for the first time to a mass audience.[79]

A big venue for Bettie Page pin-ups was *Bizarre* magazine, founded in 1954 by fetish artist John Coutts, known as John Willie.[80] Published in London and distributed widely in the United States, *Bizarre* gave rise to a host of fetish magazines such as *Bizarre Life* that, although they represented subculture tastes, were sold at mainstream kiosks in big cities because they were not pornography: none of the models went 'pink,' to use the trade expression for exposing the perineum. Instead, they appealed to mass-market fetish tastes. In 1957 John Sutcliffe, an English aeronautical engineer with a personal taste for rubber clothing, founded the magazine *Atomage* as a feature site for the new garments he was designing with a technique he had invented for bonding rubber. Sutcliffe's work made practical the fetish image of encasing literally the entire body in rubber garments, with assorted straps, zippers, padlocks, belts, and boots. From this point, the dominatrix look became a practical reality for average people: by around 1960 one English manufacturer was selling about a thousand masks and hoods a year to 'decent respectable solid citizens in all walks of life.'[81]

It was Sutcliffe's work that inspired *The Avengers*, an English television show that in 1961 opened the floodgates for fetish-SM images. Starring Patrick Macnee as the suave John Steed and, after 1965, stage actress Diana Rigg opposite him as the leather-catsuited Emma Peel, the series debuted on the

U.K.'s commercial system, ITV. It went through six cycles, terminating in 1969, although Rigg had bowed out in 1967. In 1976–7 the concept was reprised as *The New Avengers*. *The Avengers* became the template for the many power-babe series of the 1970s and after, such as *Charlie's Angels*.[82] Yet Diana Rigg, an accomplished and self-possessed actor, was anything but a babe. And the sight of her, dressed from head to toe in leather and wasting guys with deadly karate chops night after night, brought, for the first time in history, leather fetish into the living rooms of Mr and Ms America. Although the show's producers tried to downplay the kink themes in their public relations, insisting that its charm involved a Victorian gentleman and a twenty-first-century woman, the huge international audience riveted to the screen included many fetish fanciers. It gave Diana Rigg 'a saucy image, all black leather and erotic,' as she later said. 'But I was utterly confused by it. How do you write back to someone who says in really lubricious terms that they love you in black leather.' Rigg solved the problem by having her mother respond to all correspondents.[83]

In the 1960s, porn films started catering much more to mixed audiences in living rooms rather than to older men in Legion Hall smokers. The films routinely began offering more SM and more garter-belt, high-heeled fetishism.[84] Chic dominatrixes started to become cult figures, the most famous being Monique Von Cleef, who from her Manhattan apartment in late 1964 began running ads in an SM publication called *Flair*. She was astonished at the volume of the response. By January 1965, 'I had 8,734 letters in my files.'[85] The back-up in the demand for this kind of sex was clearly enormous.

The proliferation of SM in 1970s porn videos is noteworthy, given the traditional avoidance of the subject among American porn producers. SM had once been 'extremely rare in the classic stag film,' according to Al Di Lauro and Gerald Rabkin, specialists in sex-film history. One could find plenty of 'soft fladge' in British porn films, but the hitting of women in such

U.S. films had always been taboo.[86] The authors believed that
SM reached American films in the 1970s because porn producers were otherwise running out of taboos. But a more
likely explanation is that, in most SM scenarios, it's women
who are striking men. In any event, the standard American
porn film in the 1970s included, according to porn producer
Dave Friedman in 1974 (*My Tale Is Hot*, *The Master Piece*), 'a
heterosexual scene, an S-M scene, a lesbian scene; [it's] the
oldest thing in show business, something for everybody.'[87]
The point is that, by the 1970s SM scenes had come to be part
of the gamut that 'everybody' expected.

Everybody didn't rent porn films in those years. Yet mass-
market publishing was placed on bedside tables, and Gerald
and Caroline Green's *S-M: The Last Taboo*, published in 1973,
was said to be the first mass-market discussion of the subject.
So suburban readers were learning that 'Tight black glacé kid
– in boots and gloves – is a *sine qua non* of much s-m. The
creak of leather, with its inexorable sense of compression of
flesh, can produce a delectable *frisson* in many.' The authors
insisted they weren't 'encouraging old ladies to go out and
buy birches.' (An ageist comment if ever there was one: why
shouldn't 'old ladies' be as interested as anybody else?) Instead, the Greens aimed their volume right at the marriage
bed, hoping to 'allow s-m as a polymorphous play activity
preliminary to sex, instead of stigmatizing it as perversion.'[88]
It was also in the 1970s that Betty Dodson, author of the later
mass-market success *Sex for One*, herself discovered SM and
evidently encouraged members of her masturbation workshops to get into fetish wear and role playing. Dodson practised in front of a mirror wearing 'nothing but a big studded
belt and cowboy boots,' or 'a black leather dildo harness,
with or without the dildo.' By 1987 her repertoire included
'John in the Park,' 'The Fuck Bar,' and 'The Cruel Mistress.'[89]
We are not talking dirty old men locked in the bathroom here:
this is mainstream material.

As the popularity of SM images spread in the 1970s and
after, it is clear that two groups were developing: the dab-

blers, who liked mainly the images they saw in the bedroom mirror, and the serious players in the subculture. The dabblers include perhaps one American male in seven, one female in ten. The *Janus Report*, a nationwide survey conducted in the early 1990s, found that 14 per cent of men and 11 per cent of women had some lifetime acquaintance with SM. (For fetishes, it was 11 per cent of the men and 6 per cent of the women.)[90]

These are not large percentages, yet in terms of fetish fantasies the trend seems to be up. For the white American college males who had mainly come of age in the interwar years interviewed by Kinsey and associates, only 3.7 per cent of the 3,582 interviewed reported any interest in 'bizarre fantasies' (including fetishism) for purposes of masturbation.[91] By the mid-1980s, when *Woman* magazine in Britain conducted a sex survey (asking female readers to pass on a questionnaire to their husbands and male friends), the figures were much higher: 11 per cent said they had fantasies about their partner wearing 'special clothes,' choosing from a list that included high heels, leather, and rubber.[92] There are many reasons why these two surveys are not exactly comparable. Yet these data at least suggest that SM-fetish fantasies may have been on the rise. After reviewing a series of microsurveys on the popularity of SM in American society, two scholars concluded in 1987 that, 'It is clear that millions of people in the United States are involved in behaviors that most would classify as S/M.'[93]

Yet the SM subculture as such may be somewhat smaller. There are people who make these practices a way of life and who associate with the like-minded, just as aviation enthusiasts hang out together. Among them, the bottoms greatly outnumber the tops. For example, among the 300 dues-paying members of the Till Eulenspiegel Society in New York, founded in 1976 and considered the oldest of the aficionado clubs, a majority of the male members – when quizzed in the 1980s – were heterosexual and submissive; among the female members, who constituted one-third of the total, it was fifty-

fifty.[94] Yet in the subculture, switching roles is highly common: one study found that fewer than 10 per cent of those surveyed were exclusive tops or bottoms.[95] Contrary to popular impression, it is the bottoms who really control the scene not the tops, who strut about in leather cracking whips and only pretending to be in control. Says Ehrenreich, 'In the S/M configuration, the sadist is burdened with the responsibility for directing a scene, turning sex into little more than a spectator sport ... Paradoxically, the passive masochist is always at the center of attention, the consumer in an S/M scene: The sadist is only catering to his or her desires.'[96]

Nor are the scenes primarily focused upon pain. One analysis of 120 males and 40 females who filled out questionnaires in insider magazines, found that only 51 per cent of the men and 34 per cent of the women were interested in pain (by this is meant serious pain); spanking was the preferred activity (79 per cent of males and 80 per cent of females), followed by the psychodrama of 'master-slave relationships,' then oral sex (in which the top presumably 'commands' the bottom to perform it). The wilder activities, such as 'torture' and 'golden showers' (one person urinating on another), were far down the list.[97]

The SM subculture lies quite at the margin of America's sexual spectrum, rejecting the 'vanilla' sex that all the others presumably practise in favour of a lifestyle in which the partners go to the supermarket together dressed in their leathers and where the bottom often follows the top partner in the street by three paces. Yet themes that originated in this subculture have gone on to captivate the American mainstream.

First of all, leather fetish has become mainline fashion. It was not always so. Before 1900, leather was considered good for horseback journeys, like heavy wools. As John Donne said in 1635:

> For one night's revels, silk and gold we choose.
> But, in long journeys, cloth and leather use.[98]

As far as one can determine, leather did not become a high-fashion theme until the French designer Erté flirted with it very briefly during the First World War. In 1916 he sketched for *Harper's Bazaar* 'the Amazon of Tomorrow,' two women in chamois leather riding jodhpurs and boots and gauntlets. The look is strappy and spurred, a preview of what would become fashion kink half a century later but was doubtless considered, during a terrible war, an eccentric lapse. Erté's historic drawings had no follow-up.[99]

Erté toyed once again with leather in the 1950s in designing outfits for a show at the Folies Pigalle: 'I had made most of the costumes from leather or animal skins, and the unusual combination of these materials with bodies in various degrees of nakedness created an effect of violent sexuality.'[100] Unlike 'the Amazons' of 1916, however, this Erté caprice may have had a follow-up. Erté moved in the same *haut-gay* Parisian world as the young designer Yves Saint-Laurent, and it was in 1960 that Saint-Laurent, the House of Dior's chief designer, introduced leather to the world of high, evening fashion.

A word of preface first. Leather had not been totally absent from the fashion scene. American designer Bonnie Cashin had shown boots (with tweed suits) as early as 1943.[101] And during the 1950s leather did occasionally crop up in journals such as *Harper's Bazaar*. But it was almost invariably suede or kidskin sportswear in pastel shades, and, with the exception of outerwear, never black. In 1960 things changed dramatically. Several designers offered pastel leather 'sweater' and slacks combos in their spring collections, and by September fashion writer Nancy White announced in *Harper's* that 'Leather is everywhere.'[102] Yet the big move occurred in the fall collections of 1960. In September Saint-Laurent offered, in what would be his last collection for Dior, a mink-edged black alligator jacket for evening wear that one fashion writer called 'the farthest-out leather garment in the world.' The fashion house Heim was showing a leather chemise dress for evening. By October 1960 *Vogue* was cheering of the Paris collections, 'Leather? They loved it,' predicting great success for the new fashion material in the United States as well.[103]

This sudden eruption of leather was an extraordinary development. It had begun in Paris, among the fashion community that had already projected so much of the sexual excitement of the twentieth century's first half; and it leapt to the United States, which would scorch the fashion scene with sexuality for the next fifty years. It is tempting to think that leather's sudden coming out drew on fetish themes that had been slowly maturing at a subterranean level on both sides of the Atlantic since the end of the First World War. Now leather had exploded full blast upon the media stage.

1960 was the beginning. For the 1961–2 season Balenciaga set off the then fashionable *Jules et Jim* look (named after the movie) with flat leather boots to the knee. Models sported grey cardigan V-neck suits over black leather sweaters. Black high-heeled boots set off the outfit.

'Boots, boots, and more boots are marching up and down,' thrilled *Harper's Bazaar* in 1963. Saint-Laurent's boots – he was said to 'bring leather indoors and [to] show women how to dress for their boots' – ran up to the thigh. It was only 1963, yet one of Saint-Laurent's models, in thigh-high black alligator boots, a black ciré smock, black gloves, and a black leather helmet with attaching choker, looked almost like the underground image of a dominatrix.[104] In 1964 *Harper's* ran a David Bailey photo of actress Jean Shrimpton dressed in a heavy fur, black gloves, and high, glistening, black leather boots shoved right in the viewer's face:[105] Wanda had come back, this time not for a bizarre provincial Austrian nobleman but for the high-end fashion market.

So leather arrived on people's backs pulled from above and pushed from below. As Yves Saint-Laurent was putting the finishing touches on his fall 1960 collection, in August 1960 the Beatles, an unknown group from Liverpool, were arriving in the sex district of Hamburg dressed in mauve jackets and grey crocodile shoes. German kids then, in remembrance perhaps of the army officers and fliers of the

Second World War – or the Wild One – were already dressing in black leather, and Beatle Stuart Sutcliffe acquired a beautiful blonde girlfriend, Astrid, who went around in a leather jacket and 'very tight-fitting tailored leather trousers.' Paul McCartney's girlfriend, Dorothy Rohne, came over from Liverpool, and McCartney bought her a leather skirt 'so she'd look like Brigitte [Bardot],' after whom they all lusted. Astrid then got Stuart a leather suit to match her own, and the other Beatles all liked them so much they had a tailor on the Reeperbahn, Hamburg's main sex street, make matching black leather suits for all of them, coming together visually as a group. When the Beatles returned to Liverpool in 1961, they brought the black leather look back to England,[106] without, as far as one knows, any suggestion of fetishism.

Meanwhile, in her shop Bazaar on King's Road in London, around 1962 designer Mary Quant was introducing the leather look – black leather boots up to the knee and black leather coats – for the 'mod' scene in London. And as she opened a second shop in the neighbouring district of Knightsbridge, all of the six or so ex-debs working for her wore 'high black leather boots, black stockings and black leather coats.' (It was only in 1965 that Quant introduced the white mid-calf boots called 'go-go boots.') 'Swinging London,' then caught up in 'Beatlemania,' swung in a semi-fetish mode.[107]

Normally with fashion, a look will drift in and then drift out again. But after the 1960s the popularity of leather just continued to accelerate. There was never a drifting out of style, nor was there right up to the new millennium. On Christmas Eve Day, 2000, a *New York Times* story on the great increase in the consumption of leather clothing began, 'Americans are buying animal hides like Hell's Angels.'[108] The look clearly spoke to people at some deep subliminal level, laced in somehow with their new appreciation of the sexual body as a whole. The fashionable fetish garb derived not from appeals to those who wanted to whip one another but from the power of the icon itself. It was the leather imagery rather than the SM practices that were becoming fashionable, and for reasons having nothing to do with exchange of control but with total body sex. Leather spoke to the whole body more strikingly than did wool.

In the 1980s and after, however, fashion did begin to expropriate explicit SM images. High-fashion photographer Helmut Newton, known for the hard kink edge in much of his work, drove around Paris with a set of chains in his car trunk for use in shoots.[109] Several designers began dressing up paraphernalia from the dungeon for the runway. John Galliano once used a Bettie Page image for a launch in Paris.[110] In 1984 Jean-Paul Gaultier designed the kind of cone bra that Madonna would sport on her Blonde Ambition Tour in 1990. Most prominent of these designers drawing on subculture themes was Versace, known for his creative use of leather, denim, and metal mesh, and for cathecting an explicit sexiness onto the well-bred understatement of the fashion world. Even when he was designing for houses such as Callaghan and Complice, Versace experimented with such forms of body enhancement as big shoulders. But once he was master of his own house, Versace started in on leather. His first collection in 1979 featured a black leather kimono. In 1982 he melded metal and leather in men's and women's coats, and in the year of his famous bondage collection, 1992, the models wore gauntlets, chokers, and chains on their boots.[111] (*Harper's Bazaar* noted of the leather-loaded fall collection of a number of fashion houses, 'Straps and laces: It seems that designers took out a restraining order this season.')[112]

At the time of his death in 1997, Versace had become a guiding light for a whole new generation of gay designers who were openly mining homosexual and SM culture for their creativity. John Bartlett, who drew on archetypes of sailors and policemen for his men's line, found, however, that the same themes for women didn't work as well. 'The first collection was very butch,' he said, 'but I've moved past that.'[113] Yet the point is not that designers offered these images because they were gay, but because – sensitized perhaps by pre-exposure in the gay subculture – they realized that the 'Park Avenue Dominatrix,' as someone called her, would be a hit.

By the beginning of the twenty-first century, SM had come into vogue as a mainline sexual taste. What are your visions of 'perfect sex'? a popular women's magazine asked its readers in 1997. 'Being handcuffed to the bed, in candlelight, listening to jazz, while my boyfriend makes love to me – achieving orgasm,' one reader answered. And the editors printed the response rather than binning it.[114] Five hundred years of SM defined as flogging had been blown away. In July 1999 *Redbook*, as close to the heartland of American women's sexuality as it is possible to get, OK'd the wild side, addressing 'eroticist' readers, 'What you long for is kink, trash, anything taboo – handcuffs, toys, private strip shows, *Nine and a Half Weeks* [a novel and movie about SM].'[115] In its Christmas issue of 1999 *Redbook* gave prominent play to handcuffs, as guys 'confessed' to 'the sexiest gift she ever gave me.' Rob, age thirty-two, replied, 'I would definitely say **handcuffs**. It was her way of showing me that she was up for a little adventure.'[116]

For generations, home parties for products such as Tupperware or Avon make-up have been suburban institutions. Held now in the evenings so that working wives in the neighbourhood can attend, the format is friendly sociability folded around a commercial pitch. Thirty-year-old Karen Williams of Aragon, Georgia, works for one of them, a Tennessee outfit that sells lotions and the like. Tonight she's in Roswell, Georgia, a guest of Clara P. who's staging the party. Ten women have gathered in the living room to find 'some fun new things to spice up my marriage,' as one of them says. On offer are blindfolds, furry handcuffs, and the kind of 'love swing' that used to hang in SM bars in the pre-HIV days for purposes of fist fucking. Not that the guests will necessarily be fist fucking. 'I think this is great,' says Lori C., twenty-nine. 'There's no men, no children, and Karen makes it fun.'[117] Another sales organization called Tasteful Treasures, in addition to lotions, lingerie, and massage oils, offered handcuffs and a whip key chain, billed as 'novelty items.'[118] There were perhaps twelve companies that staged such home parties.

At least one firm, Seasonal Inspiration, had a 'bondage division,' where cute little key chains gave way to the basic paraphernalia of the scene. Seasonal Inspiration did house parties, too, where the women could buy a 'Beginners B&D Kit,' with leather wrist restraints, whip, leather paddle, collar, leash, and blindfold. For more advanced players, full hoods, ball gags, and penis rings were also available.[119]

By the beginning of the new millennium, middle-class America had galloped past the decades of outrage that used to envelop SM and fetish. Just as homosexuality became accepted as part of the spectrum of normal sexuality after the Stonewall riots in New York in 1969, SM and fetish were becoming accepted in living rooms in small towns in Georgia. These husbands and wives would not flog each other mercilessly with whips dipped in vinegar, as in fifteenth-century Italy. They would experiment excitedly with the voluntary exchange of power, and in the process thrill to the discovery that their arms tied to the bed, or their legs restrained to a metal bar by straps at each end, or their luscious black leather profiles by candlelight in the bedroom mirror represented sexual sensations as positive for them as the missionary position had been for others in past centuries. It was too late for older generations with their more circumscribed views of pleasure such as 'J,' author of *The Sensuous Woman*, who had hissed in 1969, 'If he wants to resort to whips and chains ... get professional help.'[120] Desire was driving the body relentlessly forwards.

CHAPTER TEN

Epilogue

'Soul and body, body and soul – how mysterious they were!' says Lord Henry in Oscar Wilde's *Picture of Dorian Gray*. 'There was animalism in the soul, and the body had its moments of spirituality ... Who could say where the fleshy impulse ceased, or the psychical impulse began?'[1]

That was in 1890. A century later we know the outcome of the story. This book describes the victory of the fleshy impulse, of desire. But if desire has won, what has really been achieved? Is there a price that we as a society have had to pay for elevating total body sex to the erotic norm and for freeing people to act more or less unconstrainedly on neural impulses? For women, let us say, is the culmination of human history listening to a Sex Pistols record while wearing a leather jacket with a tube of KY Jelly in the pocket?

One must be careful about saying that the human passions have asserted themselves in place of reason. There is really no evidence that we are any more dedicated to sensation today than at any other time in history. After all, in 1823 the English radical politician Francis Place described his father as 'governed almost wholly by his passions and animal sensations.' 'These were few, mostly relating to sturdiness and dissoluteness. Drinking, whoring, gaming, fishing and fighting,' clucked Place, were the pleasures of his father.[2] Casanova, trying to explain why he was constantly falling in and out of love, said, '*Hélas*! We love without the guidance of reason, and reason isn't any the more involved after we have ceased to love.'[3] Conservatives across the centuries have deplored the upper hand of passion over reason in the common people, using this supposed inability to choose order as justification for authoritarian rule.

What this book is saying is that people are asserting sexual pleasure over community, rather than over reason. The victory of total body sex over the repressiveness of Christian Europe, over want, disease, and stench represents the elevation of privatizing kinds of choices that end up taking people out of contact with society. Opting for the privacy of the bedroom behind locked doors, for the anonymity of the big city as opposed to the village community, for oral, anal, and extramarital sex in the face of religious fury – all are choices that are anti-communitarian though by no means irrational. What costs have these choices had for our society?

In a classic article in 1995, Harvard political scientist Robert D. Putnam noted the rise of 'bowling alone.' It struck him that between 1980 and 1993 the total number of bowlers in America had increased by 10 per cent while membership in organized bowling leagues had been plummeting. For Putnam, bowling alone became emblematic of a general decline in civic engagement and in American willingness to invest free time in 'social capital,' meaning membership in community organizations and the like. Between 1967 and 1993, 'among the college-educated, the average number of group memberships per person fell from 2.8 to 2.0,' a decline of 26 per cent. Among those less well educated the declines were similar or even greater. Putnam blamed the huge post-1950s increase in television watching for this civic crisis.[4] The article – and the following book of that title[5] – provoked a well-deserved outpouring of concern about declining social participation: fewer friends, less going out in the evening, and lessening voter participation in elections.

Declining civic engagement is another way of describing the withdrawal of individuals to the intimacy of their private lives – 'cocooning' as a pop phrase has it. The concept of

cocooning is virtually without historical precedent. Writing
in the 1930s, Virginia Woolf recalled that life in those days
was with people. She described the world of her parents'
sisters: 'It was the life of families, of groups. It was a web, a
net, spreading wide and enmeshing every sort of cousin,
dependant, and old retainer.' The myriad aunts would gather,
'cluster in chorus,' said Woolf, 'and rejoice and sorrow and
eat Christmas dinner together, and grow very old and remain
very upright ...'[6] By contrast, in the United States, the amount
of time spent socializing dropped by 1.5 hours a week between 1965 and 1985, from 8.2 hours to 6.7.[7] Where were
Virginia Woolf's aunts?

The percentage of households contributing to the arts declined from 9.6 per cent in 1989 to 8.1 per cent in 1993.[8] The
proportion of people going to church regularly declined from
around 50 per cent in 1958 to 40 per cent in the early 1990s.[9]
People willing to attend a political rally dropped by 36 per
cent between 1973 and 1993, to attend a meeting on town or
school affairs by 39 per cent, to work for a political party by
56 per cent.[10] All of these phenomena are very real, and of
great concern.

But is television the whole story, or even the main story? Is
it possible that deeper forms of hedonism push us to watch
television at night rather than going to PTA meetings? To
terminate marriages rapidly rather than endure the prospect
of lifelong heartburn? To marry later or to defer it entirely?

The story in this book permits us to extend the analysis a
little beyond television. Even though TV watching may be
part of the story, it's not responsible for sexual disaffiliation
in a couple or for rising adolescent crime rates. The crisis of
civic participation and social stability has a number of sources.
One of them is pretty clearly the growing sensualization of
human sexuality: that we expect a far more delicious encounter with our own bodies and the bodies of others than any
past generation. It is also clear that this kind of sexual inten-
sity contributes to some of the other phenomena that Putnam
and the 'bowling alone' crowd are concerned about. Accord-

ing to the General Social Survey of the University of Chicago, a database that follows some 10,000 individuals over time, in 1998 there was a negative relationship between sex and church attendance. As a demographic journal commented, 'Those who attend religious services at least once a week are less sexually active.' Even more interesting is that high rates of sex are associated with suspiciousness of others: 'The most sexually active Americans are also more likely than average to say they do not regard other people as fair or trustworthy.' Again, sex as antisocial. Finally, the more sexually active someone is, the less likely he or she is to be involved in the community. Comment the editors, 'Perhaps sex is one of the psychological tactics people use to escape from a less-than-satisfying community.'[11] Or vice versa: the more intense the sex life, the less the interest in community activities.

This kind of disaffiliation is not entirely the consequence of an absorbing sex life. Other forms of hedonism unrelated to TV viewing are also on the rise. Pharmacological hedonism is increasing among American teenagers. For adolescents, cigarette smoking was 27 per cent higher in 1999 than in 1991. Alcohol use is on the rise among students in grades 9 to 12: by 1999, 37 per cent of the nation's grade 12 girls participated in binge drinking, 50 per cent of the grade 12 boys. In 1999, 50 per cent more high school students were smoking marijuana than in 1990.[12] These changes have little to do with either television or sex. Hedonic behaviour of many kinds is on the rise in our society.

It is easy to rehearse such statistics with a finger waggle of disapproval, but that's not the message of this book. The adolescents who make most of these choices are not necessarily wicked. The point is that the choices are hedonistic, exactly as TV watching and total body sex are hedonistic options in a world that also offers puritanical options of self-denial.

Where does all this pleasure seeking come from? In this book we have seen that there are deeper hedonic variables that lurk in the shadows. Some of these, such as sexual gratification, spring from unleashed human biology. Others, such as a lesser interest in the soul and its vicissitudes, arise from the relentless secularization of our society since the end of the Eisenhower years. Yet together, these hedonic changes are creating a society oriented towards personal gratification in a way that previous generations could never have imagined.

The young men and women from the TV series *Sex and the City*, aching for sex after three-day respites and manipulating their vibrators until the onset of carpal tunnel syndrome – they tell us that at the threshold of the twenty-first century we're playing in a new ball game. People lust openly, frequently, and publicly. And they act on the basis of desire in a way that would have been inconceivable even a hundred years ago. There is an exquisiteness about this responsiveness to desire that is historically very startling. We don't want to make desire responsible for too much, in the way that some observers have incriminated television. But we must at least be mindful that it is driving us forward.

Notes

Chapter 1 Introduction

1 'TAP's Impotence Drug to Be Filed This Summer,' *Scrip*, 14 May 1999, 22

2 Robert Halsband, ed., *The Complete Letters of Lady Mary Wortley Montagu* (Oxford: Clarendon, 1967), vol. 3: 198–9; letter of 13 Jan. 1759 to Sir James Stewart.

3 Jean-Jacques Rousseau, *Les confessions* (written 1769) (new ed. Paris: Gallimard, 1959), 188.

4 Quoted in Avraam Koen, *Atoms, Pleasure, Virtue: The Philosophy of Epicurus* (New York: Lang, 1995), 98, 100.

5 Robert Latham and William Matthews, eds, *The Diary of Samuel Pepys* (Berkeley: University of California Press, 1970), vol. 3: 294.

6 Quoted in Herbert Marcuse, *Eros and Civilization* (1955) (reprint Boston: Beacon Press, 1966), 192–3.

7 John Locke, *An Essay Concerning Human Understanding* (1690) (reprint London: Dent, 1961), vol. 1: 120.

8 *Mary Wortley Montagu Letters*, vol. 3: 198.

9 Jeremy Bentham, *An Introduction to the Principles of Morals and Legislation* (1789), ed. by J.H. Burns and H.L.A. Hart (Oxford: Clarendon, 1996), 11.

10 Leslie A. Marchand, ed., *Byron's Letters and Journals* (London: Murray, 1979), vol. 9: 46.

11 D.H. Lawrence, *Lady Chatterley's Lover* (1928), ed. by Michael Squires (Cambridge: Cambridge University Press, 1993), 310–11.

12 Virginia Woolf, 'On Being Ill' (1930), in Woolf, *Collected Essays* (London: Hogarth Press, 1967), vol. 4, quotations 193–4.

13 Sigmund Freud, 'Drei Abhandlungen zur Sexualtheorie,' in Freud, *Gesammelte Werke* (Frankfurt-am-Main: Fischer, 1949), vol. 5: 91–2. Here Freud extends a view already familiar in European culture, that childhood sexuality was not necessarily centred upon the genitals. In 1896 French sexologist Marc-André Raffalovich had written, 'Sexuality and sensuality are not yet localized at 8, 9, 10, or 11.' Later, said Raffalovich, the boy's desire acquires a genital focus. But then, 'When adolescence eventuates, these physical desires once more become resorbed and decentralized.' *Uranisme et unisexualité* (Paris: Masson, 1896), 132. On other pre-Freudians to write of infantile 'perversity,' see Frank Sulloway, *Freud, Biologist of the Mind* (New York: Basic Books, 1979), 318 of paperback edition. Sulloway does not include Raffalovich.

14 Sigmund Freud, 'Meine Ansichten über die Rolle der Sexualität in der Ätiologie der Neurosen,' *Gesammelte Werke*, vol. 5: 156.

15 See on Norman O. Brown, Paul Robinson, *The Freudian Left* (New York: Harper, 1969), 228–31.

16 Salvador Dali, *Secret Life* (1942), Eng. trans. (London: Vision Press, 1961), 2.

17 Prosper Lucas, *Traité philosophique et physiologique de l'hérédité naturelle dans les états de santé et de maladie du système nerveux* (Paris: Baillière, 1847), vol. 1: 475.

18 See Peter Paemaekers and Christine Van Broeckhoven, 'Comment – Genes and Temperament, a Shortcut for Unravelling the Genetics of Psychopathology?' *International Journal of Neuropsychopharmacology* 1 (1998): 169–71; Edward Shorter, *A History of Psychiatry* (New York: Wiley, 1997), 240–5.

19 James Olds and Peter Milner, 'Positive Reinforcement Produced by Electrical Stimulation of the Septal Area and Other Regions of Rat Brain,' *Journal of Comparative and Physiological Psychology* 47 (1954): 419–27.

20 James Olds and M.E. Olds, 'Positive Reinforcement Produced by Stimulating Hypothalamus with Iproniazid and Other Compounds,' *Science* 127 (16 May 1958): 1175–6.

21 Helen E. Fisher, 'Lust, Attraction, and Attachment in Mamma-lian Reproduction,' *Human Nature* 9 (1998): 23–52.

22 Jaak Panksepp, *Affective Neuroscience: The Foundations of Human and Animal Emotions* (New York: Oxford University Press, 1998), 228.

23 William James, *The Varieties of Religious Experience: A Study in Human Nature* (New York: Modern Library, 1902), 15–16.

24 Oscar Wilde, *The Picture of Dorian Gray* (1890) (new ed. New York: Modern Library, 1998), 31.

25 Nadine Weidman, 'Heredity, Intelligence and Neuropsychol-ogy: Or, Why *The Bell Curve* Is Good Science,' *Journal of the History of the Behavioral Sciences* 33(2) (1997): 141–4.

26 Interviewed in David Healy, ed., *The Psychopharmacologists* (London: Chapman and Hall, 1998), vol. 2: 396.

Chapter 2 Sex, a Baseline

1 Steven Ziplow, *The Film Maker's Guide to Pornography* (New York: Drake, 1977), 18.

2 Diane Ackerman, *A Natural History of the Senses* (New York: Random House, 1990), xvi.

3 Peter Green, ed. and trans., *Ovid: The Erotic Poems* (London: Penguin, 1982), 90–2.

4 A.-J. Pons, ed. and trans., *Lucien. Dialogues des courtisans* (Paris: Quantin, 1881), v.

5 Alexander Nehamas and Paul Woodruff, trans. and eds, *Plato Symposium* (Indianapolis: Hackett, 1989), 48–9. Plato may have invented Diotima as a character; how much of the Symposium actually occurred is a moot point.

6 J.A. Pott and F.A Wright, trans. and eds, *Martial: The Twelve Books of Epigrams* (London: Routledge [1925]), book one, XLVI, 16.

7 John R. Clarke, *Looking at Lovemaking: Constructions of Sexuality in Roman Art, 100 B.C.–A.D. 250* (Berkeley: University of Cali-fornia Press, 1998), 25, fig. 3; 31, fig. 5.

8 Clarke, *Roman Art*, plates 14 and 15, plus the discussion on 235.

9 Clarke, *Roman Art*, 220–5.

10 Paul Englisch, *Geschichte der erotischen Literatur* (Stuttgart: Püttmann, 1927), 55–6.

11 Ovid, *Erotic Poems*, 211–12.

12 This is a distinction that many students of sexuality have made, however coloured their values by the attitudes of their time. Thus German sexologist and psychiatrist Albert Eulenburg distinguished between 'quantitative anomalies of the sex drive,' such as satyriasis and nymphomania, and 'qualitative anomalies,' such as what he considered sexual perversions. Eulenburg, *Sexuale Neuropathie* (Leipzig: Vogel, 1895), 90, 96.

13 Jerome Cardan [Cardano], *The Book of My Life* (1575), Eng. trans. (London: Dent, 1931), 36–7, 57, 281.

14 Gustav Schilling, *Denkwürdigkeiten des Herrn von H.* (c. 1787) (reprint Leipzig: Kiepenheuer, 1983), 94.

15 Francis Lacassin, ed., *Jacques Casanova de Seingalt, Histoire de ma vie* (new ed. Paris: Laffont, 1993), quotations vol. 3: 299; vol. 2: 57.

16 Casanova, *Histoire de ma vie*, vol. 1: 6.

17 Robert Latham and William Matthews, eds, *The Diary of Samuel Pepys* (new ed. Berkeley: University of California Press, 1974), vol. 8: 389–90.

18 Pepys, *Diary*, vol. 8: 588

19 Pepys, *Diary*, vol. 9: 184.

20 Pepys, *Diary*, vol. 7: 135–6.

21 Christian F. Gellert, *Tagebuch aus dem Jahre 1761*, 2nd ed. (Leipzig: Weigel, 1863), quotations 2, 40–1, 49, 87.

22 J.D. Marshall, ed., *The Autobiography of William Stout of Lancaster* (Manchester: Manchester University Press, 1967), 103–4.

23 Roland Barthes, ed., *Brillat-Savarin: Physiologie du goût* (1826) (Paris: Hermann, 1975), 43.

24 J.M. Rigg, trans., *Giovanni Boccaccio, The Decameron* (London: Everyman, 1930); on floor shaking, vol. 1: 177; for woman on top, vol. 1: 39; vol. 2: 236.

25 Casanova, *Histoire de ma vie*, vol. 1: 766.

26 Pepys, *Diary*, vol. 7: 142; vol. 8: 39; vol. 9: 132; vol. 9: 312.

27 Pepys, *Diary*, vol. 7: 389.

28 R. Howard Bloch, 'Modest Maids and Modified Nouns: Obscenity in the Fabliaux,' in Jan M. Ziolkowski, ed., *Obscenity:*

Social Control and Artistic Creation in the European Middle Ages (Leiden: Brill, 1998), 293–307, quotation 293.

29 Stephen Haliczer, *Sexuality in the Confessional: A Sacrament Profaned* (New York: Oxford University Press, 1996), 157–9.

30 'Luisa Sigea Toletana' [pseudonym for Nicolas Chorier], Donald A. McKenzie, Eng. trans. and ed., *Dialogues on the Arcana of Love and Venus* (c. 1660) (Lawrence, KA: Coronado Press, 1974), quotations 16, 54.

31 Robert Darnton, *The Corpus of Clandestine Literature in France, 1769–1789* (New York: Norton, 1995), 202, 208.

32 John Cleland, *Fanny Hill, or Memoirs of a Woman of Pleasure* (1749) (reprint London: Penguin, 1985), see esp. 50, 76–7, 205.

33 Pisanus Fraxi [Henry Ashbee], *Bibliography of Prohibited Books* (1885) (reprint London: Jack Brussel, 1962), vol. 3: 408–15.

34 Pepys, *Diary*, vol. 5: 264.

35 Agnolo Firenzuola, *On the Beauty of Women* (1541), trans. and ed. by Konrad Eisenbichler and Jacqueline Murray (Philadelphia: University of Pennsylvania Press, 1992), quotations 30, 33. 'Celso' is speaking.

36 Pierre de Bourdeilles ['Brantôme'], *Les dames galantes* (reprint Paris: Garnier, 1965), 155, 159–60. On male concepts of female beauty in the sixteenth century see Jean-Louis Flandrin and Marie-Claude Phan, 'Les métamorphoses de la beauté féminine,' *L'Histoire* 68 (June 1984): 48–57; and Flandrin, 'Soins de beauté et recueils de secrets,' in *Les soins de beauté: Moyen Age, Débuts des temps modernes: Actes du IIIe Colloque International Grasse (26–8 April 1985)* (Nice: Centre d'études médiévales, Université de Nice, 1987), 13–29.

37 Jean-Jacques Rousseau, *Les confessions* (reprint Paris: Gallimard, 1959), 113.

38 Casanova, *Histoire de ma vie*, vol. 1: 587.

39 Willard Bissell Pope, ed., *The Diary of Benjamin Robert Haydon* (Cambridge, MA: Harvard University Press, 1960), vol. 1: 336. Later, however, Haydon does enthuse about 'full exquisite thighs' (495).

40 John Warrington, ed., *More's Utopia*, rev. ed. (London: Dent, 1951), 99.

41 Helen Gardner, ed., *John Donne, The Elegies and the Songs and*

Sonnets (Oxford: Clarendon, 1965), letter, xviii; quotation from poem, 15.

42 Pepys, *Diaries*, vol. 2: 43; vol. 8: 128; vol. 9: 439.

43 Brantôme, *Dames galantes*, 170.

44 Indispensable on the history of masturbation is Thomas Laqueur's *Solitary Sex: A Cultural History of Masturbation* (New York: Zone Books, 2003), although the conclusions of the present work differ somewhat from his. For other scholarly accounts of the history of masturbation see Jean-Louis Flandrin, *Les amours paysannes (XVIe–XIXe siècle)* (Paris: Flammarion, 1970), 160–5; Edward Shorter, *The Making of the Modern Family* (New York: Basic Books, 1975), 98–102, where I argued that a real increase in the frequency of masturbation occurred in the eighteenth and early nineteenth centuries. I am now more agnostic on the question.

45 Casanova, *Histoire de ma vie*, vol. 2: 672.

46 Rousseau, *Les confessions*, 152–5.

47 Anon. Review of Tissot's book *L'onanisme*, in *Journal de médecine, chirurgie*, 12 (1760), 483–94, quotation 483–4; G. Cless and G. Schübler, *Versuch einer medizinischen Topographie [der Stadt] Stuttgart* (Stuttgart: Sattler, 1815), 46.

48 M.R.D. Foot, ed., *The Gladstone Diaries* (Oxford: Clarendon, 1968), vol. 1: 276, 334, 351; vol. 2: 322.

49 Mary Wollstonecraft, *A Vindication of the Rights of Woman* (1792) (reprint London: Dent, 1929), 156.

50 Dafydd Johnston, 'Erotica and Satire in Medieval Welsh Poetry,' in Ziolkowski, ed., *Obscenity*, 60–72, quotation 69–70.

51 Ann Rosalind Jones, *The Currency of Eros: Women's Love Lyric in Europe, 1540–1620* (Bloomington: Indiana University Press, 1990), 171.

52 *Mémoires de Mme Roland* (Paris: Bibliothèque Nationale, 1883), vol. 3: 105, 111, 115.

53 For details of Mme de Graffigny's erotic life see English Showalter, ed., *Correspondance de Madame de Graffigny* (Oxford: Voltaire Foundation, 1985), vol. 1: 184–5.

54 Haliczer, *Sexuality in the Confessional*, 122, 128; the woman in question was cited in a religious manual.

55 Casanova, *Histoire de ma vie*, vol. 1: 359.

56 Medical evidence might represent a fourth source of information on the sexual attitudes and practices of women (it certainly
illumines the values of the physicians themselves). Many other
historians have relied upon such evidence in assessing female
sexuality, and it may be useful at least to comment on the
subject here. Briefly, the doctors' evidence is so mixed as to be
unusable. There were physicians who felt women to be veri-
table fountains of desire, others who considered their female
patients totally unresponsive. It is almost impossible to discern
a central trend, or majority opinion, in the considerable medical
literature before 1850 on female sexuality. There were certainly
numerous physicians who encountered desirous women in
their practices. Johann Storch, a gynecologist in Gotha, Germany, wrote in 1751 that it was better to permit hired wet
nurses living in the employer's home to have occasional conjugal visits than to ban sex entirely: 'They should not pine away
secretly for their husbands, which could be much more dangerous [for their milk] than moderate intercourse.' How about
prohibiting intercourse to nursing mothers? Storch said indig-
nantly, 'Middle-class women [*frei erzogene Weiber*] are not accustomed to letting their passion be reigned in.' On another
occasion Storch, meditating about the cause of a deadly pelvic
infection, noted that the husband's penis had been especially
large, 'and as he engaged in coitus very powerfully – and she,
for her part, did not fail to respond to him –, the inflammation
was created on the inner portion of the cervix.' Johann Storch,
Von Weiber-Kranckheiten (Gotha: Mevius, 1746–53), quotations
vol. 7: 67, 97; vol. 8: 177. Felix Platter, by contrast, city health
officer of Basel in the early seventeenth century, evidently saw
mainly women who were indifferent to intercourse and derived
no pleasure from the sexual act. 'A nobleman told me of the
case of his wife.' He had married her as a young woman many
years previously and had enjoyed a 'moderate' amount of
intercourse with her. But at some point her willingness evapo-
rated, 'and since then she cannot be persuaded in the slightest,
and even confesses that she has never had the least pleasure

from it nor has she even experienced a frisson. Now she feels nothing at all ... and accommodates him only as a favour.' The nobleman was said to have tried many medications. Platter told of another case, a woman who had been a virgin until her marriage at forty (it was her husband's second marriage) 'and has never felt a trace of desire, either in nocturnal encounters nor in any other manner.' Platter found it remarkable that both women 'still love their husbands immoderately and that the husbands accept the situation, even though their libidos in this unsatisfactory situation are only partially satisfied.' Felix Platter, *Observationes: Krankheitsbeobachtungen* (1st Latin ed. 1614), trans. into German (Berne: Huber, 1963), vol. 1: 161. Perhaps the doctors are like the four blind men, each describing a different part of the elephant, none having a comprehensive overview of the complex world of female sexuality. Perhaps they report differently according to their own prejudices and predilections. Perhaps they see mainly pathology, which, by definition, is different from the normal experiences of average people that we try to capture in the present volume. In any event, the route of medical evidence is unpromising for the history of female sexuality.

57 Boccaccio, *Decameron*, quotation, vol. 2: 119.
58 Englisch, *Geschichte der erotischen Literatur*, 558.
59 Annie Le Brun and Jean-Jacques Pauvert, eds, *Oeuvres complètes du Marquis de Sade* (Paris: Pauvert, 1987), 'Histoire de Juliette,' vol. 9: 377.
60 Wollstonecraft, *Vindication Rights of Woman*, 102.
61 Wollstonecraft, *Vindication Rights of Woman*, 32, 56, 145, 147.
62 See Diane Jacobs, *Her Own Woman: The Life of Mary Wollstone-craft* (New York: Simon and Schuster, 2001), 111f.
63 Diana Robin, ed., *Laura Cereta, Collected Letters of a Renaissance Feminist* (Chicago: University of Chicago Press, 1997), 37–9.
64 W. Butler-Bowdon, ed., *The Book of Margery Kempe, 1436* (London: Cape, 1936), 30–1.
65 Douglas G. Greene, ed., *The Meditations of Lady Elizabeth Delaval* (Gateshead: Northumberland Press, 1978), 37, 47, 61, 79–80, 204.

66 Heinz Herz, ed., *Liselotte von der Pfalz: Briefe der Herzogin Elisabeth Charlotte von Orléans an ihre Geschwister* (Leipzig: Koehler, 1972), 167, 205, 241.

67 Edward Jenkins, ed., *The Cavalier and His Lady: Selections from the Works of the First Duke and Duchess of Newcastle* (London: Macmillan, 1872), quotations from her work 'A True Relation of My Birth, Breeding and Life ...' (1656), pp. 31–71, quotations pp. 46, 71.

68 Robert Halsband, ed., *The Complete Letters of Lady Mary Wortley Montagu* (Oxford: Clarendon, 1965), vol. 1: 66, 155.

69 *Mary Wortley Montagu Letters*, vol. 1: 53, 96; vol. 3: 27, 44.

70 Lars E. Troide and Stewart J. Cooke, eds, *The Early Journals and Letters of Fanny Burney* (Oxford: Clarendon, 1994), vol. 3: 295.

71 Jacques Solé, *L'amour en Occident à l'époque moderne* (Paris: Michel, 1976), 155.

72 Brantôme, *Dames galantes*, 5.

73 John W. Baldwin, *The Language of Sex: Five Voices from Northern France around 1200* (Chicago: University of Chicago Press, 1994), 53; a tale from a medieval French *fabliau*.

74 Brantôme, *Dames galantes*, 151: 'les entretienent de beaux et lascifs discours, de mots follastres et paroles lubriques.'

75 Quoted from *Le Papillotage* (Rotterdam, 1769), in Jean Hervez, *Les sociétés d'amour au XVIIIe siècle* (Paris: Daragon, 1906), 5–6. 'As changeable as fashion ... women find a new lover': quotation is Hervez himself, not the anonymous eighteenth-century author.

76 *Le Papillotage*, quoted in Hervez, 7.

77 Brantôme, *Dames galantes*, 192, 200.

78 Quoted in Elizabeth Colwill, 'Pass as a Woman, Act like a Man: Marie Antoinette as Tribade in the Pornography of the French Revolution,' in Jeffrey Merrick and Bryant T. Ragan, Jr, eds, *Homosexuality in Modern France* (New York: Oxford University Press, 1996), 54–79, quotation 69.

79 Byron, *Letters*, vol. 7: 43.

80 Donatien Alphonse François de Sade, *Voyage d'Italie*, ed. by Maurice Lever (Paris: Fayard, 1995), vol. 1: 72.

81 Sade, *Voyage d'Italie*, vol. 1: 72.

82 Luigi Valmaggi, *I cicisbei: Contributo alla storia del costume italiano nel. Sec. XVIII* (Turin: Chiantore, 1927), 154–5.

83 On the role of female desire in the system see ibid., 139–41.

84 *Mary Wortley Montagu Letters*, vol. 2: 496.

85 Aristocratic French women also knew the system of 'chevalier servant,' yet not in the Italian form of permanent male concubine. Hervez suggests that the chevalier servant at the eighteenth-century court served more as a kind of procurer (*procurateur*) of pretty boys for circles of women. See Hervez, *Sociétés d'amour*, 21–2, on the circle around la princesse de Bouillon.

Chapter 3 A Baseline for Gays and Lesbians

1 Julien Green, *Jeunesse* (Paris: Plon, 1974), 203.

2 Quoted in Noël Greig, ed., *Edward Carpenter: Selected Writings, vol. 1: Sex* (London: GMP, 1984), 18.

3 See Brigitte Eriksson, 'A Lesbian Execution in Germany, 1721: The Trial Records,' *Journal of Homosexuality* 6 (1980): 27–40, and Louis Crompton, 'The Myth of Lesbian Impunity: Capital Laws from 1270 to 1791,' in that same issue, 11–25. The point is not that 'Sexual relations between women were either ignored or dismissed,' as Judith C. Brown argues. It is that they were not tolerated once they were discovered. That a large body of legislation on the subject did not exist is irrelevant. Brown, 'Lesbian Sexuality in Medieval and Early Modern Europe' (1985), reprinted in Martin Duberman et al., eds, *Hidden from History: Reclaiming the Gay and Lesbian Past* (New York: Penguin, 1989), 67–75, quotation 70.

4 André Gide, *Corydon* (1911), enlarged ed. (Paris: Gallimard, 1920), 24, 27.

5 Owing to the influence of Michel Foucault, the social-constructionist view has predominated within gay studies until recently. For a summary of the debate between the 'essentialists' (inborn) and the 'social constructionists,' see Franz X. Eder et al., eds, *Sexual Cultures in Europe: National Histories* (Manchester: Manchester University Press, 1999), 4–5. For a typical social-

constructionist argument see Rudi C. Bleys, *The Geography of Perversion: Male-to-Male Sexual Behavior Outside the West and the Ethnographic Imagination, 1750–1918* (New York: New York University Press, 1995), 7: 'The longterm change from an act-orientated definition [anyone committing sodomy on man or woman] to an "identity"-oriented definition is now generally known as "the construction of modern homosexuality."' Alfred Kinsey was a social constructionist *avant la lettre*, believing, in the words of his biographer, that, 'In the end, whether a person got involved with one sexual outlet or another was largely a matter of chance.' James H. Jones, *Alfred C. Kinsey: A Public/ Private Life* (New York: Norton, 1997), 532.

6 Rictor Norton, *The Myth of the Modern Homosexual: Queer History and the Search for Cultural Unity* (London: Cassell, 1997), 22.

7 Phyllis Grosskurth, *John Addington Symonds: A Biography* (London: Longmans, 1964), 270–1.

8 Paul Näcke, 'Ein Besuch bei den Homosexuellen in Berlin,' *Archiv für Kriminalanthropologie und Kriminalistic* 15 (1904), reprinted in Magnus Hirschfeld, *Berlins Drittes Geschlecht* (1904) (Berlin: Rosa Winkel, 1991), 165–94, quotation 189.

9 Donald Webster Cory [Edward Sagarin], *The Homosexual in America: A Subjective Approach* (New York: Greenberg, 1951), 66–72.

10 Cory, *Homosexual in America*, 13.

11 See Michel Foucault, *Histoire de la sexualité, vol. 1: La volonté de savoir* (Paris: Gallimard, 1976). Lillian Faderman, for example, considers the existence of butch-femme couples theoretically impossible before the sexologists describe them: 'The women who attended such functions [drag balls in New York in the 1890s] were perhaps the first conscious "butches" and "femmes." There could be no such social equivalents for women who loved women before the sexologists turned their attention to them, since earlier they had had no awareness of themselves as a group.' *Odd Girls and Twilight Lovers: A History of Lesbian Life in Twentieth-Century America* (New York: Columbia University Press, 1991), 59.

12 Paul Näcke, 'Die Diagnose der Homosexualität,' *Neurologisches*

Centralblatt 27 (1909): 338–51, quotation 342. Näcke said that
most gay men first felt same-sex strivings 'around the time of
puberty' (343). See also his 'Einteilung der Homosexuellen,'
Allgemeine Zeitschrift für Psychiatrie 65 (1908): 109–28, at 118.

13 Ritch C. Savin-Williams, '... *And Then I Became Gay': Young
Men's Stories* (New York: Routledge, 1998), 15, table 1.2.

14 Dean Hamer, *The Science of Desire: The Search for the Gay Gene
and the Biology of Behavior* (New York: Simon and Schuster,
1994), 65. See also Dean H. Hamer et al., 'A Linkage between
DNA Markers on the X Chromosome and Male Sexual Orientation,' *Science* 261 (1993): 321–7.

15 Rictor Norton, ed., *My Dear Boy: Gay Love Letters through the
Centuries* (San Francisco: Leyland, 1998), 16.

16 Quoted in Norton, *Myth Modern Homosexual*, 276.

17 Joanne Glasgow, ed., *Your John: The Love Letters of Radclyffe Hall*
(New York: New York University Press, 1997), 50–1.

18 Claudie Lesselier, 'Silenced Resistances and Conflictual Identities: Lesbians in France, 1930–1968,' *Journal of Homosexuality* 25
(1993): 105–25, quotation 118.

19 Janet Lever, 'Lesbian Sex Survey,' *The Advocate*, 22 Aug. 1995:
22–30; see 28.

20 Del Martin and Phyllis Lyon, *Lesbian/Woman* (1972) (rev. ed.
Volcano, CA: Volcano Press, 1991), 74.

21 On 'childhood gender nonconformity' (CGN) see Richard C.
Pillard and J. Michael Bailey, 'A Biological Perspective on
Sexual Orientation,' *Psychiatric Clinics of North America* 18(1)
(March 1995): 71–84, esp. 73–4.

22 Johann Ludwig Casper, 'Über Nothzucht und Päderastie und
deren Ermittelung Seitens des Gerichtsarztes,' *Vierteljahrsschrift
für gerichtliche und öffentliche Medicin* 1 (1852): 21–78, esp. 62. In
his later textbook, Casper emphasized the inborn nature of a
good deal of homosexuality while allowing that some was
acquired as well 'as a result of oversaturation in the natural
pleasures of sex.' Casper, *Practisches Handbuch der gerichtlichen
Medicin*, 5th ed. (posthumous edition edited by Carl Liman)
(Berlin: Hirschwald, 1871), vol. 1: 180–1.

23 On Krafft-Ebing see Harry Oosterhuis, *Stepchildren of Nature:*

Krafft-Ebing, Psychiatry, and the Making of Sexual Identity (Chicago: University of Chicago Press, 2000).

24 Richard von Krafft-Ebing, 'Zum Verständnis der konträren Sexualempfindung,' *Jahrbuch für sexuelle Zwischenstufen* 3 (1901): 1–36, quotations 2. Krafft-Ebing did not, however, revise his previous opinions in the twelfth edition of his sexology text *Psychopathia sexualis*, published in 1902, the preface of which he signed in December, weeks or days before his death (perhaps he was too weak to do so). The subsequent editions of *Psychopathia sexualis* were unchanged, and the fourteenth, published in 1912, was reprinted in the 1990s. Richard von Krafft-Ebing, *Psychopathia sexualis* (reprint Munich: Matthes and Seitz, 1997), see, for example, 225.

25 Havelock Ellis and John Addington Symonds, *Sexual Inversion* (London: Wilson and Macmillan, 1897), xiv, 106–7, 129.

26 L.S.A.M. v. Römer, 'Die erbliche Belastung des Zentralnervensystems bei Uraniern, geistig gesunden Menschen und Geisteskranken,' *Jahrbuch für sexuelle Zwischenstufen* 7(1) (1905): 67–81, see esp. 69–70. Römer presented more of his data in his *Die uranische Familie: Untersuchungen über die Ascendenz der Uranier* (Leizpig and Amsterdam: Verlag von Maas and Van Suchtelen, 1906).

27 Edward M. Miller, 'Homosexuality, Birth Order, and Evolution: Toward an Equilibrium Reproductive Economics of Homosexuality,' *Archives of Sexual Behavior* 29 (2000): 1–34, quotation 16.

28 Franz J. Kallmann, 'Twin and Sibship Study of Overt Male Homosexuality,' *American Journal of Human Genetics* 4 (1952): 136–53, quotation 143.

29 J. Michael Bailey et al., 'Genetic and Environmental Influences on Sexual Orientation and Its Correlations in an Australian Twin Sample,' *Journal of Personality and Social Psychology* 78 (2000): 524–36.

30 See Richard C. Pillard and J. Michael Bailey, 'Human Sexual Orientation Has a Heritable Component,' *Human Biology* 70 (1998): 347–65; 356, table 2. In a study of a U.S. national sample, Kenneth S. Kendler and co-workers found 'nonheterosexual sexual orientation' to be concordant in 31.6 per cent of monozy-

gotic twin pairs and in 8.3 per cent of dizygotic. 'Sexual Orientation in a U.S. National Sample of Twin and Nontwin Sibling Pairs,' *American Journal of Psychiatry* 157 (2000): 1843–6; see 1845, table 1.

31 Frederick L. Whitam et al., 'Homosexual Orientation in Twins: A Report on 61 Pairs and Three Triplet Sets,' *Archives of Sexual Behavior* 22 (1993): 187–206.

32 For an overview, see Ray Blanchard, 'Birth Order and Sibling Sex Ratio in Homosexual Versus Heterosexual Males and Females,' *Annual Review of Sex Research*, 8 (1997): 27–67.

33 Martin L. Lalumière et al., 'Sexual Orientation and Handedness in Men and Women: A Meta-Analysis,' *Psychological Bulletin* 126 (2000): 575–92.

34 Terrence J. Williams et al., 'Finger-length Ratios and Sexual Orientation,' *Nature* 404 (2000): 455–6.

35 Simon LeVay, 'A Difference in Hypothalamic Structure between Heterosexual and Homosexual Men,' *Science* 253 (1991): 1034–7.

36 Magnus Hirschfeld, 'Das Ergebnis der statistischen Untersuchungen über den Prozentsatz der Homosexuellen,' *Jahrbuch für sexuelle Zwischenstufen* 6 (1904): 107–78, see esp. 128–35 on the micro-milieux; 136, 147–54 on the questionnaire data.

37 In the United States only about 3 per cent of adult men and 1 per cent of women reported having any same-sex sexual activity within the past year; in Britain the figures were considerably lower. See Edward O. Laumann et al., *The Social Organization of Sexuality: Sexual Practices in the United States* (Chicago: University of Chicago Press, 1994), 295, fig. 8.1, and discussion on 297.

38 Hans Licht [Paul Brandt], *Sittengeschichte Griechenlands* (1925–8) (rev. reprint ed. Stuttgart: Günther, 1960), 291–2, 310–11.

39 Alexander Nehamas and Paul Woodruff, trans. and eds, *Plato, Symposium* (Indianapolis: Hackett, 1989), 27.

40 John R. Clarke, *Looking at Lovemaking: Constructions of Sexuality in Roman Art, 100 B.C.–A.D. 250* (Berkeley: University of California Press, 1998), 38. The gemstone is from the late Hellenistic period and carries a Greek inscription.

41 Licht [Brandt], *Sittengeschichte*, 342. 'Bürschen-Dreht-Euch.'

42 Robert Aldrich, *The Seduction of the Mediterranean: Writing, Art*

and Homosexual Fantasy (London: Routledge, 1993), 17; as the author notes, 'vase paintings mostly show women or satyrs performing fellatio on men.'

43 J.A. Pott and F.A. Wright, trans., *Martial: The Twelve Books of Epigrams* (London: Routledge, 1920), XLVIII, 'The Poet's Needs,' 60. There is much additional evidence of this in addition to Martial.

44 Clarke, *Looking at Lovemaking*, 83.

45 Aldrich, *Seduction of the Mediterranean*, 29.

46 Clarke, *Looking at Lovemaking*, 83.

47 John Boswell, *Christianity, Social Tolerance, and Homosexuality: Gay People in Western Europe from the Beginning of the Christian Era to the Fourteenth Century* (Chicago: University of Chicago Press, 1980), 73.

48 See Licht [Brandt], *Sittengeschichte*, on Sappho and her circle, 227–9.

49 Terence DuQuesne, trans. and ed., *Sappho of Lesbos: The Poems* (Oxford: Darengo, 1990), 45 (XVIII), 52 (XIX).

50 This account represents the combined version of the translation of A.-J. Pons, Lucien: *Dialogues des courtisanes* (Paris: Quantin, 1881), 21–5; and Licht [Brandt], *Sittengeschichte*, 225–6.

51 John Boswell's account makes clear that early medieval society was largely uncensorious of homosexual behaviour; yet contemporaries, and Boswell himself, take for granted that anal intercourse is meant. *Christianity, Social Tolerance*, 180–5. 'Sodomy,' as Boswell points out, embraced 'any emission of semen not directed exclusively toward the procreation of a legitimate child within matrimony.' It included as well much heterosexual activity (202).

52 Bernd-Ulrich Hergemöller, 'Grundfragen zum Verständnis gleichgeschlechtlichen Verhaltens im späten Mittelalter,' in Rüdiger Lautmann and Angela Taeger, eds, *Männerliebe im alten Deutschland* (Berlin: Rosa Winkel, 1992), 9–38, quotations 20–1.

53 Michael Rocke, *Forbidden Friendships: Homosexuality and Male Culture in Renaissance Florence* (New York: Oxford University Press, 1996), 93. Unlike anal sex, in fellatio the younger man was the inserter.

54 Rictor Norton, 'England's First Pornographer,' www.infopt
.demon.co.uk/wilmot.htm, 5.

55 Rictor Norton, *Mother Clap's Molly House: The Gay Subculture in
England, 1700–1830* (London: GMP, 1992), 107–8.

56 Michael Rey, 'Parisian Homosexuals Create a Lifestyle, 1700–
1750: The Police Archives,' *Eighteenth Century Life* 9 (1985),
179–91, see 183–4.

57 Pott and Wright, trans., *Martial: The Twelve Books of Epigrams*,
XLII, 58.

58 Jean-Jacques Rousseau, *Les confessions* (written 1769) (new ed.
Paris: Gallimard, 1973), 104.

59 Heinz Herz, ed., *Liselotte von der Pfalz. Briefe der Herzogin
Elisabeth Charlotte von Orléans an ihre Geschwister* (Leipzig:
Koehler, 1972), 344.

60 Norton, *Myth Modern Homosexual*, 242.

61 E. William Monter, 'Sodomy and Heresy in Early Modern
Switzerland,' *Journal of Homosexuality* 6 (1980): 41–53, see 51 n6.
Needless to say, in Calvinist Geneva, a city with a population of
under 20,000, there was no 'continuous subculture.'

62 Heinz ed., *Liselotte*, 171–2, 320.

63 Rey, 'Parisian Homosexuals,' 186.

64 Michael D. Sibalis, 'Paris,' in David Higgs, ed., *Queer Sites: Gay
Urban Histories since 1600* (London: Routledge, 1999), 10–37, see
17.

65 Quoted in Pisanus Fraxi [Henry Spencer Ashby], *Bibliography of
Prohibited Books* (1879) (reprint Kila, MT: Kessinger, nd), vol. 2:
408–9. Bloch, *Sex Life of Our Time*, identifies the author of the
quoted passage as Paul Lacroix (515). My translation from the
French.

66 Norton, *Myth Modern Homosexual*, 243.

67 Information from Norton, *Mother Clap's Molly House*, 50–1, 54,
169, 184.

68 Gert Hekma, 'Amsterdam,' in Higgs, ed., *Queer Sites*, 61–88, see
67. Despite this evidence, Hekma doubts that a 'homosexual
identity' existed before the 1950s. 'Most homosexual acts till
that time were perpetrated by men who sought sexual pleasure
and did not care much about the gender of their partner' (68).

The notion that men were ever indifferent to their partner's gender, to say nothing of until the 1950s, strikes me as extremely unlikely.

69 Dirk Jaap Noordam, 'Sodomy in the Dutch Republic, 1600–1725,' in Kent Gerard and Gert Hekma, eds, *The Pursuit of Sodomy: Male Homosexuality in Renaissance and Enlightenment Europe* (New York: Harrington Park, 1989), 207–28, see 215–17.

70 D.A. Coward, 'Attitudes to Homosexuality in Eighteenth-century France,' *Journal of European Studies* 10 (1980): 231–54, see 234.

71 William Lithgow, *The Totall Discourse of the Rare Adventures and Painefull Peregrinations* ... (1632) (reprint Glasgow: MacLehose, 1906), 38.

72 Rocke, *Forbidden Friendships*, 5, 13, 95, 102–3, 115, 120. On Venice, see Guido Ruggiero, *The Boundaries of Eros: Sex Crime and Sexuality in Renaissance Venice* (New York: Oxford University Press, 1985), who finds that by the fifteenth century 'homosexuality [became] a style and a way of life that it had not been before' (137).

73 According to Anthony M. Scacco, 'The Sexual Assaults that occur within prisons and jails cannot be categorized as homosexual attacks, rather they are assaults by heterosexually-oriented males on other males for political reasons, i.e. in order to show power or dominance over other human beings.' *Rape in Prison* (Springfield, IL: Thomas, 1975), 67. See also George L. Kirkham, 'Homosexuality in Prison,' on 'jockers' (aggressors) and 'pressure punks' (passive recipients). In James M. Henslin, ed., *Studies in the Sociology of Sex* (New York: Appleton, 1971), 325–49, esp. 338–45.

74 Rocke, *Forbidden Friendships*, 29, 162, 191.

75 Randolph Trumbach, 'London,' in Higgs, ed., *Queer Sites*, 89–111, see 90.

76 Trumbach summarizes the outlines of this argument in *Sex and the Gender Revolution*, vol. 1: 3–9; see also Rocke, *Forbidden Friendships*, 87–8; Bryant T. Ragan, Jr, 'The Enlightenment Confronts Homosexuality,' in Jeffrey Merrick and Ragan, eds, *Homosexuality in Modern France* (New York: Oxford University

Press, 1996), 8–29: 'With the birth of the "new sodomite," sodomitical subcultures developed in many West European cities, including Paris ... They often called each other by feminine nicknames ... and adopted effeminate mannerisms' (12).

77 Licht [Brandt], *Sittengeschichte*, 341–2.

78 Hergemöller, in *Männerliebe*, 32.

79 Norton, *My Dear Boy*, 68.

80 Norton, *Mother Clap's Molly House*, 101–4.

81 Jeffrey Merrick, 'The Marquis de Villette and Mademoiselle de Raucourt,' in Merrick, ed., *Homosexuality Modern France*, 30–53, see 44.

82 See Judith C. Brown, *Immodest Acts: The Life of a Lesbian Nun in Renaissance Italy* (New York: Oxford University Press, 1986) on 'sodomy' between females (anal sex is not meant) as 'the sin which cannot be named' (19).

83 Havelock Ellis attempts a brief chronicle of the dildo in *Sexual Inversion* (London: Wilson and Macmillan, 1897), 77 n1.

84 On the deep historical continuity of lesbian culture see Judy Grahn, *Another Mother Tongue: Gay Words, Gay Worlds* (Boston: Beacon, 1984), 33–5, 96–7, 152–7.

85 Brown, *Immodest Acts*, 120.

86 Merrick, 'Villette-Raucourt,' 44.

87 Lillian Faderman, *Surpassing the Love of Men: Romantic Friendship and Love between Women from the Renaissance to the Present* (New York: Morrow, 1981): 'Love between women has been primarily a sexual phenomenon only in male fantasy literature. "Lesbian" describes a relationship in which two women's strongest emotions and affections are directed toward each other. Sexual contact ... may be entirely absent' (17–18). The author believes that sexual love between women began to emerge only late in the nineteenth century as a result of the feminist movement (187–9, 204f.).

88 Jill Liddington, ed., *Female Fortune: Land, Gender, and Authority: The Anne Lister Diaries and Other Writings, 1883–36* (London: Rivers Oram Press, 1998) 102.

89 Helena Whitbread ed., *I Know My Own Heart: The Diaries of*

Anne Lister, 1790–1840 (New York: New York University Press, 1992), 273.

90 See Paul Englisch, *Geschichte der erotischen Literatur* (Stuttgart: Püttmann, 1927), 429–33.

91 Francis Lacassin, ed., *Jacques Casanova de Seingalt, Histoire de ma vie* (new ed. Paris: Laffont, 1993), vol. 1: 761.

92 Norton, *Myth Modern Homosexual*, 204.

93 *I Know My Own Heart*, 273.

94 Faderman believes butch-femme pairing a socially imposed recent creation, 'because women were emulating the only examples of domestic situations available to them in a patriar-chal culture.' *Surpassing the Love of Men*, 323; see also 456 n36. For the opposite view – butch-femme as an age-old 'dyke' tradition – see Grahn, *Another Mother Tongue*, 46, 145–6.

95 Susie Bright interview, in Andrea Juno, ed., *Angry Women* (New York: Juno Books, 1991), 194–221, quotation 211.

96 *I Know My Own Heart*, 48, 151, 267.

97 The Anne Listers of this world in the 1820s give the complete lie to Lillian Faderman's view of the 1890s that 'the sexologists gave many of them [butches and femmes] a concept and a descriptive vocabulary for themselves, which was as necessary in forming a lesbian subculture as the modicum of economic independence they were able to attain ...' *Odd Girls*, 59.

98 Pierre Viguié, ed., *Mémoires de Madame de la Guette* (first pub. 1681) (Paris: Jonquières, 1929), esp. xv, xvi, 3.

99 P.M. Wise, 'Case of Sexual Perversion,' *Alienist and Neurologist* 4 (1883): 87–91. Wise considered her 'erotomania' also part of her insanity, but he did say that in the two years she had been at Willard Asylum in Willard, New York, 'Dementia has been progressive and she is fast losing her memory and capacity for coherent discourse' (90).

Chapter 4 Hindrances

1 Georg Queri, *Bauernerotik und Bauernfehme in Oberbayern* (Munich: Piper, 1911), 38. 'Wär's nit in mein Bett noch so guat schlaffa / aber dee Teufelsflöh gebn koan Ruah / hab ja mit

eahna dee ganze Nacht z schaffa/zreissen mir s Leilach und d
Deck'n dazua / hoassts allweil: kratz amal, kratz amal / im
Arsch und überall, überall / bissn und bissn, bissn muass sei!'

2 Ulrich Bräker, *Lebensgeschichte und natürliche Ebentheuer* [sic]
des Armen Mannes im Tockenburg (1788) (reprint ed. Basel:
Birkhäuser, 1945), vol. 1: 86.

3 I am grateful to Prof. Reinhard Spree for sharing his unpublished
10 per cent sample of the patients in this hospital. 'Krätze.'

4 Francis Lacassin, ed., *Jacques Casanova de Seingalt, Histoire de ma
vie* (1789) (rev. ed. Paris: Laffont, 1993), vol. 1: 24–5.

5 Robert Latham and William Matthews, eds, *The Diary of Samuel
Pepys* (Berkeley: University of California Press, 1976), vol. 9: 424.

6 Pepys, *Diary*, vol. 8: 133; 1667.

7 Michel de Montaigne, *Journal de voyage en Italie* (1774) (new ed.
Paris: Garnier, 1942), 216.

8 Tobias Smollett, *Travels through France and Italy* (1766) (reprint
Oxford: Oxford University Press, 1981), 203–4.

9 M.R.D. Foot, ed., *The Gladstone Diaries* (Oxford: Clarendon,
1968), vol. 2: 448.

10 John Beresford, ed., *The Diary of a Country Parson: The Reverend
James Woodforde* (London: Oxford University Press, 1926), vol. 2:
29, 253.

11 Peter Salovey et al., *Reporting Chronic Pain Episodes on Health
Surveys*, National Center for Health Statistics. Vital Health
Statistics 6(6) (1992): 1.

12 Jacob Zeitlin, trans. and ed., *The Essays of Michel de Montaigne*
(New York: Knopf, 1936), vol. 3: 292–3.

13 Jean-Jacques Rousseau, *Les confessions* (new ed. Paris: Gallimard, 1973), 517–18.

14 Montaigne, *Essays*, vol. 3: 289.

15 Albert Köbele, *Ortssippenbuch Wollbach* (Grafenhausen bei Lahr:
Selbstverlag des Herausgebers, 1962), 272, no. 1508, plus cross-
references.

16 U.S. Bureau of the Census. *Historical Statistics of the United
States, Colonial Times to 1970, Bicentennial Edition, part 2* (Washington, DC: Government Printing Office, 1975), 56–7.

17 Elizabeth Arias, 'United States Life Tables, 2000,' *National Vital
Statistics Reports* 51 (3) (19 Dec. 2002): 7, 9.

18 Beth-Zion Abrahams, trans. and ed., *The Life of Glückel of Hameln, 1646–1724, Written by Herself* (New York: Yoseloff, 1963), 11, 80, 104.

19 Luke 12: 19–20.

20 Caroline Walker Bynum, *Fragmentation and Redemption: Essays on Gender and the Human Body in Medieval Religion* (New York: Zone, 1992), 189.

21 Quoted in Eberhard Winkler, *Die Leichenpredigt im deutschen Luthertum bis Spener* (Munich: Kaiser, 1967), 53.

22 Anton Linsenmayer, *Geschichte der Predigt in Deutschland von Karl dem Grossen bis zum Ausgange des vierzehnten Jahrhunderts* (1886) (reprint Frankfurt: Minerva, 1969), 476.

23 John W. Baldwin, *The Language of Sex: Five Voices from Northern France around 1200* (Chicago: University of Chicago Press, 1994), 174.

24 Earl Jeffrey Richards, trans., *Christine de Pizan. The Book of the City of Ladies (1405)* (New York: Persea, 1982), 52, 54, 155, 256.

25 Winkler, *Leichenpredigt*, 96. Many of these homilies were offered at the graveside, yet the Sunday morning message could not have been much different.

26 A. Freybe, *Das Memento mori in deutscher Sitte* (Gotha: Perthes, 1909), 40, 46.

27 Annie Le Brun and Jean-Jacques Pauvert, eds, *Oeuvres complètes du Marquis de Sade* (Paris: Pauvert, 1987), 'Histoire de Juliette,' vol. 8: 59–60.

28 Louis Marie Lavergne, *Topographie médicale de Lamballe et de ses environs en 1787* (Léhon: Entre-Nous, 1959), 27–8.

29 K.H. Lübben, *Beiträge zur Kenntniss der Rhön in medizinischer Hinsicht* (Weimar: Wagner, 1881), 45–6.

30 Schraube, 'Medicinisch-topographische Skizze des Kreises Querfurt,' *Monatsblatt für medicinische Statistik und öffentliche Gesundheitspflege* 8 (20 Aug. 1864): 63–4.

31 Georg Wilhelm Consbruch, *Medicinische Ephemeriden nebst einer medicinischen Topographie der Grafschaft Ravensberg* (Chemnitz: Hofmann, 1793), 46.

32 Henriette Dussourd, *Au même pot et au même feu: Étude sur les communautés familiales agricoles du Centre de la France* (Moulins: Pottier, 1962), 44–5.

33 Eugène Olivier, *Médecine et santé dans le pays de Vaud au XVIIIe siècle* (Lausanne: Payot, 1962), vol. 1: 563–5.

34 Robert Halsband, ed., *The Complete Letters of Lady Mary Wortley Montagu* (Oxford: Clarendon, 1965), 255.

35 According to scholar Lauri Kuusanmäki, quoted in Matti Sarmela, *Reciprocity Systems of the Rural Society in the Finnish-Karelian Culture Area with Special Reference to Social Intercourse of the Youth* (Helsinki: Academia Scientiarum Fennica, 1969), 43.

36 Franz Xaver Mezler, *Versuch einer medizinischen Topographie der Stadt Sigmaringen* (Freiburg: Herder, 1822), 189; written 1810.

37 Martine Segalen, 'Le mariage, l'amour et les femmes dans les proverbes populaires français' (pt 2), *Ethnologie française* 6 (1976): 33–88. Thus in the Franche-Comté district, 'En juillet et en août, ni femmes ni choux,' 63.

38 G.R. Quaife, *Wanton Wenches and Wayward Wives: Peasants and Illicit Sex in Early Seventeenth Century England* (London: Croom Helm, 1979), 78–9.

39 According to folklorist Paul Sébillot, quoted in Martine Segalen, *Mari et femme dans la société paysanne* (Paris: Flammarion, 1980), 50.

40 The doctors, following ancient texts, believed that women had to experience sexual pleasure in order to conceive. Jean Liébaut, in his sixteenth-century gynecology textbook, wrote, 'The woman receives more pleasure and contentment from this natural combat [sex] than the man. For the uterus, having received from Nature an incredible desire to conceive and to procreate, is so avid for virible semen, desires it so much ... to suck and retain it, that only a small quantity of matter is required for this use and common purpose.' Jean L. Liébaut, *Thrésor des remèdes secrets pour les maladies des femmes*, rev. ed. (Paris: Robert, 1597), 529–30. These views may be considered male fantasies.

41 Abel Hugo, *France pittoresque* (Paris: Delloye, 1835), vol. 2: 29.

42 Ibid., vol. 1: 299.

43 E.-J. Savigné, *Moeurs, coutumes, habitudes il y a plus d'un siècle des habitants de ... Saint-Romain-en-Galles* (Vienne: Ogeret, 1902), 11.

44 Armand Cassan, *Statistique de l'arrondissement de Mantes* (Mantes: Forcade, 1833), 56–7.

45 Warren Derry, ed., *The Journals and Letters of Fanny Burney (Madame d'Arblay)* (Oxford: Clarendon, 1982), vol. 9: 250.

46 Quoted in Octave Uzanne, *Son altesse la femme* (Paris: Quantin, 1885), 303.

47 Alfred W. Crosby, 'Smallpox,' in Kenneth Kiple, ed., *The Cambridge World History of Human Disease* (New York: Cambridge University Press, 1993), 1010.

48 *Mary Wortley Montagu Letters*, vol. 1: 182 nl.

49 Hector Fleischmann, *Les demoiselles d'amour du Palais-Royal* (Paris: Bibliothèque des curieux, 1911), 139.

50 Charles-Augustin Sainte-Beuve, *Mes poisons* (reprint Paris: Jalard, 1965), 72.

51 On these statistics see Edward Shorter, *Women's Bodies: A Social History of Women's Encounter with Health, Ill-Health, and Medicine* (1982) (republ. Brunswick, NJ: Transaction, 1991), 97–102.

52 Carl N. Degler, *At Odds: Women and the Family in America from the Revolution to the Present* (New York: Oxford University Press, 1980), 225.

53 Heinrich Fasbender, *Geschichte der Geburtshilfe* (1906) (reprint Hildesheim: Olms, 1964), 36.

54 Guillaume Mauquest de la Motte, *Traité complet des acouchements* (1715) (new ed. Leiden: Langerak, 1729), 71.

55 Jacques Gélis 'Sages-femmes et accoucheurs: L'obstétrique populaire aux XVIIe et XVIIIe siècles,' *Annales ESC* 32 (1977): 927–57, quotation 931–2.

56 Casanova, however, read this logic the other way: pregnancy is so dangerous that women must enjoy sex enormously if they are willing to risk it. 'The pleasure that I experienced when a woman whom I loved has made me happy [sexually] is certainly great, but I know that I would not have wanted it if, in order to get it, I should have had to expose myself to the risk of becoming pregnant. The woman exposes herself to the risk even after she has given birth several times. Thus she finds that the pleasure is worth the pain' ['que le plaisir vaut la peine'], *Histoire de ma vie*, vol. 3: 651.

Chapter 5 Why Not the Romantics?

1 Alfred de Musset, *La confession d'un enfant du siècle* (1836) (reprint Paris: Gallimard, 1973), 38–9 ff.
2 Ibid., 109.
3 Lars E. Troide, ed., *The Early Journals and Letters of Fanny Burney* (Oxford: Clarendon, 1988), vol. 1: 1.
4 Joyce Hemlow and Althea Douglas, eds, *Journals and Letters of Fanny Burney* (Oxford: Clarendon, 1972), vol. 2: 136.
5 Burney, *Early Journals*, vol. 1: 127.
6 Friedrich Hebbel, *Tagebücher, 1835–43* (Munich: Deutscher Taschenbuch Verlag, 1984), vol. 1: 12.
7 Willard Bissell Pope, ed., *The Diary of Benjamin Robert Haydon* (Cambridge, MA: Harvard University Press), vol. 1: 443, 493.
8 Haydon, *Diary*, vol. 2: 10–11.
9 Burney, *Early Journals*, vol. 2: 62–3. On talk of Omai in the Burney home see Kate Chisholm, *Fanny Burney: Her Life, 1752–1840* (London: Chatto, 1998), 37–8.
10 David Baumgardt, ed., *Seele und Welt: Franz Baader's Jugendtagebücher, 1786–1792* (Berlin: Wegweiser-Verlag, nd), 43.
11 A quip of the Marquis de Ségur, quoted in Élisabeth de Gramont, *Mémoires, vol. 2: Les marronniers en fleurs* (Paris: Grasset, 1929), 42. 'Le plus fort battement de coeur du 18e siècle.'
12 Eugène Asse, ed., *Lettres de Mlle. de Lespinasse* (Paris: Charpentier, 1876), 147.
13 Lespinasse, *Lettres*, 13, 39, 110, 112, 118, 173, 217. For an introduction to her life, see le Marquis de Ségur, *Julie de Lespinasse* (Paris: Calmann-Lévy, 1905).
14 Arsène Houssaye, *Les confessions: Souvenirs d'un demi-siècle, 1830–1880* (Paris: Dentu, 1885), vol. 2: 92.
15 Charles F. Dupêchez, ed., *Mémoires, souvenirs et journaux de la Comtesse D'Agoult (Daniel Stern)* (Paris: Mercure de France, 1990), vol. 1: 196f., 308, 317.
16 Bernard Gagnebin et al., eds, *Jean-Jacques Rousseau: Les confessions* (written 1769, first published 1789) (Paris: Gallimard, 1959), 129, 281, 321, 502, 530, 537, 538.

17 *Mémoires de Mme Roland* (Paris: Bibliothèque nationale, 1883), vol. 4: 21–2.
18 Théophile Gautier, *Mademoiselle de Maupin* (1835) (augmented ed. Paris: Garnier, 1966), 131. The sentence was completed, 'that I cannot tolerate the idea of being for a month or two without a woman.'
19 Philippe M. Monnier, ed., *Henri-Frédéric Amiel, Journal intime* (Lausanne: L'Age d'Homme, 1976), vol. 1: 146, 157.
20 Haydon, *Diary*, vol. 2: 79, 325.
21 Leslie A. Marchand, ed., *Byron's Letters and Journals* (London: John Murray, 1973), vol. 1: 232 n1.
22 Byron, *Letters*, vol. 1: 107, 208.
23 One Byron biographer finds that he was not a woman-killer at all. According to Phyllis Grosskurth, 'It is doubtful if he was even particularly highly sexed and his periods of debauchery were sporadic. Sex he seemed to regard as an inevitable culmination of the more exciting foreplay of dangerous flirtation ...' *Byron: The Flawed Angel* (Toronto: Macfarlane Walter and Ross, 1997), 185–6.
24 Byron, *Letters*, vol. 10: 128.
25 George Moore, *Confessions of a Young Man* (1888) (reprint London: Heinemann, 1937), 40–1.

Chapter 6 The Great Breakout

1 Lawrence to Edward Garnett, 8 July 1912. James Boulton, ed., *The Letters of D.H. Lawrence* (Cambridge: Cambridge University Press, 1979), vol. 1: 425.
2 Frieda Lawrence, *'Not I, but the Wind ...'* (Toronto: Macmillan, 1934), 35.
3 Armand Dubarry, *Les invertis* (Paris: Chamuel, 1896), 8.
4 Virginia Woolf, *Mr Bennett and Mrs Brown* (London: Hogarth, 1924), 4.
5 Jeanne Schulkind, ed., *Virginia Woolf. Moments of Being* (Brighton: University of Sussex Press, 1976), from Woolf's paper 'Old Bloomsbury,' c. 1922, 157–79, quotations 173–4.

6 Alain Corbin, 'Coulisses,' in Corbin et al., eds, *De la Révolution à la Grande Guerre*, vol. 4 of Philippe Ariès and Georges Duby, eds, *Histoire de la vie privée* (Paris: Seuil, 1987), 544.

7 Randolph Trumbach raises the intriguing possibility of a 'new heterosexuality' for eighteenth-century Englishmen, in which they might have felt driven to acquire women as sexual conquests for social reasons, an essentially quantitative development. See his *Sex and the Gender Revolution, vol. 1: Heterosexuality and the Third Gender in Enlightenment London* (Chicago: University of Chicago Press, 1998), 231 and passim. See also Michel Frey, 'Du mariage et du concubinage dans les classes populaires à Paris (1846–1847),' *Annales ESC* 38 (1978): 803–29, see 814; Edward Shorter, *The Making of the Modern Family* (New York: Basic, 1975), passim.

8 Woolf *Mr. Bennett*, 5.

9 U.S. Bureau of the Census, *Historical Statistics of the United States, Colonial Times to 1970, Bicentennial Edition, Part 1* (Washington, DC: GPO, 1975), Ser. B 126–135: 56. Data are for Massachusetts only, as nationwide life-expectancy statistics for the United States do not exist before 1900.

10 Adna Ferrin Weber, *The Growth of Cities in the Nineteenth Century* (1899) (reprint Ithaca: Cornell University Press, 1963), 40, 47, 73.

11 From Constantin Guys, quoted in Arthur Symons, *From Toulouse-Lautrec to Rodin, with Some Personal Impressions* (London: Lane, 1929), 126.

12 André de Fouquières, *La courtoisie moderne* (Paris: Horay, 1952), 20.

13 Alain Corbin, *Les filles de noce: Misère sexuelle et prostitution (19e et 20e siècles)* (Paris: Aubier Montaigne, 1978), 282.

14 Magnus Hirschfeld, *Berlins Drittes Geschlecht* (1904) (reprint Berlin: Rosa Winkel, 1991), 13.

15 Michael D. Sibalis, 'Paris,' in David Higgs, ed., *Queer Sites: Gay Urban Histories since 1600* (London: Routledge, 1999), 10–37, see 12–13.

16 Émile Zola, *Nana* (1880) (reprint ed. Paris: Garnier-Flammarion, 1968), 214, 217.

17 Henri Baudrillart, *Les populations agricoles de la France: Maine, Anjou, Touraine* ... (Paris: Guillaumin, 1888), 120.

18 D.-N. Bonnet, *Treize années de pratique à la Maternité de Poitiers* (Poitiers: Oudin, 1857), 8.

19 Iwan Bloch, *The Sexual Life of Our Time* (German ed. 1907), Eng. trans. (London: Rebman, 1908), 291–2.

20 Walter Scott Patton, *Insects, Ticks, Mites and Venomous Animals, Part II (Public Health)* (Croydon: Grubb, 1931), 327; Arthur M. Greenwood, 'The Danish Treatment of Scabies,' *Journal of the American Medical Association* 82 (9 Feb. 1924): 466–7; see also Reuben Friedman, *The Story of Scabies* (New York: Froben, 1947), vol. 1: 223–4.

21 Alexander Wood, 'Treatment of Neuralgic Pains by Narcotic Injections,' *British Medical Journal* 2 (28 Aug. 1858): 721–3, at a meeting of the British Medical Association in Edinburgh; his first report was 'New Method of Treating Neuralgia by the Direct Application of Opiates to the Painful Points,' *Edinburgh Medical and Surgical Journal* 82 (1855): 265–81.

22 Milt Freudenheim, '2nd Chance for Aspirin Is Also One for Bayer,' *New York Times*, 9 Aug. 1997: 21.

23 Charles Baudelaire, *Le spleen de Paris* (Paris: Scripta manent, 1925), 26.

24 August Strindberg, *Die Beichte eines Toren*, German trans. from Swedish (written 1887–8; 1st German ed., 1893; no Swedish ed.) (retranslated Munich: Müller, 1910), 26. The book traces in novel form 'Axel' Strindberg's first marriage. On the real-life events corresponding to the novel (in English *A Fool's Apology*) see Olof Lagercrantz, *August Strindberg* (1979), Eng. trans. (New York: Farrar Straus Giroux, 1984), 54–68 et seq.

25 Natalie Barney, *Traits et portraits* (Paris: Mercure de France, 1963), 205.

26 Peter Gardella, *Innocent Ecstasy: How Christianity Gave America an Ethic of Sexual Pleasure* (New York: Oxford University Press, 1985), 77–8, 138.

27 U.S. Bureau of the Census, *Statistical Abstract of the United States: 1999* (119th ed.) (Washington, DC: National Technical Information Service, 1999), 71, table 89. Data for June 1998.

28 The Gallup Poll, *Public Opinion 1935–1971* (New York: Random House, nd), 712. Poll date, 23 Jan. 1948.

29 Michael S. Teitelbaum, *The British Fertility Decline: Demographic Transition in the Crucible of the Industrial Revolution* (Princeton: Princeton University Press, 1984), 115, table 6.1, which gives an overview of European marital fertility rates.

30 Ibid., 208.

31 Quoted in Angus McLaren, *Birth Control in Nineteenth-century England* (London: Croom Helm, 1978), 135.

32 J.R. Ackerley, *My Father and Myself* (London: Bodley Head, 1968), 49. The author was Peter's brother.

33 Katharine Bement Davis, *Factors in the Sex Life of Twenty-two Hundred Women* (New York: Harper, 1929), 76; see also ch. 2.

34 Robert Latou Dickinson, *A Thousand Marriages: A Medical Study of Sex Adjustment* (Baltimore: Williams and Wilkins, 1931), 249.

35 On the history of abortion as a means of birth control see Edward Shorter, *Women's Bodies: A Social History of Women's Encounter with Health, Ill-Health and Medicine* (1982) (reprint New Brunswick, NJ: Transaction, 1991), ch. 8.

36 Corbin, 'Coulisses,' 551.

37 Lisa Palac, *The Edge of the Bed: How Dirty Pictures Changed My Life* (Boston: Little Brown, 1998), 93.

38 Peter Green, ed. and trans., *Ovid: The Erotic Poems* (London: Penguin, 1982), book two (5): 118.

39 Francis Lacassin, ed., *Jacques Casanova de Seingalt, Histoire de ma vie* (new ed. Paris: Laffont, 1993), vol. 1: 360, 739.

40 Christopher Nyrop, *The Kiss and Its History*, Eng. trans. William Frederick Harvey (London: Sands, 1901), 13, 23, and passim.

41 Henry T. Finck, *Romantic Love and Personal Beauty* (London: Macmillan, 1887), vol. 1: 380. Interestingly, even a relative sexual avant-gardist such as Iwan Bloch is silent on the subject of tongue kissing. *Sexual Life of Our Time*, 31–6.

42 Paul H. Gebhard and Alan B. Johnson, *The Kinsey Data: Marginal Tabulations of the 1938–63 Interviews Conducted by the Institute for Sex Research* (Philadelphia: Saunders, 1979), 251, table 202. Kinsey broke his data down by male/female, then for each college/non-college, with separate tabulations for blacks,

making it difficult to get an overview. Non-college whites had
the lowest rates of tongue kissing. He interviewed no non-
college blacks.

43 Casanova, *Histoire de ma vie*, vol. 1: 738–9.

44 Bloch, *Sexual Life of Our Time*, 31.

45 Gilbert V. Hamilton, *A Research in Marriage* (New York: Boni,
1929), 176, table 121.

46 See Geoff Mains, 'The Molecular Anatomy of Leather,' in Mark
Thompson, ed., *Leatherfolk: Radical Sex, People, Politics, and
Practice* (Boston: Alyson, 1991), 37–43, esp. 40.

47 J.M. Rigg, trans., *Giovanni Boccaccio, The Decameron* (London:
Everyman, 1930), vol. 1: 72–3; second day, third story.

48 See Hans Peter Duerr, *Der Mythos vom Zivilisationsprozess, vol. 4:
Der erotische Leib* (Frankfurt-am-Main: Suhrkamp, 1997), 28, 53,
199.

49 Gebhard, *Kinsey Data*, 253, table 204.

50 Maurice Rat, ed., *Brantôme, Les dames galantes* (new ed. Paris:
Garnier, 1965), 169–70.

51 Stephen Haliczer, *Sexuality in the Confessional: A Sacrament
Profaned* (New York: Oxford University Press, 1996), 159, 170.

52 Trumbach, *Sex and the Gender Revolution*, 157.

53 E. Pelkonen, *Über volkstümliche Geburtshilfe in Finnland* (Helsinki: Finnische Literatur-Gesellschaft, 1931), 56. 'Mit dem
Hinterteil wird gedroschen, mit dem Munde gesät.'

54 Anon. ('Spectator'), 'Erotische Ausdruckweisen der Sorrentiner
Landbevölkerung,' *Anthropophyteia Jahrbücher* 7 (1910): 46–53,
quotation 50.

55 Quoted in Kathryn Norberg, 'The Libertine Whore: Prostitution
in French Pornography from Margot to Juliette,' in Lynn Hunt,
ed., *The Invention of Pornography: Obscenity and the Origins of
Modernity, 1500–1800* (New York: Zone, 1993), 225–52, quotation 242.

56 Cited in Henry S. Ashbee ('Pisanus Fraxi'), *Bibliography of
Prohibited Books* (1885) (reprint New York: Jack Brussel, 1962),
vol. 3: 187. Ashbee accepts the letters as genuine.

57 Richard Ellmann, ed., *Selected Letters of James Joyce* (New York:
Viking, 1975), 181.

58 Adolf Frisé, ed., *Robert Musil Tagebücher* (new ed. Reinbek bei Hamburg: Rowohlt, 1983), vol. 1: 773.

59 Thomas P. Riggio et al., eds, *Theodore Dreiser, American Diaries, 1902–1926* (Philadelphia: University of Pennsylvania Press, 1982), 289, 291.

60 Gebhart, *Kinsey Data*, 371, table 322; 372, table 323; 'in first marriage.'

61 Peter Knight, 'The History of Sex in Cinema, Part 17: The Stag Film,' *Playboy* Nov. 1967: 154–8, 170–89, see 180.

62 Palac first made the comment in 1992 in a short-lived magazine entitled *Future Sex*. She quotes it again in *Edge of the Bed*, 100.

63 Helen Gardner, ed., *John Donne, The Elegies and the Songs and Sonnets* (Oxford: Clarendon, 1965), 19.

64 Robert Hobart Cust, trans., *The Autobiography of Benvenuto Cellini* (New York: Dodd, Mead, 1961), 382–3.

65 Haliczer, *Sexuality in the Confessional*, 170.

66 Margaret C. Jacob, 'The Materialist World of Pornography,' in Hunt, ed., *Invention of Pornography*, 157–202; see 197, fig. 4.10

67 Trumbach, *Sex and the Gender Revolution*, 107; see also 157.

68 Gilbert Lely, *Vie du marquis de Sade* (1952–7) (rev. ed. Paris: Pauvert, 1965), 182–5. The author thinks that the prostitutes were lying about refusing Sade, yet given that anal intercourse was not part of a prostitute's standard menu at that time, I see no inherent reason to doubt their truthfulness.

69 Brantôme, *Dames galantes*, 169.

70 Casanova, *Histoire de ma vie*, vol. 2: 650.

71 Ibid.

72 Peter Wagner, ed., *John Cleland, Fanny Hill, or Memoirs of a Woman of Pleasure* (new ed. London: Penguin, 1985), 192–3.

73 Ashbee, *Bibliography*, vol. 1: 115–16.

74 Nicolas Chorier ('Luisa Sigea Toletana'), *Dialogues on the Arcana of Love and Venus* (Lawrence, KA: Coronado Press, 1974), 165.

75 Gert Schiff, ed., *Johann Heinrich Füssli: Abbildungen* (Zurich: Berichthaus, 1973), 125, drawing, 548. 'Rollenaustausch.'

76 William Lithgow, *The Totall Discourse of the Rare Adventures and Painefull Peregrinations of Long Nineteene Yeares Travayles ...* (1632) (reprint Glasgow: MacLehose, 1906), 23.

77 Chorier, *Dialogues Arcana Love*, 136–7.
78 Annie Le Brun and Jean-Jacques Pauvert, eds., *Oeuvres complètes du Marquis de Sade* (Paris: Pauvert, 1987), 'Histoire de Juliette, Pt IV,' vol. 9: 138.
79 Michael Rocke, *Forbidden Friendships: Homosexuality and Male Culture in Renaissance Florence* (New York: Oxford University Press, 1996), 130–1.
80 A representative sample of the Veneto region of Italy in the mid-1970s found that only 14 per cent of married men and 9 per cent of married women said they practised anal sex occasionally or 'frequently.' Giovanni Caletti, *Il comportamento sessuale degli italiani* (Bologna: Calderini, 1976), 197.
81 On peasants using anal intercourse for birth control see Anon., 'Sorrentiner Landbevölkerung,' 48.
82 Sigmund Freud to Friedrich S. Krauss, 26 June 1910, printed in 'Nachwort des Herausgebers,' *Anthropophyteia Jahrbücher* 7 (1910): 471–7 (the letter itself is at 472–4), quotation 473.
83 Ellmann, ed., *Joyce Selected Letters*, 184.
84 Michael Squires, ed., *D.H. Lawrence, Lady Chatterley's Lover* (new ed. Cambridge: Cambridge University Press, 1993), 223.
85 Peter Weiermair, ed., *Erotic Art from the 17th to the 20th Century: The Döpp Collection* (Zurich: Stemmle, 1995), 215.
86 Philippe Alméras, *Céline entre haines et passion* (Paris: Laffont, 1994), 115, 117–19.
87 Gebhard, *Kinsey Data*, 383, table 334.
88 Hamilton, *Research in Marriage*, 188, table 137. Of 100 men asked if they had ever entered their wives' rectums, 7 said yes and 6 said, 'No, but I have had the impulse to do so (188, table 138).
89 I am grateful to Susan Bélanger, who visited the ISR for me and undertook these tabulations, analysing, among the total 50,000 images in the collection, all of the oral- and anal-sex images for heterosexuals, as well as all gay-and-lesbian sex variants. The 'lesbian' material was largely valueless, in that virtually all of it was produced for male consumption rather than representing genuine lesbian erotic self-images. At the ISR, Kath Pennavaria and curator Jennifer Pearson generously facilitated this, for them, rather burdensome research.

90 Fulgence Raymond and Pierre Janet, *Les obsessions et la psy-chasthénie* (Paris: Alcan, 1902), vol. 2: 190. In Janet's view the fatigue caused by masturbation lay at the root of the patient's general absence of will.

91 Wolfgang Kersten, ed., *Paul Klee Tagebücher, 1898–1918* (Berne: Paul-Klee-Stiftung, 1988), 21.

92 Haakon M. Chevalier, ed. and trans., *The Secret Life of Salvador Dali* (London: Vision, 1942), 125.

93 Siegfried Bernfeld, *Trieb und Tradition im Jugendalter: Kultur-psychologische Studien an Tagebüchern* (Leipzig: Bart, 1931), 99, 104.

94 M.J. Exner, *Problems and Principles of Sex Education: A Study of 948 College Men* (New York: Association Press, 1922), 16, 18.

95 Katharine Bement David, 'A Study of Certain Auto-Erotic Practices,' *Mental Hygiene* 8 (1924): 668–723; see esp. 674–6.

96 Hamilton, *Research in Marriage*, 436.

97 Quoted in Lynn Garafola, *Diaghilev's Ballets Russes* (New York: Oxford University Press, 1989), 59.

98 Emory Holloway, ed., *Walt Whitman: Complete Poetry and Selected Prose and Letters* (London: Nonesuch, 1967), 89–90.

99 Edwin Haviland Miller, *Walt Whitman's 'Song of Myself'* (Iowa City: University of Iowa Press, 1989), 14, 18.

100 Musil, *Tagebücher*, vol. 1: 35, 161–2.

101 Townsend Ludington, ed., *The Fourteenth Chronicle: Letters and Diaries of John Dos Passos* (Boston: Gambit, 1973), 31.

102 Nina Hamnett, *Laughing Torso: Reminiscences* (London: Constable, 1932), 19.

103 Mary J. Serrano, trans., *Marie Bashkirtseff: The Journal of a Young Artist, 1860–1884* (New York: Cassell, 1889), 178.

104 Bashkirtseff, *Journal*, 162.

105 Sibilla Aleramo [pseud. for Rina Faccio], *Una Donna* (1906) (reprint Milan: Feltrinelli, 1994), 29.

106 Valentine de Saint-Point, 'Futurist Manifesto of Lust' (1913), trans. and reprinted in Umbro Apollonio, ed., *Futurist Manifestos* (London: Thames and Hudson, 1973), 70–4. The futurists have received a bit of an unfair reputation as anti-feminists, despite the ill-chosen wording of one of the manifestos of

futurist leader Filippo Tommaso Marinetti. Many futurists quite liked the new woman. In one of his plays, the futurist dramatist Umberto Boccioni has 'the woman' say impatiently to the critic who can only criticize and not create, 'You've been neutered. How boring you must be in bed!' Zeno Birolli, ed., *Umberto Boccioni, Gli scritti editi e inediti* (Milan: Feltrinelli, 1971), 226.

107 Mary Roberts Rinehart, *My Story* (New York: Farrar, 1931), 74.

108 Matthew J. Bruccoli, ed., *The Notebooks of F. Scott Fitzgerald* (New York: Harcourt Brace, 1945), 69–70.

109 Martha Graham, *Blood Memory* (New York: Doubleday, 1991), 59.

110 G. Mercer Adam, *Sandow on Physical Training* (New York: Tait, 1894), 13, 44–5, 56

111 Patricia Anderson, *When Passion Reigned: Sex and the Victorians* (New York: Basic, 1995), 50, 59.

112 Lars E. Troide, ed., *The Early Journals and Letters of Fanny Burney* (Oxford: Clarendon, 1988), vol. 1: 292.

113 Colette, *Claudine en ménage* (Paris: Mercure, 1902), 67.

114 Cl. Pichois and R. Forbin, eds, *Colette: Lettres de la vagabonde* (Paris: Flammarion, 1961), 59. On the boxing lessons see Claude Francis and Fernande Gontier, *Creating Colette*, Eng. trans. (South Royalton, VT: Steerforth Press, 1998), vol. 1: 314.

115 Joris-Karl Huysmans, *À rebours* (1884) (new ed. Paris: Charpentier, 1908), 137. It could be argued that 'Miss Urania' was a caricature, lampooned by the homosexual Huysmans; yet the image of her as powerful and muscular is a gripping one.

116 Alméras, *Céline*, 117.

117 Karl Beckson, ed., *The Memoirs of Arthur Symons: Life and Art in the 1890s* (University Park, PA: Pennsylvania State University Press, 1977), 17–18, 70, 72, 138, 144.

118 Albert Eulenburg, *Sexuale Neuropathie: Genitale Neurosen und Neuropsychosen der Männer und Frauen* (Leipzig: Vogel, 1895), 79.

119 See Weiermair, *Erotic Art*, passim.

120 Lawrence, *Lady Chatterley's Lover*, 234–5.

Chapter 7 The Great Breakout for Gays and Lesbians

1 Oscar Wilde, *The Picture of Dorian Gray* (1890) (reprint New York: Modern Library, 1998), 25

2 Ibid., 87–8.

3 Alain Corbin, 'Coulisses,' in Michelle Perrot., ed., *Histoire de la vie privée: vol. 4: De la Révolution à la Grande Guerre* (Paris: Seuil, 1987), 589.

4 This interpretation is suggested by Andrew Warwick, 'Exercising the Student Body: Mathematics and Athleticism in Victorian Cambridge,' in Christopher Lawrence and Steven Shapin, eds, *Science Incarnate: Historical Embodiments of Natural Knowledge* (Chicago: University of Chicago Press, 1998), 288–326, see 312.

5 Richard Buckle, *Diaghilev* (New York: Atheneum, 1979), 146.

6 Magnus Hirschfeld, *Berlins Drittes Geschlecht* (1904) (reprint Berlin: Rosa Winkel, 1991), 101–2.

7 According to Ackerley's biographer, Peter Parker, *Ackerley: A Life of J.R. Ackerley* (New York: Farrar Straus Giroux, 1989), 134.

8 J.R. Ackerley, *My Father and Myself* (London: Bodley Head, 1968), 128–30.

9 Havelock Ellis and John Addington Symonds, *Sexual Inversion* (1897) (reprint New York: Arno, 1975), 51, 117–18.

10 Samuel M. Steward, *Chapters from an Autobiography* (San Francisco: Grey Fox, 1980), 51. Lord Alfred did, however, confide that occasionally 'he [Wilde] "sucked" me.' Yet Bosie denied sodomitic relations between the two of them, which is the main point. Douglas Murray, *Bosie: A Biography of Lord Alfred Douglas* (New York: Hyperion, 2000), 33.

11 Roger Sawyer, *Roger Casement's Diaries, 1910: The Black and the White* (London: Pimlico, 1997), 42–3.

12 Numa Praetorius [pseud.], 'Homosexuelle Pissoirinschriften aus Paris,' *Anthropophyteia: Jahrbücher für folkloristische Erhebungen* ... 8 (1911): 410–22, esp. 416–17.

13 Marc-André Raffalovich, *Uranisme et unisexualité* (Paris: Masson, 1896), 118–24, 137–8

14 Paul Näcke, 'Der Kuss Homosexueller,' *Archiv für Kriminal-Anthropologie* 17 (1904): 177–8, quotation 177.

15 Paul Näcke, 'Einteilung der Homosexuellen,' *Allgemeine Zeitschrift für Psychiatrie* 65 (1908): 109–28, esp. 114.

16 Hirschfeld, *Berlin Drittes Geschlecht*, 98.

17 Max Katte, 'Die virilen Homosexuellen,' *Jahrbuch für sexuelle Zwischenstufen* 7 (i) (1905): 87–106, quotation 89. See also Iwan Bloch, *The Sexual Life of Our Time* (1907), Eng. trans. (London: Rebman, 1908), 509.

18 Sharon R. Ullman, *Sex Seen: The Emergence of Modern Sexuality in America* (Berkeley: University of California Press, 1997), 63–6.

19 Claude Hartland, *The Story of a Life* (1901) (reprint San Francisco: Grey Fox, 1985), passim.

20 Gilbert V. Hamilton, *A Research in Marriage* (New York: Boni, 1929), 492, table 443.

21 Paul H. Gebhard and Alan B. Johnson, *The Kinsey Data: Marginal Tabulations of the 1938–1963 Interviews Conducted by the Institute for Sex Research* (Philadelphia: Saunders, 1979), 549, table 499; 555, table 505. These data, of course, are for the entire sample, yet the majority were born between 1910 and 1924. As for giving anal sex, 18.7 per cent of gay males said this occurred in more than 40 per cent of their sex encounters (556, table 506). In photographs of gay-male sex at the Institute for Sex Research in Bloomington, Indiana, the 380 images depicting gays between the 1880s and 1950s represented anal sex as about half of the total, oral-genital and tonguing making up the rest (group sex, masturbation, and petting are excluded from these tabulations). There is no discernible trend.

22 An anonymous source, quoted in Iwan Bloch, *Odoratus Sexualis: A Scientific and Literary Study of Sexual Scents and Erotic Perfumes* (New York: Panurge, 1934), 122.

23 For a wonderful account of hygienic improvements from the late nineteenth century on, see Siegfried Giedion, *Mechanization Takes Command* (1948) (reprint New York: Norton, 1969), 628f.

24 Cecil Woolf, ed., *Baron Corvo, Frederick Rolfe, The Venice Letters* (1974) (London: Woolf, 1987), 35. Amadeo and his friends, themselves homoerotically inclined, disliked anal sex but loved deep kissing (62).

25 See Phyllis Grosskurth, *John Addington Symonds* (London: Longmans, 1964), 276.

26 See F. Valentine Hooven, *Beefcake: The Muscle Magazines of America* (Cologne: Benedikt Taschen, 1995), passim.

27 Greg Mullins, 'Nudes, Prudes, and Pigmies: The Desirability of Disavowal in *Physical Culture,' Discourse* 15 (Fall 1992): 27–48, see 47 n2.

28 See Rictor Norton, 'The Beginnings of Beefcake' (1999), www.infopt.demon.co.uk/beefcake.htm, 9.

29 Donald Vining, *A Gay Diary, Vol. 2: 1946–1954* (New York: Pepys Press, 1980), 440.

30 Norton, 'Beefcake,' 7.

31 David Leddick, *Naked Men: Pioneering Male Nudes, 1935–1955* (New York: Universe, 1997), 22, 28, 36, 41, 45.

32 John Glassco, *Memoirs of Montparnasse* (Toronto: Oxford University Press, 1970), 54.

33 Bloch, *Sexual Life of Our Time*, 498.

34 Oscar Méténier, *Vertus et vices allemands* (Paris: Michel, 1904), 85–90.

35 Jean Weber, interviewed in Gilles Barbedette and Michel Carassou, *Paris Gay 1925* (Paris: Presses de la Renaissance, 1981), 62–9, quotation 67.

36 André Koeniguer, 'Venise, Sodome de l'Adriatique,' *Arcadie* 288 (1977): 629–35, quotations 632, 634.

37 George Chauncey, *Gay New York: The Making of the Gay Male World, 1890–1940* (New York: Flamingo, 1994), 106.

38 'Harold,' quoted in David K. Johnson, 'The Kids of Fairytown: Gay Male Culture on Chicago's Near North Side in the 1930s,' in Brett Beemyn, ed., *Creating a Place for Ourselves: Lesbian, Gay, and Bisexual Community Histories* (New York: Routledge, 1997), 97–117, 107.

39 'Kepner,' quoted in Douglas Sadownick, *Sex between Men: An Intimate History of the Sex Lives of Gay Men Postwar to Present* (New York: HarperSanFrancisco, 1996), 43.

40 Gebhard and Johnson, *Kinsey Data*, 581, table 531; 603–8, tables 553–8.

41 André Gide, *Corydon* (1911) (new ed. Paris: Gallimard, 1920),

28, 36, 38; for a brief account of Ulrichs and other sexologists see David F. Greenberg, *The Construction of Homosexuality* (Chicago: University of Chicago Press, 1988), 408 and passim. On the relatively small number of effeminate gays in Germany see Paul Näcke, 'Die Diagnose der Homosexualität,' *Neurologisches Centralblatt* 27 (1909): 338–51, esp. 341, and Hirschfeld, *Berlin Drittes Geschlecht* 51–2.

42 Vining, *Gay Diary*, vol. 2: 378–9, entry of 26 June 1952.

43 John Loughery, *The Other Side of Silence: Men's Lives and Gay Identities: A Twentieth-Century History* (New York: Holt, 1998), 6.

44 Ibid., 40.

45 Ina Russell, ed., *Jeb and Dash: A Diary of Gay Life, 1918–1945* (Boston: Faber, 1993), 74, 91.

46 Louis-Charles Royer, *L'amour en Allemagne* (Paris: Eds de France, 1930), 91.

47 Russell, *Jeb and Dash*, 90.

48 Mary MacLane, *I, Mary MacLane: A Diary of Human Days* (New York: Stokes, 1917), 199, 209, 277.

49 Ibid., 246.

50 Colette, *Le pur et l'impur* (Paris: Aux armes de France, 1941), 29–30.

51 Ibid., 26, 87–8, 131–2.

52 Diana Frederics [pseud.], *Diana: A Strange Autobiography* (1939) (reprint New York: Arno, 1975), 69, 83, 98–9, 242, 246.

53 Émile Zola, *Nana* (1880) (reprint Paris: Garnier-Flammarion, 1968), 312.

54 'Léo Taxil' [Gabriel-Antoine Jogand-Pàges], *La corruption fin-de-siècle* (Paris: Noirot, 1891), 263.

55 'Police Seize Novel by Radclyffe Hall,' *New York Times* 12 Jan. 1929: 3.

56 Alfred C. Kinsey et al., *Sexual Behavior in the Human Female* (1953) (New York: Pocket Books, 1965), 493, table 131.

57 Katharine Bement Davis, *Factors in the Sex Life of Twenty-two Hundred Women* (New York: Harper, 1929), 245, 247, 298.

58 Yvette Guilbert, *La chanson de ma vie (Mes mémoires)* (Paris: Grasset, 1927), 78. 'Comment, Louise, tu nies que tu m'aimes? Tu t'em ... bêtes [sic] pourtant pas quand tu m'friandes!'

59 'Taxil' [Jogand-Pagès], *La corruption*, 265. 'Les petites agenouillées.'

60 Colette, *Le pur et l'impur*, 109; Natalie Clifford Barney, *Aventures de l'esprit* (1929) (reprint New York: Arno, 1975), 22: 'L'amour, débarrassé de sa fonction ... peut cependant se prêter à des variations infinies.' Barney's work is filled with such exclamations.

61 Ellis and Symonds, *Sexual Inversion*, 98.

62 The aquarelles are reproduced in Peter Weiermair, ed., *Erotic Art from the 17th to the 20th Century: The Döpp-Collection* (Zurich: Stemmle, 1995), 182, 184. I have not seen Wegener's original work, which may have been influenced by the tastes of her husband, Einar, who began to cross-dress in the 1920s and in 1930 became the first person ever to have a sex-change operation, after which she divorced him. See Kenneth Tindall, 'Gerda Wegener,' www.gerda.utopian.net.

63 Kinsey, *Sexual Behavior Human Female*, 492, table 130.

64 Royer, *L'amour en Allemagne*, 138–9.

65 See Elizabeth Lapovsky Kennedy and Madeleine D. Davis, *Boots of Leather, Slippers of Gold: The History of a Lesbian Community* (New York: Routledge, 1993), 5–8.

66 Devendra Singh et al., 'Lesbian Erotic Role Identification: Behavioral, Morphological, and Hormonal Correlates,' *Journal of Personality and Social Psychology* 76 (1999): 1035–49.

67 Brassaï [Gyula Halasz], *The Secret Paris of the '30s*, Eng. trans. (London: Thames and Hudson, 1976), np.

68 Ruth Roellig, 'Einführung zu "Berlins lesbische Frauen," 1928,' in Adele Meyer, ed., *Lila Nächte: Die Damenklubs im Berlin der Zwanziger Jahre* (Berlin: Edition Lit, 1994), 17.

69 Ibid., 20.

70 Roellig, 'Die Zauberflöte,' in Meyer, *Lila Nächte*, 55.

71 Diana Souhami, *Mrs Keppel and her Daughter* (New York: St Martin's, 1996), 127, 131, 140, 220.

72 Vern Bullough and Bonnie Bullough, 'Lesbianism in the 1920s and 1930s: A Newfound Study,' *Signs: Journal of Women in Culture and Society* 2 (1977): 895–904, esp. 900.

73 See Kate Summerscale, *The Queen of Whale Cay* (New York: Viking, 1997), passim.

Chapter 8 Towards Total Body Sex

1 Paul H. Gebhard and Alan B. Johnson, *The Kinsey Data: Marginal Tabulations of the 1938–1963 Interviews Conducted by the Institute for Sex Research* (Philadelphia: Saunders, 1979), 251, table 202. I averaged the percentages for white male and female college graduates.

2 James R. Browning et al., 'Sexual Motives, Gender, and Sexual Behavior,' *Archives of Sexual Behavior* 29 (2000): 135–53, 144, table 4.

3 'J' [Terry Garrity], *The Sensuous Woman* (New York: Lyle Stuart, 1969), 127.

4 Keith L. Justice, *Bestseller Index* (Jefferson, NC: Mcfarland, 1998), 161.

5 Edward O. Laumann et al., *The Social Organization of Sexuality: Sexual Practices in the United States* (Chicago: University of Chicago Press, 1994), 106–7.

6 *Durex Global Survey* (1996): 5, table 2; 7, table 3.

7 Samuel S. Janus and Cynthia L. Janus, *The Janus Report on Sexual Behavior* (New York: Wiley, 1993), 95, table 3.39.

8 J. Abma et al., *Fertility, Family Planning, and Women's Health: New Data from the 1995 Survey of Family Growth*. National Center for Health Statistics. Vital Health Statistics 23 (19) (1997): 31, table 20.

9 A.P. MacKay et al., *Adolescent Health Chartbook. Health, United States, 2000* (Hyattsville, MD: National Center for Health Statistics, 2000), 75, fig. 25.

10 David Frum, *How We Got Here. The 70's: The Decade That Brought You Modern Life (for Better or Worse)* (New York: Basic, 2000), 195.

11 Laumann, *Social Organization of Sexuality*, 130, table 3.8A.

12 Ibid., 208, table 5.9A. Similar trends are apparent for those unions beginning with cohabitation.

13 Kinsey Collection of Photographs, Institute for Sex Research, no. 34648.

14 Gebhard and Johnson, *Kinsey Data*, 253 table 204. 'Some' plus 'much.'

15 Charles White, *The Life and Times of Little Richard* (1984), rev. ed. (New York: Da Capo, 1994), 84.
16 'J' [Garrity], *Sensuous Woman*, 110, 113.
17 Laumann, *Social Organization of Sexuality*, 98, table 3.6, quotation 102.
18 Gebhard and Johnson, *Kinsey Data*, 371–2, tables 322, 323.
19 Arthur Knight and Hollis Alpert, 'The History of Sex in Cinema,' *Playboy* Nov. 1967, 154–8, 170–89, statistics 180.
20 Steven Ziplow, *The Film Maker's Guide to Pornography* (New York: Drake, 1977), 31.
21 Trevor Cole, 'Canuck Speciality?' *Globe and Mail* 1 Apr. 2000: R6.
22 Jack Morin, *Anal Pleasure and Health* (1981), 2nd ed. (Burlingame, CA: Down There Press, 1986), 1.
23 Laumann, *Social Organization of Sexuality*, 99 table 3.6.
24 Gebhard and Johnson, *Kinsey Data*, 383, table 334, responses 'little,' 'some,' or 'much.'
25 Susie Bright interview, in Andrea Juno, ed., *Angry Women* (New York: Juno Books, 1991), 194–221, quotation 216.
26 Janice I. Baldwin and John D. Baldwin, 'Heterosexual Anal Intercourse,' *Archives of Sexual Behavior* 29 (2000): 357–73; 647 remained in the sample, including 23 bisexual and 8 homosexual students who had engaged in both vaginal and anal intercourse.
27 Pamela Lister, '5,000 Married Men Confess What Keeps Sex (With You) Hot,' *Redbook* June 1999: 98–101, 126, quotation 100.
28 Susan Bakos, 'Secrets of Sexy Wives,' *Redbook* Sept. 1999: 121, 142, quotation 142.
29 Al Di Lauro and Gerald Rabkin, *Dirty Movies: An Illustrated History of the Stag Film, 1915–1970* (New York: Chelsea, 1976), 98.
30 Ziplow, *Film Maker's Guide to Pornography*, 16.
31 See 'Romantic Porn in the Boudoir,' *Time* 30 Mar. 1987: 63.
32 Laurence O'Toole, *Pornocopia: Porn, Sex, Technology and Desire* (London: Serpent's Tail, 1998), 81.
33 Tristan Taormino, *The Ultimate Guide to Anal Sex for Women* (San Francisco: Cleis, 1998), 78.

34 'J,' *Sensuous Woman*, 38–9.
35 Laumann, *Social Organization of Sexuality*, 82, table 3.1. Single persons outside relationships, however, masturbate most frequently of all.
36 Carol Tavris and Susan Sadd, *The Redbook Report on Female Sexuality* (New York: Delacorte, 1975), 96.
37 Gebhard and Johnson, *Kinsey Data*, 206, table 157.
38 Betty Dodson, *Sex for One: The Joy of Selfloving* (1974) (reprint New York: Three Rivers, 1996), 82, 84.
39 Karen V. Kukil, ed., *The Journals of Sylvia Plath, 1950–1962* (London: Faber, 2000), 13–15, 20.
40 Elizabeth Siegel Watkins, *On the Pill: A Social History of Oral Contraceptives, 1950–1970* (Baltimore: Johns Hopkins University Press, 1998), 62.
41 See on this Andrea Tone's well-researched book *Devices and Desires: A History of Contraceptives in America* (New York: Hill and Wang, 2001), ch. 10.
42 Quoted in Barry Miles, *Paul McCartney: Many Years from Now* (New York: Holt, 1997), 118–19.
43 Deirdre English, Amber Hollibaugh, and Gayle Rubin, 'Talking Sex: A Conversation on Sexuality and Feminism,' *Socialist Review* 11(4) (Jul/Aug. 1981): 43–62, quotation 46.
44 Naomi Wolf interview with Tad Friend, 'Yes,' *Esquire* Feb. 1994: 48–9, quotation 49.
45 Annie Le Brun and Jean-Jacques Pauvert, ed, *Oeuvres complètes du Marquis de Sade* (Paris: Pauvert, 1987), 'Histoire de Juliette,' vol. 8: 509.
46 Deirdre Carmody, 'Helen Gurley Brown to Give Cosmopolitan Reins to Successor,' *New York Times* 17 Jan. 1996: C6.
47 Barbara Ehrenreich, Elizabeth Hess, Gloria Jacobs, *Re-making Love: The Feminization of Sex* (New York: Anchor, 1986), 60.
48 Susie Bright, 'Introduction,' in Lisa Palac, *The Edge of the Bed: How Dirty Pictures Changed My Life* (Boston: Little Brown, 1998), ix. See also Bright interview in Juno, *Angry Women*, 216.
49 Linda Williams, *Hard Core: Power, Pleasure, and the 'Frenzy of the Visible'* (Berkeley: University of California Press, 1989), 31.
50 Rossana Campo, *L'attore americano* (Milan: Feltrinelli, 1997),

127–8. I am grateful to Patrizia Guarnieri for calling this to my attention.

51 Cook's Diary, Feb. 1997, posted on 'Open Pages,' http://diary.base.org.

52 'The New Ideal of Beauty,' *Time* 30 Aug. 1982: 72–7, quotation 72.

53 Sallie Tisdale, *Talk Dirty to Me* (New York: Doubleday, 1994), 215.

54 See Leslie Heywood, *Bodymakers: A Cultural Anatomy of Women's Body Building* (New Brunswick, NJ: Rutgers University Press, 1998), 27–8.

55 Holly Brubach, 'The Athletic Esthetic,' *New York Times Magazine*, 23 June 1996: 48–51, quotation 50.

56 Shirley Castelnuovo and Sharon R. Guthrie, *Feminism and the Female Body: Liberating the Amazon Within* (Boulder, CO: Lynne Reinner, 1998), 57.

57 Bill Stoneman, 'Weighty Trends for Fitness Marketers,' *American Demographics* April 1999: 24.

58 Donald Vining, *A Gay Diary, Vol. 1, 1933–1946* (New York: Pepys Press, 1979), 311, 469, 486, 489.

59 Donald Vining, *A Gay Diary, Vol. 2, 1946–54* (New York: Pepys Press, 1980), 23–4, 75, 106–7.

60 Donald Vining, *A Gay Diary, Vol. 4, 1967–1975* (New York: Pepys Press, 1983), 276, 331, 351, 394.

61 Laud Humphreys, *Tearoom Trade: Impersonal Sex in Public Places* (1970) (rev. ed. Chicago: Aldine, 1975), quotation 6; see also 10, 13, 108–9.

62 James H. Jones, *Alfred C. Kinsey: A Public/Private Life* (New York: Norton, 1997), 496–7.

63 Edward William Delph, *The Silent Community: Public Homosexual Encounters* (Beverley Hills: Sage, 1978), 127.

64 Edmund White, *States of Desire: Travels in Gay America* (New York: Dutton, 1980), 265–6.

65 John Loughery, *The Other Side of Silence: Men's Lives and Gay Identities: A Twentieth-Century History* (New York: Holt, 1998), 357.

66 Paul Näcke, 'Quelques détails sur les homo-sexuels de Paris,' *Archives d'anthropologie criminelle* 20 (1905): 411–14, see 412.

67 On the history of the American bathhouse scene, see Loughery, *Other Side of Silence*, 356–64, quotation 359.

68 Ibid., 356–7.

69 Karla Jay and Allen Young, *The Gay Report: Lesbians and Gay Men Speak Out about Sexual Experiences and Lifestyles* (New York: Summit, 1977), 501.

70 Quoted in James Miller, *The Passion of Michel Foucault* (New York: Simon and Schuster, 1993), 264.

71 Donald Webster Cory [Edward Sagarin], *The Homosexual in America: A Subjective Approach* (New York: Greenberg, 1951), 138.

72 Philip Blumstein and Pepper Schwartz, *American Couples* (New York: Morrow, 1983), 196, fig. 27; 273, figs 46, 47.

73 E. White, *States of Desire*, 267.

74 Kinsey Collection, Institute of Sex Research, no. 44020.

75 Jay and Young, *Gay Report*, 440. Fifty per cent of the gay-male respondents to a 1994 magazine poll said that they loved nipple play. Janet Lever, 'The 1994 Advocate Survey of Sexuality and Relationships: The Men,' *The Advocate* 23 Aug. 1994: 16–24, see 20.

76 Delph, *Silent Community*, 144.

77 Daniel Harris, *The Rise and Fall of Gay Culture* (New York: Hyperion, 1997), 100–1.

78 John Preston, *Mr. Benson* (1983) (reprint New York: Badboy, 1992), 11–12.

79 Jay and Young, *Gay Report*, 456, 464.

80 Laumann, *Social Organization of Sexuality*, 318. The figures for 'active' and 'receptive' are so close, for both oral and anal, that reporting them separately is unnecessary. Couples clearly practise reciprocity.

81 Loughery, *Other Side of Silence*, 393.

82 George Chauncey, *Gay New York: The Making of the Gay Male World, 1890–1940* (London: HarperCollins, 1995), 358.

83 Loughery, *Other Side of Silence*, 214.

84 C. White, *Little Richard*, 30.

85 Tom Burke, 'The New Homosexuality,' *Esquire* Dec. 1969: 178, 304–17, quotation 305.

86 Seymour Kleinberg, 'Where Have All the Sissies Gone?' *Christopher Street* 2 (Mar. 1978): 4–17, quotation 6.

87 E. White, *States of Desire*, 45–6. White was hostile to these trends.

88 Jay and Young, *Gay Report*, 375–6.

89 Ibid., 570.

90 Martin P. Levine, *Gay Macho: The Life and Death of the Homo-sexual Clone* (New York: New York University Press, 1998), 55–6, 50–1.

91 Pat Califia, *Macho Sluts* (Los Angeles: Alyson, 1988), 13.

92 Lillian Faderman, *Odd Girls and Twilight Lovers: A History of Lesbian Life in Twentieth-Century America* (New York: Columbia University Press, 1991), 60–1.

93 Jeanne Cordova, 'Butches, Lies, and Feminism,' in Joan Nestle, ed., *The Persistent Desire: A Femme-Butch Reader* (Boston: Alyson, 1992), 272–92, quotation 282.

94 Bonnie Zimmerman, *The Safe Sea of Women: Lesbian Fiction, 1969–1989* (Boston: Beacon, 1990), 96–7.

95 Karla Jay, 'Introduction,' in Jay, ed., *Lesbian Erotics* (New York: New York University Press, 1995), 6.

96 Martin Duberman, *Stonewall* (New York: Dutton, 1993), 177–8.

97 Jane Juffer, *At Home with Pornography: Women, Sex, and Every-day Life* (New York: New York University Press, 1998), 123; Jill Nagle, 'First Ladies of Feminist Porn: A Conversation with Candida Royalle and Debi Sundahl,' in Nagle, ed., *Whores and Other Feminists* (New York: Routledge, 1997), 156–66, quota-tion 164.

98 Cherry Smyth, *Damn Fine Art by New Lesbian Artists* (London: Cassell, 1996), 23.

99 English, Hollibaugh, and Rubin, 'Talking Sex,' 48.

100 Blumstein and Schwartz, *American Couples*, 196, 273. The Laumann data show considerably greater gay-lesbian equality in number of partners per month. Yet in their tables it is impossible to separate out the lesbian and gay couples; and the figures on mean number of partners per month include sex with both men and women. Thus a lesbian-inclined woman living with a husband would have quite high scores. *Social Organization of Sexuality*, 317, table 8.5.

101 Judy Grahn, *Another Mother Tongue: Gay Words, Gay Worlds* (1984) (rev. ed. Boston: Beacon, 1990), 210.

102 Ibid., 210.

103 Jane DeLynn, 1991 interview with WKCR FM, posted on www.janedelynn.com.

104 Stephanie Nolen, 'Bathhouse Raid Angers Lesbian Community,' *Globe and Mail* 16 Sept. 2000: A27.

105 Grant Cogswell, 'There's a Whole World Underground,' *The Stranger* 9, 28 (30 Mar.–5 Apr. 2000). At www.thestranger.com/2000–03–30/feature.

106 DeLynn 1991 interview.

107 Grahn, *Another Mother Tongue*, 5, 36.

108 Elizabeth Lapovsky Kennedy and Madeline D. Davis, *Boots of Leather, Slippers of Gold: The History of a Lesbian Community* (New York: Routledge, 1993), 196–9, 203.

109 Jay and Young, *Gay Report*, 396.

110 Janet Lever, 'Lesbian Sex Survey,' *The Advocate* 22 Aug. 1995: 22–30, see 26. Seventy-five per cent of the 2,525 respondents to a questionnaire said they 'loved' oral sex.

111 Jay and Young, *Gay Report*, 388.

112 Lever, 'Lesbian Sex Survey,' 26.

113 J.M. Sundet et al., 'Prevalence of Risk-Prone Sexual Behaviour in the General Population of Norway,' in Alan F. Fleming et al., eds, *The Global Impact of AIDS* (New York: Liss, 1988), 53–60: 59, table 11. No figure was given for lesbians with only women partners.

114 Josey Vogels, 'Fun in the Anal Zone,' *Now* 20–6 July 2000: 24.

115 Joan Nestle, 'The Femme Question,' in Nestle, ed., *Persistent Desire*, 138–46, quotation 141.

116 Ibid., 142–3.

117 Jay and Young, *Gay Report*, 527.

118 JoAnn Loulan, *The Lesbian Erotic Dance* (San Francisco: Spinsters, 1990), question 113 at 259. In *The Advocate* survey in 1995, '29 per cent fall into the classic butch-femme pairing.' Lever, 'Lesbian Sex Survey,' 28.

119 See Pat Califia and Robin Sweeney, *The Second Coming: A Leatherdyke Reader* (Los Angeles: Alyson, 1996), passim.

Chapter 9 SM and Fetish

1 Kathleen Beckett, 'Versace Rocks On,' *Harper's Bazaar*, Nov. 1992: 169–71, 193; quotation 171.

2 Havelock Ellis, 'Love and Pain' (1903), in *Studies in the Psychology of Sex* (1913) (2nd enlarged ed. Philadelphia: Davis, 1928), vol. 3: 66–188, quotation 185.

3 See Irving Bieber, 'Sadism and Masochism,' in Silvano Arieti, ed., *American Handbook of Psychiatry* (New York: Basic, 1966), vol. 3: 256–70, quotation (Bieber speaking) 259. Interestingly, psychiatry today continues to see 'sexual sadism' and 'sexual masochism' as sex deviations, or 'paraphilias,' despite the fact that large numbers of otherwise normal people derive pleasure from them. See American Psychiatric Association, *Diagnostic and Statistical Manual of Mental Disorders, 4th ed. Text Revision (DSM-IV-TR)* (Washington, DC: American Psychiatric Association, 2000), 572–4. Many citizens will be surprised to discover that their behaviour corresponds to an illness that may include as symptoms a taste for 'restraint (physical bondage), blindfolding (sensory bondage), paddling, spanking ...' et cetera, this at a time when the safe practice of SM is now being taught in workshops on university campuses. One recalls that the American Psychiatric Association also considered homosexuality an illness until its members voted otherwise in 1973, and that 'hysteria' was once deemed as frequent in women as the common cold. Psychiatry, in other words, has always stood as a bulwark for the most conservative aspects of social opinion.

4 Ellis, 'Love and Pain,' 82. According to Ellis, '[Man's] certain pleasure in manifesting his power over a woman by inflicting pain upon her is an outcome and survival of the primitive process of courtship, and an almost or quite normal constituent of the sexual impulse in man' (83).

5 Thomas S. Weinberg and G.W. Levi Kamel, 'S&M: An Introduction to the Study of Sadomasochism,' in Weinberg, ed., *S&M: Studies in Dominance and Submission* (Amherst, NY: Prometheus, 1995), 15–24, quotation 19.

6 Kathy Acker interview, in Andrea Juno, ed., *Angry Women* (New York: Juno Books, 1991), 177–85, quotation 180.

7 According to one survey in the early 1990s, 69 per cent of single men and 74 per cent of single women agreed with the proposition that 'Sex and intimacy are two different things.' Samuel S. Janus and Cynthia L. Janus, *The Janus Report on Sexual Behavior* (New York: Wiley, 1993), 141, table 5.1. On the historical limits of romantic love in the life of the couple, see Edward Shorter, *The Making of the Modern Family* (New York: Basic, 1975), passim.

8 Maurice North, *The Outer Fringe of Sex: A Study in Sexual Fetishism* (London: Odyssey, 1970), 69–70.

9 This is Valerie Steele's interpretation. She writes, 'To the extent that fetish fashion is popular with women, in large part this is because it adds the idea of power to femininity.' *Fetish: Fashion, Sex and Power* (New York: Oxford, 1996), 185.

10 Giovanni Pico della Mirandola, *Disputationes adversus astrologiam divinatricem ... a cure di Garin* (1495) (reprint Florence: Vallecchi, 1946), 413 (the volume contains a parallel Italian translation). 'Un abitudine contratta da bambino.'

11 Peter Wagner, ed., *John Cleland, Fanny Hill, or Memoirs of a Woman of Pleasure* (1748–9) (new ed. London: Penguin, 1985), 181.

12 Paul Näcke, 'Kriminologische und sexologische Studien,' *Archiv für Kriminalanthropologie* 47 (1912): 237–78, see 245. Paul Garnier, 'Le sadi-fétichisme,' *Annales d'hygiène publique* ser. 3, 43 (1900): 97–121, see 100. Ellis, 'Love and Pain,' 136.

13 Norman Breslow et al., 'On the Prevalence and Roles of Females in the Sadomasochistic Subculture: Report of an Empirical Study,' *Archives of Sexual Behavior* 14 (1985): 303–17, quotation 310.

14 John Boswell, *Christianity, Social Tolerance, and Homosexuality: Gay People in Western Europe from the Beginning of the Christian Era to the Fourteenth Century* (Chicago: University of Chicago Press, 1980), 80 n91. 'Hans Licht' found no sign of SM in ancient Greece, he says. 'Sadistische oder masochistische Szenen habe ich in der altgriechischen Literatur nirgends gefunden.' Hans Licht [Paul Brandt], *Sittengeschichte Griechenlands* (1925–8) (new ed. Stuttgart: Günther, 1960), 349.

15 Ellis, 'Love and Pain,' 129.

16 F.A., 'Beiträge zur Geschichte des Frauenzimmers,' *Anthropophyteia Jahrbücher* 9 (1912): 244–9, quotation 247.

17 Pico della Mirandola, *Disputationes*, 413.
18 Rictor Norton, *Mother Clap's Molly House: The Gay Subculture in England, 1700–1830* (London: GMP, 1992), 68.
19 Randolph Trumbach, *Sex and the Gender Revolution, Vol. 1: Heterosexuality and the Third Gender in Enlightenment London* (Chicago: University of Chicago Press, 1998), 158–60.
20 *Almanach des adresses des demoiselles de Paris ... ou calendrier du plaisir* (1791), reprinted by Hector Fleischmann as *Les demoiselles d'amour du Palais-Royal* (Paris: Bibliothèque des curieux, 1911), 135, 136, 164. Such ads, five in number, represented only 1 per cent of the 510 total entries in the almanac.
21 Carl Felix von Schlichtegroll, *Sacher-Masoch und der Masochismus* (Dresden: Dohrn, 1901), 66.
22 Luisa Sigea Toletana [Nicolas Chorier], *Dialogues on the Arcana of Love and Venus* (c. 1660), translated into modern English by Donald A. McKenzie from the 1752 Elzevir edition (Lawrence, KA: Coronado Press, 1974), 112–13, 117.
23 On Johann Kirsten, *Lottchens Reisen ins Zuchthaus* (1778) see Hugo Hayn and Alfred N. Gotendorf, *Bibliotheca Germanorum Erotica et Curiosa* (Munich: Müller, 1913), vol. 2: 298. On W. Reinhard, *Lenchen im Zuchthause* (1840), evidently written late in the eighteenth century, see Hayn and Gotendorf, 303; W. Reinhard, *Nell in Bridewell* (Paris: Society of British Bibliophiles, 1900), quotation 95.
24 Summarized by Pisanus Fraxi [Henry Ashbee], *Bibliography of Prohibited Books* (1879) (reprint Kila, MT: Kessinger, nd), vol. 1: 371–3.
25 Cleland, *Fanny Hill*, 183–7.
26 Annie Le Brun and Jean-Jacques Pauvert, *Oeuvres complètes du Marquis de Sade* (Paris: Pauvert, 1987), 'Histoire de Juliette,' vol. 8: 540.
27 Sade, 'Histoire de Juliette,' *Oeuvres*, vol. 9: 445–6.
28 Krafft-Ebing died just after this twelfth edition was prepared in 1902. The quotation here is from Richard von Krafft-Ebing, *Psychopathia sexualis*, 14th ed. (1912), ed. by Alfred Fuchs (reprint ed. Munich: Matthes and Seitz, 1997), 165.
29 Sade, 'Histoire de Juliette,' vol. 8: 99–100.

30 Sade, 'Histoire de Juliette,' vol. 8: 104–5.

31 Brantôme, *Les dames galantes* (1566) (reprint Paris: Garnier, 1960), 36–7.

32 Ann Rosalind Jones, *The Currency of Eros: Women's Love Lyric in Europe, 1540–1620* (Bloomington: Indiana University Press, 1990), 100–1. Translation is Jones's.

33 Gert Schiff, ed., *Johann Heinrich Füssli: Abbildungen* (Zurich: Berichthaus, 1973), 125. No. 547, 'Herrin und Sklave'; no. 549, 'Symplegma eines gefesselten nackten Mannes und zweier Frauen.'

34 Émile Zola, *Nana* (1880) (new ed. Paris: Garnier-Flammarion, 1968), 413–14.

35 Krafft-Ebing used the terms 'sadism' (which he did not coin) and 'masochism' (which he did) in the sixth edition of *Psychopathia sexualis* (1891). These quotations from the 12th ed. (1902): 151–3.

36 Krafft-Ebing, *Psychopathia sexualis*, 12th ed. (1902), 161.

37 Richard von Krafft-Ebing, *Psychopathia sexualis: Eine klinisch-forensische Studie* (Stuttgart: Enke, 1886).

38 Ellis, 'Love and Pain,' 128, 148.

39 Richard Ellmann, ed., *Selected Letters of James Joyce* (New York: Viking, 1975), 188–9.

40 James Joyce, *Ulysses* (1922) (reprinted with corrections London: Penguin, 1971), 492.

41 Schlichtegroll, *Sacher-Masoch*, 199–200.

42 Edith Cadivec, *Confessions and Experiences*, Eng. trans. (New York: Grove, 1971), 114–19. German original, *Bekenntnisse und Erlebnisse* (Hellerau: privately published, 1931). The other volume was her *Eros: The Meaning of My Life*, Eng. trans. (New York: Grove, 1969). German original *Eros, der Sinn meines Lebens* (Hellerau: privately published, 1932).

43 Thomas P. Riggio et al., eds, *Theodore Dreiser, American Diaries, 1902–1926* (Philadelphia: University of Pennsylvania Press, 1982), 347, 376.

44 Dominique Aury, *Literary Landfalls* (1958), Eng. trans. (London: Chatto and Windus, 1960), 75. Aury in turn was a pseudonym for the author's real family name, which was never revealed.

45 Pauline Réage [Dominique Aury], *Story of O*, Eng. trans. (London: Olympia, 1970), quotation from Corgi ed., 8.

46 John De St Jorre, 'The Unmasking of O,' *New Yorker* 1 Aug. 1994: 42–50; sales information on 42.

47 Réage, *Story of O*, 53

48 G.R., ed., *L'Anti-Justine de Restif de la Bretonne* (orig. 1798) (reprint Paris: Bibliothèque privée, 1969), see esp. 26–31, 60, 71, 77, 78, and a lush example on 146–7.

49 See Liz Stanley, ed., *The Diaries of Hannah Cullwick, Victorian Maidservant* (New Brunswick: Rutgers University Press, 1984) for the impressions of one of the cleaning women herself.

50 Steele, *Fetish*, 57–90.

51 Jean-Martin Charcot and Valentin Magnan, 'Inversion du sens génital' (pt 2), *Archives de neurologie* 4 (1882): 296–322, esp. 306; most of the article deals with homosexuals.

52 On Sacher-Masoch's life see Albrecht Koschorke, *Leopold von Sacher-Masoch: Die Inszenierung einer Perversion* (Munich: Piper, 1988). For details on Angelica/Wanda's flogging of Sacher-Masoch, see her autobiography, Wanda von Sacher-Masoch, *Meine Lebensbeichte: Memoiren* (Berlin: Schuster, 1906), 95–6, 137–8, 140–1.

53 Leopold von Sacher-Masoch, *Venus im Pelz* (1870) (reprint Cologne: Könemann, 1996), 28, 30, 46, 94.

54 Alfred Binet, 'Le fétichisme dans l'amour,' *Revue philosophique* 24 (1887): 143–274.

55 Krafft-Ebing, *Psychopathia sexualis*, 6th ed. (1891), 98–108.

56 Marion Delorme, *Allerlei Fetische* (Paris: Leipziger Verlag, c. 1900, confiscated 1912). Cited in Hayn and Gotendorf, *Bibliotheca Germanorum*, vol. 2: 285.

57 Hayn and Gotendorf, *Bibliotheca Germanorum*, vol. 2: 310.

58 Gaétan Gatian de Clérambault, 'Passion érotique des étoffes chez la femme,' *Archives d'anthropologie criminelle de médecine légale* 23 (1908): 439–70, quotations 467, 470. 'Gatian' begins the surname.

59 Ellmann, *Joyce Selected Letters*, 172.

60 See Gaylyn Studlar, 'Masochism, Masquerade, and the Erotic Metamorphoses of Marlene Dietrich,' in Jane Gaines and Char-

lotte Herzog, eds, *Fabrications: Costume and the Female Body* (New York: Routledge, 1990), 229–49; list of films on 235.

61 Inevitably, there will be exceptions to a generalization of this magnitude, yet they are tiny. In *Fanny Hill*, for example, John Cleland creates an 'elderly gentleman' who gives Fanny a dozen pairs of white kid gloves, on the condition that he bite off their fingers' ends (190).

62 Romi [no first name available], *Maisons closes dans l'histoire, l'art, la littérature et les moeurs* (Paris: Serg, nd [1965]), 2 vols. The text notes that most first-class houses had their 'torture chambers,' yet the author considered SM a bizarre perversion and makes no reference to leather as such (see vol. 2: 94–5).

63 For details on Menken and Swinburne, see Wolf Mankowitz, *Mazeppa: The Lives, Loves and Legends of Adah Isaacs Menken* (London: Blond and Briggs, 1982), quotations 216, 219. For the text of 'Dolores (Notre-Dame des Sept Douleurs)' see Edmund Gosse and Thomas James Wise, eds, *The Complete Works of Algernon Charles Swinburne, vol. 1: Poetical Works* (London: Heinemann, 1925), 284–98.

64 Wanda von Sacher-Masoch, *Meine Lebensbeichte*, 156.

65 An 1870 caricature shows a booted and otherwise naked Empress Eugénie lying on a table: it is a critique of the lewdness of the Second Empire, but many women normally wore boots in those days, and it's unclear if the drawing is meant to have a kink edge. See Eduard Fuchs, *Geschichte der erotischen Kunst* (1908) (reprint Berlin: Guhl, 1977), 370.

66 Émile Zola, *Thérèse Raquin* (1868) (new ed. Paris: Charpentier, 1886), 91.

67 Krafft-Ebing, *Psychopathia sexualis*, 6th ed. (1891), 90.

68 Cited in Peter Mendes, *Clandestine Erotic Fiction in English, 1800–1930: A Bibliographical Study* (Aldershot: Scolar Press, 1993), 393.

69 Steele, *Fetish*, 51, 70–1.

70 Peter Weiermair, ed., *Erotic Art from the 17th to the 20th Century: The Döpp Collection* (Zurich: Stemmle, 1991), 99.

71 Louis-Charles Royer, *L'amour en Allemagne* (Paris: Eds de France, 1930), 92–6.

72 On usage of the term 'dominatrix' in pornography before the First World War see Hayn and Gotendorf, *Bibliotheca Germanorum*, vol. 2: 282; for example, R. Bröhmeck, *Dominatrix. Roman-Zyclus* (Paris: Leipziger Verlag, c. 1906–8), 5 vols, among which were: vol. 1, *Der Sklave der schönen Despotin*; vol. 2, *Frau Lehrerin*; vol. 3, *Der Fuss im Nacken*, and so forth.

73 Kinsey Collection, Institute for Sex Research, nos 62203, 65706; see also 62219.

74 Alan Mac Clyde, *Le cuir triomphant* (Paris: Librairie Générale, nd [early 1930s]). In the Kinsey Collection, donated by U.S. Customs in 1958. The contents represent such variations as 'pony girl.' See in the ISR as well, Alan Mac Clyde, *La Madone du Cuir Verni* (Paris: Librairie artistique, nd [early 1930s]); and J. Van Styk, *L'infernale dominatrice* (Paris: Jardin d'Eros, [1935]).

75 David Kunzle, *Fashion and Fetishism* (Totowa, NJ: Rowman and Littlefield, 1982), 7.

76 Chris Gosselin and Glenn Wilson, *Sexual Variations: Fetishism, Sado-masochism and Transvestism* (London: Faber, 1980), 65. The sample is described on 32.

77 William A. Rossi, *The Sex Life of the Foot and Shoe* (New York: Saturday Review Press/Dutton, 1976), 165.

78 Barbara Ehrenreich, Elizabeth Hess, Gloria Jacobs, *Re-making Love: The Feminization of Sex* (New York: Doubleday, 1986), 124.

79 This information from Karen Essex and James L. Swanson, *Bettie Page: The Life of a Pin-up Legend* (Los Angeles: General, 1996), 143–71; plus several Bettie Page websites such as www.fantasies.com/bettie/bettie.shtml.

80 Essex and Swanson, *Bettie Page*, 171.

81 'The Rubber Man,' in *Shiny Rubber Vintage Special, 1975–1995* (nd, late 1990s), 9–13; C.J. Trail-Hill, 'The Psychology of Rubber, part II,' dated June 1964: the manuscript was consulted at the Institute for Sex Research, quotation 153. The author was owner of the Natural Rubber Company in London.

82 Gareth Humphreys, 'John Steed – You're Needed: A History of the Avengers,' http://nyquist.ee.valbenta.ca/~dawe/avengers.

83 'Quotes from the Avengers,' http://nyquist.ee.valbenta .ca/~dawe/avengers.

84 Arthur Knight and Hollis Alpert, 'The Stag Film,' *Playboy* Nov. 1967: 154–8, 170–89, see 180.

85 Monique Von Cleef, *The House of Pain* (Secaucus, NJ: Lyle Stuart, nd [1970?]), 162.

86 Al Di Lauro and Gerald Rabkin, *Dirty Movies: An Illustrated History of the Stag Film, 1915–1970* (New York: Chelsea House, 1976), 97–8.

87 Quoted in Kenneth Turan and Stephen F. Zito, *Sinema: American Pornographic Films and the People Who Make Them* (New York: Praeger, 1974), 43.

88 Gerald Green and Caroline Green, *S-M: The Last Taboo* (New York: Grove, 1973), 163, 186.

89 Betty Dodson, *Sex for One: The Joy of Selfloving* (New York: Three Rivers, 1987), 135, 137.

90 *The Janus Report*, 115, 122.

91 Paul Gebhard and Alan B. Johnson, *The Kinsey Data: Marginal Tabulations of the 1938–1963 Interviews Conducted by the Institute for Sex Research* (Philadelphia: Saunders, 1979), 229, table 180.

92 Deidre Sanders, *The Woman Report on Men* (London: Sphere, 1987), 101.

93 Charles Moser and Eugene E. Levitt, 'An Exploratory-Descriptive Study of a Sadomasochistically Oriented Sample' (1987), reprinted Weinberg, ed., *S&M: Studies in Dominance and Submission*, 93–112, quotation 95.

94 Ehrenreich, Hess, and Jacobs, *Re-making Love*, 127–8.

95 Moser and Levitt, 'Exploratory Study,' 100.

96 Ehrenreich, Hess, and Jacobs, *Re-making Love*, 128–9.

97 Norman Breslow et al., 'On the Prevalence and Roles of Females in the Sadomasochistic Subculture: Report of an Empirical Study,' *Archives of Sexual Behavior* 14 (1985): 303–17, 315, table 13.

98 John Donne, 'The Anagram,' in Helen Gardner, ed., *John Donne, The Elegies and the Songs and Sonnets* (Oxford: Clarendon, 1965), 21–2, quotation 22.

99 Charles Spencer, *Erté* (London: Studio Vista, 1970), 70.

100 Erté, *Things I Remember: An Autobiography* (London: Peter Owen, 1975), 149.

101 Enid Nemy, 'Bonnie Cashin ... Is Dead at 84,' *New York Times* 5 Feb. 2000: A14.

102 *Harper's Bazaar* Feb. 1960: 145; Sept. 1960: 196.

103 *Vogue* 1 Sept. 1960: 224, 282; 15 Oct. 1960: 123.

104 This chronology is based on Georgina Howell, *In Vogue: Six Decades of Fashion* (London: Book Club Associates, 1979), 275–83.

105 Howell, *In Vogue*, 252.

106 Barry Miles, *Paul McCartney: Many Years from Now* (New York: Holt, 1997), 63–71.

107 See Mary Quant, *Quant by Quant* (London: Cassell, 1965), 98–9.

108 Leslie Kaufman and Craig S. Smith, 'Millions of Chinese Pigs Fuel a Fashion Boom in the West,' *New York Times* 24 Dec. 2000: 1.

109 'Chain Reactions,' *Vogue* Sept. 1992: 537; see 532.

110 Essex and Swanson, *Bettie Page*, 262.

111 For an overview, see Amy M. Spindler, 'Versace's Errors Showed Him a Way,' *New York Times* 5 Aug. 1997: B8.

112 'Black Leather,' *Harper's Bazaar* Aug. 1992: 77.

113 Constance C.R. White, 'John Bartlett: On the Fringe No More,' *New York Times* 17 Feb. 1998: A20.

114 Beth Howard, '*Shape* Readers on Body Image and Sex: Survey,' *Shape* Sept. 1997: 118–23, 147–52, quotation 152.

115 Pamela Lister, 'His Secret Turn-ons (and Yours),' *Redbook* July 1999: 77–9, 100–2, quotation 102.

116 Kristina Dell, 'Guys Confess ...,' *Redbook* Dec. 1999: 66. Bold-faced in original.

117 Bette Harrison, 'In-home Showings for Women Aid Sales of Sensual Products,' Cox News Service, www.s-t.com/daily/11–98/11–06–98/b02li037.htm.

118 Tasteful Treasures by Mary, http://members.aol.com/_ht_a/ttreasures by mary/webpage/tasteful.html.

119 See http://members.aol.com/seakap1/index.html.

120 'J' [Terry Garrity], *The Sensuous Woman* (New York: Lyle Stuart, 1969), 131.

Chapter 10 Epilogue

1 Oscar Wilde, *The Picture of Dorian Gray* (1890) (New York: Modern Library, 1998), 65.

2 Mary Thale, ed., *The Autobiography of Francis Place* (Cambridge: University Press, 1972), 20.

3 Francis Lacassin, ed., *Jacques Casanova de Seingalt, Histoire de ma vie* (new ed. Paris: Laffont, 1993), vol. 1: 847.

4 Robert D. Putnam, 'Bowling Alone: America's Declining Social Capital,' *Journal of Democracy* 6 (1995): 65–78, quotation 72.

5 Robert D. Putnam, *Bowling Alone: The Collapse and Revival of American Community* (New York: Simon and Schuster, 2000).

6 Virginia Woolf, 'On Being Ill' (1930), reprinted in Woolf, *Collected Essays* (London: Hogarth, 1967), vol. 4: 193–203, quotation 201–2.

7 John P. Robinson and Geoffrey Godbey, *Time for Life: The Surprising Ways Americans Use Their Time* (University Park, PA: Pennsylvania University Press, 1997), 170, table 13.

8 Judith Miller, 'As Patrons Age, Future of Arts Is Uncertain,' *New York Times* 12 Feb. 1996: A1.

9 Lee Burns, *Busy Bodies: Why Our Time-obsessed Society Keeps Us Running in Place* (New York: Norton, 1993), 95.

10 Robert D. Putnam, 'The Strange Disappearance of Civic America,' *American Prospect* 24 (Winter 1996): 34–48, see 35.

11 John Robinson and Geoffrey Godbey, 'No Sex, Please ... We're College Graduates,' *American Demographics* Feb. 1998, www.americandemographics.com.

12 A.P. MacKay et al., *Adolescent Health Chartbook. Health, United States, 2000* (Hyattsville, MD: National Center for Health Statistics, 2000), 76, 79, 80. The statistics on alcohol were estimated from bar graphs.

Index